CW00431520

CLINICAL AROMATHERAPY IN NURSING

CLINICAL AROMATHERAPY IN NURSING

Jane Buckle
RGN, MA, BPhil, Cert Ed, MISPA, MIScB

A member of the Hodder Headline Group
LONDON • NEW YORK • SYDNEY • AUCKLAND

First published in Great Britain in 1997 by
Arnold, a member of the Hodder Headline Group
338 Euston Road, London NW1 3BH

© 1997 Jane Buckle

All rights reserved. No part of this publication may be reproduced or transmitted in any form
or by any means, electronically or mechanically, including photocopying, recording or any
information storage or retrieval system, without either prior permission in writing from the
publisher or a licence permitting restricted copying. In the United Kingdom such licences are
issued by the Copyright Licensing Agency: 90 Tottenham Court Road, London W1P 9HE.

Whilst the advice and information in this book is believed to be true and accurate at the time of
going to press, neither the author nor the publisher can accept any legal responsibility or
liability for any errors or omissions that may be made. In particular (but without limiting the
generality of the preceding disclaimer) every effort has been made to check essential oil
dosages; however, it is still possible that errors have been missed. Furthermore, dosage
schedules are constantly being revised and new side-effects recognized. For these reasons the
reader is strongly urged to consult the essential oil companies' printed instructions before
administering any of the oils recommended in this book.

British Library Cataloguing in Publication Data
A catalogue record for this book is available from the British Library

Library of Congress Cataloging-in-Publication Data
A catalog record for this book is available from the Library of Congress

ISBN 0 340 63177 5

Composition in 10/13pt Palatino by Phoenix Photosetting, Chatham, Kent
Printed and bound in Great Britain by JW Arrowsmith Ltd, Bristol

**For Michael,
who made it possible**

CONTENTS

FOREWORD

Few would deny that complementary therapies have captured the public imagination. Many health care professionals have been slow to respond to this interest, although this could not be said of nurses. Through my work with the Royal College of Nursing Complementary Therapies Forum I have observed significant interest of nurses in the use of essential oils in their work. Indeed, a survey conducted by the Forum indicated that aromatherapy was the most popular and commonly used complementary therapy engaged in by nurses.

Many nurses wish to extend their knowledge and skills in the use of essential oils in order to expand their therapeutic repertoire. This has created much debate on the related professional issues surrounding nurses' use of aromatherapy. In particular, there is an urgent need to examine how nurses can ensure that their practice is safe, efficacious and acceptable to patients. Nurses have been hindered in their development of this area of work by the serious lack of information that is relevant to the clinical context of their work. This book by Jane Buckle begins to address these issues by integrating information on the use of essential oils and their skilled application in trying to meet patients' needs for nursing. Due attention is given to nursing concerns such as promoting comfort and alleviating pain and anxiety in those who are sick. These areas are discussed with sensitivity and a strong vision of the potential application of aromatherapy by nurses.

Jane Buckle is particularly suited to write such a book. She combines over 20 years of clinical experience in a range of settings, and the practice of aromatherapy both in clinical settings and in private practice. She has undertaken various courses in the use of aromatherapy, and academic study in the field of complementary therapies. Jane has also worked for the Research Council for Complementary Medicine, and is currently engaged in research work in the USA. She is also involved in delivering courses to a range of health care professionals in the UK and the USA. As such, Jane is particularly well placed to combine the range of perspectives necessary to achieve a rounded, creative and critical view of the opportunities and limitations of using aromatherapy within nursing practice.

Much work still has to be done to achieve a developed standard and protocol of accepted aromatherapy practice by nurses in clinical settings. Further development is needed in the education of nurses about using essential oils in their work. Ongoing consideration is needed to review the potential for evaluating the effectiveness of essential oils in helping to meet patients' needs for nursing. Particular attention is needed to continue to organize, review and make available the evidence of the benefits and limitations of aromatherapy in clinical practice. Jane has shown leadership in beginning the important work of trying to meet the specific needs of nurses working within the health service.

Jane Buckle has made an important step in highlighting the issues and potential for extending the therapeutic range of nurses using aromatherapy to meet patient needs in an effective and sensitive way. Through this book I believe that a valuable contribution has been made to the development of integrative health care – that which combines the best of orthodox and complementary practices.

Dr Steven Ersser
Principal Lecturer in Nursing
School of Health Care Studies
Oxford Brookes University
Oxford

PREFACE

Writing this book has been a journey of discovery for me. It began with three questions. What is clinical aromatherapy? What is nursing? And how can the two work together?

Clinical aromatherapy has much to offer mankind because it reveals the softer side of a hard world – a side that involves our senses. We perceive ourselves as human *beings*, yet how many of us have forgotten how to '*be*'? Perhaps the power of speech made us forget how to touch and how to smell. But essential oils are not just 'pretty smells' – they have a direct impact on us at a psychological, physiological and molecular level. Because they have antibacterial, antifungal and antiviral properties, they could have a potentially important role to play in integrated health care. Essential oils are highly complex and concentrated compounds and, as such, their use carries a need for specialized training and control.

The recent advent of nursing diagnosis is propitious – it gives nurses the ability to analyse their caring. Clinical aromatherapy could have a part to play in nursing, not as some add-on speciality, but ultimately as an intrinsic part of nursing.

However, aromatherapy seems to have become part of nursing without any real clinical focus. There is no clear nursing perspective or obvious scientific evidence. I feel that these issues are pressing, and I have tried to address them. For clinical aromatherapy to be accepted as part of nursing, it needs to be taken much more seriously. We need evidence of clinical efficacy and safety. We need protocols and policies to protect ourselves and our patients, and we need to be cognizant of the scientific data available.

My objective is for nurses interested in using aromatherapy to have a clear clinical focus and to view aromatherapy from a *nursing* perspective. My aim is to make hospitals more hospitable places by improving the quality of our patient care and enhancing the environment in which we work.

Jane Buckle

ACKNOWLEDGEMENTS

I would like to thank Dr Ken Howells, Dr Steve Ersser, Tony Balacs and Tim Vaughn for their help in editing parts of this manuscript, Penny Simpson, Sharon MacNish and Annette Godfrey-Hardinge for their ongoing support, Dr Kim Jobst and Dr David Taylor-Reilly for their valued comments, Noreen Frisch, President of the American Holistic Nursing Association, for drawing my attention to the concept of nursing diagnosis, Caroline Stevenson for her advice on aromatherapy and homeopathy, Professor Sara-Jane Anderson for her help with nursing theory, Harriet Griffy for her research, Mary Lou Quinn for her help with obtaining reference papers, all of the co-ordinators of my course in clinical aromatherapy in the USA, especially Irene Belcher and Lori Wyzykowski who were the first, and my editors, Richard Holloway and Fiona Goodgame. Particular thanks to Shirley Price and Robert Tisserand, two leaders in the field, whose work has inspired and motivated me: I hope they will find my book of interest and use. Finally, thanks to my family and friends for allowing me time to write, and to the village of Hunter, New York, for giving me the peace and equanimity to complete what I began. Thank you all.

'The effects of aromatherapy can be medicinal as well as relaxing'
Amer Fasihi, Financial Times

'Nurses everywhere are pushing at the boundaries of care to find innovative ways of solving longstanding problems. The increased use and greater understanding of complementary therapies provide a good example of this'
Christine Hancock, President RCN

'Look with your understanding, find out what you already know, and you'll see the way to fly'
Jonathan Livingstone Seagull

Part 1

Overview

1

INTRODUCTION

In the 1995 newsletter of the Critical Care Section of the Royal College of Nursing it was announced that the Forum Annual Study for 1995 had been awarded to two nurses, Jane Blythe and Fiona McFayden, for their work on developing aromatherapy in an Intensive-Care Unit. Their work was unusual in that they were developing this aromatherapy for the benefit of relatives and staff.[1]

Aromatherapy is the fastest growing complementary therapy, and it is also the fastest growing therapy among nurses.[2] The questions 'why now?' and 'why nurses?' are fairly simple to answer. But does it work? And is it safe? Many nurses currently using aromatherapy on hospital wards do not appear to know exactly what they are using on their patients, although they have accountability.[3] It could be argued that, as yet, there is no specialized training course for nurses wishing to use clinical aromatherapy to enhance their care. Steps are afoot to address this situation, and it is hoped that there will be courses in clinical aromatherapy specifically for nurses. Details of these types of courses are referred to in Chapter 9 on organizations and training.

Some of the criticisms levelled at clinical aromatherapy have cited the paucity of research.[4] This is fair comment. Research has been mainly limited to animals or *in-vitro* systems. However, there are currently many pilot studies being conducted by nurses in hospitals world-wide. Nurses are not trained in research, and usually have little or no funding. They carry out research on aromatherapy for Bachelor or Masters degrees, or because of a personal interest. Often the patient population is small and the study modest.

Perhaps orthodox medicine might be more open to the kind of data that nurses are compiling if orthodox researchers were to look hard at their own research. A Canadian study which evaluated 4000 recent medical papers and applied 28 basic criteria that should be fulfilled in scientific papers concluded that only 40 of the 4000 papers met all of the critiera. This analysis went on to state that only 15% of medical interventions are supported by reliable scientific evidence and often statements are not supported by any evidence at all. This paper was printed in a peer-reviewed journal on medical ethics.[5]

Non-conventional medicine, which includes complementary/alternative therapies, has been around much longer than Western medicine.[6] However, with their growth in popularity there appears to be a power struggle between the 'believers in Western medicine' and the 'believers in "non-conventional medicine".' One answer could be to try and encourage these two groups to work together, but would the differences in philosophical approach allow for a comfortable marriage between them?

There is a difference between complementary therapies and alternative medicine. A complementary therapy denotes a therapy that does not stand on its own but is an adjunct to another system of healing, e.g. reflexology, healing touch. Alternative medicine has the ability to stand on its own, usually with its own diagnostic skills learned through a degree-type programme such as acupuncture, homeopathy, herbal medicine or osteopathy.

Western medicine is reductionist, specialist, and claims to be rigorously scientific, although 'most therapies applied daily in doctors' offices have never been tested by the scientific method'.[5] Many procedures carry with them serious risks and side-effects. Some hotly promoted procedures have turned out to be of little value, such as the fashion of removing the appendix, tonsils or adenoids in the 1950s and 1960s, or inserting grommets in the 1970s and 1980s.

Orthodox treatments are invasive, either in the form of surgery (to remove the 'bad' part) or drug therapy (to 'zap' invading pathogens). The philosophy is simple – a symptom or a disease process must be eliminated; only then is the patient cured. Cures are often dramatic – normal sinus rhythm is restored after asystole, blue babies turn pink, seizures stop. Treatment is generally the same for everyone, regardless of age, sex, background, diet, stress level, weight, etc. Some treatments undoubtedly save lives, but some can kill.[7]

Success is measured by how quickly the patient returns to his or her place in the work-force. Very few follow-up audits of orthodox treatment take place, and if the patient 'breaks down' again, this is classified as a new occurrence rather than as a re-occurrence. The rationale behind complementary therapies is different. Such therapies are not aimed at one specific body system as, for example, in endocrinology, and they are normally non-invasive. Practitioners are interested in the individuality of the patient and what has led them to this particular disease process, or set of symptoms,[8] and feel that when the patient is balanced, homeostasis can return, and the disease will be unable to survive. They illustrate this viewpoint by stating that that the world is full of viruses and bacteria, but that it is mainly individuals whose immunity is compromised (through emotional, spiritual or physical trauma) who tend to succumb.[9] Twenty years of orthodox research into cancer, with relatively little progress towards a cure, supports this viewpoint.[10]

Success in complementary therapies is based on a long-term view. Practitioners look at the 'patterning' of the disease process – how often the patient has been ill over his or her lifetime, and whether the incidence and severity of the disease has increased. All diseases are taken into account, not just those of the same system, as the health of the whole patient is evaluated. Patients are warned that treatment may take some time. Chronic disease does not happen overnight, and neither will it disappear overnight. Emphasis is placed on teaching the patient preventative medicine in order to avoid a relapse, and on providing support during the healing process. The patient is encouraged to rest, and not to work, whilst the repairing process is in progress. The old-fashioned idea of convalescing is stressed as important.

Is it possible for the two opposites to merge? Perhaps. I think and hope so. Possibly complementary / alternative medicine could think of itself as the yin part of medicine. Orthodox/western practitioners could consider themselves to be the yang of medicine. Together yin and yang make a circle, each needing the other to be a whole. Yang is often seen to be masculine, dominant, intrusive, and perhaps mechanical. Yin usually involves the more intuitive, feminine, 'soft' approach.

Together there could be a strong working symbiotic partnership, each bringing out the best in the other. Acute illnesses and trauma would be treated with western drugs/surgery, whilst chronic illnesses (e.g. arthritis, insomnia, and irritable bowel syndrome) could be helped by a more complementary approach.

So where would be the place of aromatherapy? Is it medicine? Is it nursing? Is it alternative? Is it complementary? The answers depend on the type of aromatherapy used and the approach of the practitioner. Clinical aromatherapy is used to help fight or prevent infection, encourage healing and promote relaxation, and can be integrated into both the medical and the nursing model. Clinical aromatherapy in nursing is complementary. Clinical aromatherapy within medicine can be alternative; in France some doctors use essential oils as an alternative to orthodox drugs.

This book is about clinical aromatherapy within nursing – in other words, the enhancement of our nursing skills in a clinical setting using the science of essential oils within the art of aromatherapy.

Approaches in aromatherapy can be herbal or chemical. Herbalists are vitalists; they believe in the synergy of plants (i.e. the whole is more than the sum of its parts). Chemists believe that it is the chemistry of a plant that endows it with its therapeutic properties. A chemist is more likely to have a reductionist viewpoint – eradicate the symptom and the patient will be cured. A herbalist might have a broader and more holistic approach to the patient, stressing their background and intrinsic make-up. Both approaches have validity, but each may only see one side of the whole picture.

Of all the complementary therapies, aromatherapy is perhaps the most misunderstood. It is maligned, misrepresented and confusing. Even the name 'aromatherapy' is a misnomer. Small wonder that orthodoxy ridicules what the perfume industry guards so well.

Until recently, aromatherapy has been closely associated with massage. Perhaps this confusion arose because aromatherapy emerged in England via the beauty therapy industry. Only now has it become sufficiently integrated into the nursing system for the massage element become less important. Touch and smell can be important tools for enhancing the way in which a nurse relates to her patients. However, I feel strongly that massage and touch, using essential, oils are quite different.

One has only to watch a masseuse and then to watch a nurse to see how different they are. Both procedures also *feel* very different. A massage can be a wonderfully invigorating or relaxing experience: all of the muscles in the body are given a work-out. Touch with essential oils (as used by a nurse on a sick patient) is given in an extremely gentle, very slow manner, more akin to stroking than to massage. The fact that aromatherapy can be used in certain situations when massage *cannot* be used underlines the difference. It would make life much simpler if we found a different word. So confused have people become that, in the USA (where I teach, and where in many States nurses are not allowed to massage their patients) I have called touch with essential oils the 'm' technique, an abbreviation for manual technique.

Outside England, aromatherapy is seen in a very different light. In France, essential oils are often given orally (in a gelule capsule or dissolved in a vegetable disperse) by medical or herbal doctors in order to combat a bacterial or viral infection. These practitioners can also give essential oils rectally or vaginally in a gelule capsule. In other parts of the world essential oils are merely inhaled. Overall, the use of essential oils, either topically, inhaled or taken internally, goes back several thousand years.

Because only one or two drops of essential oil are used and touch can be involved, aromatherapy is known for its gentleness. It is extolled in the stress management of patients.[11] It is true that by combining two powerful non-verbal communicators, namely touch and smell, aromatherapy can produce tremendous relaxation in a relatively short period of time. However, nursing is not just about relaxing patients. It is also about improving their comfort level, reducing their pain and restoring their empowerment. These descriptions are terms used in *nursing diagnosis*. Nursing diagnosis is an attempt to describe in precise language what we do as nurses. The practice which is widely accepted (and expected) in the USA is fairly new in the UK, and the subject is covered in its own section in this book. Nursing diagnosis textbooks include the word 'infection' and specifically mention the use of 'appropriate precautions to prevent infection'.[12] Nursing diagnosis also explores when medical diagnosis can be included in a nursing diagnosis statement.[12]

It is possible to use the same essential oil for relaxation and to prevent cross-infection. It is possible to use an essential oil both to promote sleep and to fight an opportunistic infection, or to soothe the pain of arthritis and kill a fungal infection at the same time. Which one of these is not nursing? Aromatherapy makes us question how wide our role as nurses really is.

During illness and following surgery, relaxation is a vital key to recovery.[13] The ability to relax can be enhanced by aromatherapy. Florence Nightingale (Figure 1.1) once said that 'the cure is in the caring'.[14] Aromatherapy allows nurses to demonstrate their caring in a deeply profound way. By helping their patients to *feel* better, nurses may help them to *get* better.

As Karilee Shames pleads in her profound book, *The Nightingale Conspiracy*, let us 'have more high-touch in our high-tech world and put more caring back into curing. Then, together, we will create a less costly, more healthy system, one that empowers us all'.[15]

There is much more to aromatherapy than stress management and caring. A drop of essential oil carries the concentrated life support system of a plant – a life support system which protects the plant from infection by parasites, fungi, bacteria and insects, and regulates its growth with hormones. It is life support systems such as these that have given us aspirin, atropine, codeine, curare, digitalis, ephedrine, ergometrine, ipecacuanha, morphine, papaveretum, podophyllium, quinine, senna, theophylline and vinblastine, to name just a few.[16] Even the contraceptive pill was originally derived from a plant – the Mexican yam.[17]

This book is not intended to be a substitute for training, but rather a handbook to indicate areas where clinical aromatherapy could be used within a clinical setting. The author believes strongly in the need for clinical training. For this reason, specific numbers of drops of essential oils and methods of use have deliberately been omitted.

There is a desperate need for a clinical focus. We need to concentrate on the nursing perspective and make a serious attempt to collate the information and evidence that already exists from nurses who are currently using essential oils. This could supply the beginnings of an extensive knowledge base – a database that records which essential oil is being used where, how, and the positive (or negative) reactions.

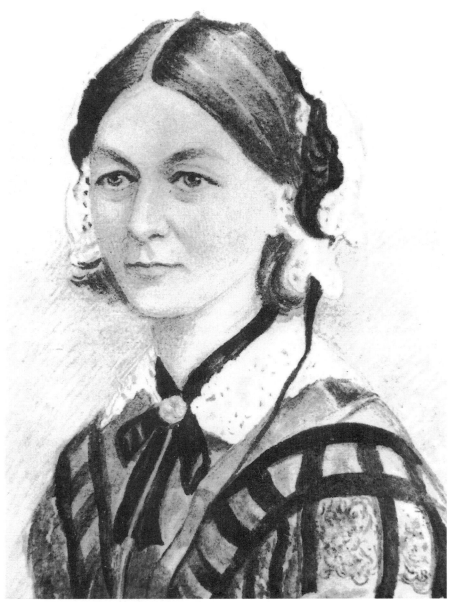

FIGURE 1.1 Florence Nightingale. Reproduced with kind permission of the Royal College of Nursing Archives.

We need to address the very real concerns of safety mentioned in the Control of Substances Hazardous to Health Regulations (COSHH) 1994 requirements and the Chemical (Hazard Information and Packing for Supply) (CHIPS 2) Regulations, and we need clear protocols and policies for nurses and hospital Trusts. With these guidelines in place, the author believes that aromatherapy could not only enhance nursing and patient care, but also prove to be cost-effective in a health care business which needs a rapid, reliable turnover. This is a book about the potential of clinical aromatherapy in nursing, written for nurses by a nurse.

REFERENCES

1. **Endacott, R.** 1995: *Royal College of Nursing: Critical Care Forum Newsletter* **Spring issue**, p. 1.

2. **Ersser, S.** 1990: Touch and go. *Nursing Standard* **4**, 39.

3. **Buckle, J.** 1992: Which lavender? *Nursing Times* **88**, 54–5.

4. **Vickers, A.** 1996: *Massage and aromatherapy: a guide for health professionals.* London: Chapman and Hall.

5. **Smith, R.** 1992: The ethics of ignorance. *Journal of Medical Ethics.* Reprinted in *Newsletter of People's Medical Society* **12**, 4–51.

6. **Vickers, A.** 1993: What is complementary medicine? In *Complementary medicine and disability.* London: Chapman and Hall.

7. **Craig, C.R. and Stitzel, R.** 1994: Lipid mediators of homeostasis and inflammation. In *Modern pharmacology*, 4th edn. New York: Little, Brown & Co, 489–99.

8. **Hildebrand, S.** 1994: Aromatherapy. In Wells, R. (ed.), *Supportive therapies in heathcare.* London: Baillière Tindall, 124–5.

9. **Gasgoigne, S.** 1993: *Manual of conventional medicine for alternative practitioners.* Richmond: Jigme Press, 16–18.

10. **Beardsley, T.** 1994: Trends in cancer epidemiology: a war not won. *Scientific American* **270**, 130–38.

11. **Kusmerik, J.** 1992: Perspectives in aromatherapy. In Toller, V. and Dodd, G. (eds), *Fragrance in the psychology and biology of perfume.* New York: Elsevier Applied Science, 277–85.

12. **Carpenito, L.J.** 1993: *Nursing diagnosis*, 3rd edn. Philadelphia, PA: J.B. Lippincott.

13. **Nightingale, F.** 1859: *Notes on nursing: what it is and what it is not.* London: Harrison & Sons.

14. **Mathers, P.** 1991: Learning to cope with the stress of palliative care. In Penson, J. and Fraser, R. (eds), *Palliative care for people with cancer.* London: Edward Arnold, 260–61.

15. **Shames, K.** 1993: *The Nightingale conspiracy*. Montclair, NJ: Enlightenment Press.

16. **Hollman, A.** 1991: *Plants in medicine for the Chelsea Physic Garden*. London: Chelsea Physic Garden.

17. **Ryman, D.** 1991: *Aromatherapy*. London: Piatkus.

2

AROMATHERAPY IN THE CONTEXT OF NURSING

CONCEPTUAL FRAMEWORK

For many years nursing has been called a profession, but it may be more accurate to describe it as an 'emerging profession with a concept of mission which is open to change'.[1] It is this ability to change which makes nursing an art as well as a science. There have been many changes since Florence Nightingale's day. The nurse's role has become increasingly technological, with more and more medical breakthroughs. Surgical procedures have become more intricate and a field of critical-care nursing has developed. Babies can now survive at 22 weeks, so neonatal nursing was born. Spare-part surgery has became so normal that donor cards vie for space with our credit cards.

However, even with all the changes there is an enduring conceptual framework underlying nursing. Two other words share the same Latin derivation as the word 'nurse'. They are 'nourish' and 'nurture'. We have nourished and nurtured our patients to the best of our ability no matter what the drug regime, the surgical operation or the hospital constraints. Nursing the world over shares a common aim – to facilitate a speedy return to health (or to a peaceful and dignified death) through nurturing the body and nourishing the soul.

How do we 'know' how to nurse? Much of what we do is based upon experience, some of what we do is learned in the classroom, and some is based on research. However, if one accepts (as many do) that nursing is a calling – a vocation – there is a prevailing belief that much of what nurses do is learned intuition. How many nurses just 'know' that a patient will not make it through the night? How many nurses just 'know' they must go into that room before a patient arrests, or 'know' that a child's temperature has just returned to normal? These are similar to the instincts of a mother for her child. It is the nurturing instinct in nursing which gives nursing the dignity of a noble profession.

Until recently, our 'body of knowledge' was derived from the experience of thousands of nurses who have gone before us, and from our own intuition.[1] However, in recent years, nursing theorists have developed frameworks to explain that experience of nursing and to put it into a theoretical context. Nursing diagnosis may not be as prevalent in the UK as it is in the USA, but this method of defining what nurses do and the rationale behind their actions can only become more evident if nursing is to progress.

There will always be resistance to change, and there will be those who ask where the body of knowledge was when Florence Nightingale anointed the brows of her soldier patients with lavender (Figure 2.1). They will ask what her nursing diagnosis, her nursing plan, would have been. Equally, there will be others who will agree with Larry Dossy, who argues that 'A body of knowledge that does not fit with prevailing ideas can be ignored as if it does not exist, no matter how scientifically valid it may be'.[2]

In today's world, nurses are being asked to define their role, so the appearance of nurse academicians is apposite as they struggle to give some kind of status to nursing. A change in status usually brings with it a change in language. This language needs to be understood by nurses, and by others outside the field of nursing, so everyone can be clear as to what nurses do, why they do it and what they hope to achieve by doing what they do.

Some might argue that this is all reductionist and mechanistic. How can the theory of nursing diagnosis have validity when every patient is different? The answer is that we need to show a clear protocol of what we do. This can only help the development and future of nursing, which lies in the ability to integrate holism, nursing theory and nursing diagnosis symbiotically. Then we can use the science of language to reveal the true art of nursing.

Behind the scientific framework of nursing there is increased discussion of the role of holism in nursing – the art or skill of the nurse to care for the whole patient, rather than for the symptoms that the patient is presenting. No complementary therapy on its own can make a nurse holistic, because holism is something which comes from within.

Aromatherapy involves smell and touch, which are basic needs – learned memories of pleasurable and comforting experiences for both nurse and patient – basic needs. So let us seek a way to nurture our patients in a truly holistic manner. Let us put some good 'scents' back into nursing and, in the process, feel good about what we do. But if we argue our case using nursing theory and nursing diagnosis, we can only make our case stronger and more valid.

THE NIGHTINGALE'S SONG TO THE SICK SOLDIER.

LISTEN, soldier, to the tale of the tender NIGHTINGALE,
　'Tis a charm that soon will ease your wounds so cruel,
Singing medicine for your pain, in a sympathising strain,
　With a jug, jug, jug of lemonade or gruel.

Singing bandages and lint; salve and cerate without stint,
　Singing plenty of both of liniment and lotion,
And your mixtures pushed about, and the pills for you served out,
　With alacrity and promptitude of motion.

Singing light and gentle hands, and a nurse who understands
　How to manage every sort of application,
From a poultice to a leech ; whom you haven't got to teach
　The way to make a poppy fomentation.

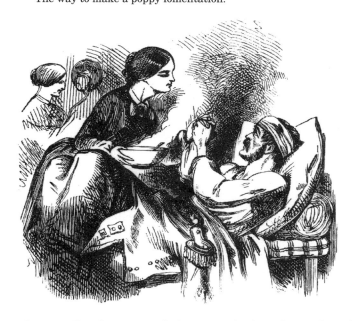

Singing pillow for you smoothed, smart and ache and anguish soothed,
　By the readiness of feminine invention;
Singing fever's thirst allayed, and the bed you've tumbled, made,
　With a careful and considerate attention.

Singing succour to the brave, and a rescue from the grave,
　Hear the NIGHTINGALE that's come to the Crimea,
'Tis a NIGHTINGALE as strong in her heart as in her song,
　To carry out so gallant an idea.

FIGURE 2.1 The Nightingale's Song to the Sick Soldier. Reproduced with kind permission of the Royal College of Nursing Archives.

We have come so far already. It is wonderful to see nurse/acupuncturists, nurse/massage therapists and nurse/aromatherapists being accepted (and paid!) as part of our National Health Service. It is incredible to see these *complementary* therapies being used as they were intended – to *complement* any system into which they are integrated – yet just a short time ago they were ridiculed as quackery.

NURSING DIAGNOSIS

For this section of the book, I have relied heavily on the standard nursing textbook *Nursing Diagnosis: Applications to Clinical Practice*.[3] In some instances I have used similar examples, followed by parallel analysis to show how aromatherapy can be part of nursing diagnosis.

According to the authors of the book *Nursing Interventions: Treatment for Nursing Diagnosis*, nursing interventions are 'any direct care treatment that a nurse performs on behalf of a client'.[4] Using this definition, all treatments initiated by a nurse are related to nursing diagnosis. So if we can show that an aromatherapy intervention could be seen to be a nursing intervention, aromatherapy would be an appropriate response to a nursing diagnosis. Many nurses feel that nursing diagnosis allows them to assess their patients and write care plans more easily.

In the USA, and increasingly here in the UK, the development of nursing diagnosis is an attempt to give focus to the specifications of nursing need by creating an exact language to analyse how the nurse is to reach the decision of what to do. Although resented by some, who may feel that this language is just what nursing does *not* need, it is arguable that nursing diagnosis is exactly what nursing *does* need – a practical tool to clarify the nature, origin and manifestations of nursing need. Nursing diagnosis can also give validity to a complementary therapy within the concept of a care plan. Gordon writes in *Nursing Diagnosis: Process and Application* that the fact that 'a nursing diagnosis is a health problem a nurse can treat does not mean that non-nursing consultants cannot be used. The critical element is whether the nurse-prescribed interventions can achieve the outcome established with the client'.[5]

Although the practice of nursing diagnosis is not yet widespread in the UK, it soon will be. Because it could be a wonderful tool for nurses wishing to use complementary therapies, I have included a section in this book showing how nurses could use nursing diagnosis to argue the validity of aromatherapy.

The term 'nursing diagnosis' was first introduced in 1953 by Fry, who was attempting to set a standardized language for nursing care plans.[3] However, nurses disliked the idea of the word 'diagnosis', feeling that it was too medical. They felt that nursing had a tradition of avoiding making statements about patients. Twenty years went by before the first meeting of the National Group for the Classification of Nursing Diagnosis was held. Eventually, in 1990, the North American Nursing Diagnosis Association (NANDA) approved the following definition of nursing diagnosis: 'Nursing diagnosis is a clinical judgment about individual, family, or community responses to actual or potential health problems/life processes. Nursing diagnosis provides the basis for selection of nursing interventions to achieve outcomes for which the nurse is accountable.'[3]

It is the independent function of a professional nurse to make a nursing diagnosis and to decide upon a course of action to be followed for the solution of the problem.[6]

The practice of nursing often interfaces with the practice of other health professionals; physicians and nurses collaborate in common areas. This can sometimes lead to a nurse having to decide on the priority between responding to a nursing or medical diagnosis. Sometimes a nurse may only attend to those patient problems which require referral to a physician for treatment, because of time constraints. Sometimes the nurse may feel that a medical diagnosis is in some way more important than her own nursing diagnosis in requiring action.

Looking at the areas of nursing diagnosis, it is obvious that they carry very generalized headings, under which more specific headings are given. There are many headings which could lend themselves to the use of aromatherapy. These could include the following:

- anxiety;
- ineffective airway clearance;
- body image disturbance;
- ineffective breathing patterns;
- ineffective breast-feeding;
- caregiver role strain;
- altered comfort;
- impaired communication;
- constipation;
- decisional conflict;
- defensive coping.

The list quoted in Lynda Juall Carpenito's book, *Nursing Diagnosis: Applications to Clinical Practice*[3] continues at length – it includes some 120 different nursing diagnosis headings on a general level, very few of which could *not* be helped with aromatherapy.

Nursing diagnosis represents a situation that is the primary responsibility of the nurse. Nurses may also indicate collaborative problems in their nursing diagnosis which would indicate that both medical and nursing interventions are required, and they can pin-point potential complications which might be collaborative problems or straightforward nursing problems.

For example, a patient with pneumonia would have the potential complications, within the collaborative area, of septic shock, paralytic ileus and respiratory insufficiency. The nursing diagnosis would be:

- activity intolerance due to compromised respiration, high risk of fluid balance deficit due to fever and hyperventilation;
- ineffective airway clearance due to pain and tracheobronchial secretions;
- altered comfort related to hyperthermia, malaise and pulmonary pathology;
- high risk for ineffective management of therapeutic regimen.

The above would be due to nutritional needs, home care needs, restrictions, signs and symptoms of complications and follow-up care.

With the specification of precise needs for nursing it is easier to see those areas where aromatherapy could be used. These would be in the nursing diagnosis of altered comfort, and ineffective airway clearance. I shall consider the first of these as a separate issue.

Nursing diagnosis of altered comfort

Because the cause of the altered comfort is listed as:

- hyperthermia;
- malaise;
- pulmonary pathology;

then anything which is going to alleviate those causes could help to enhance the comfort level of the patient. Malaise might respond to an essential oil with calming and soothing properties. Hyperthermia might respond to tepid sponging using a floral water which contained an essential oil known to be cooling. Pulmonary pathology might respond to an essential oil known to be bronchodilating, which also had antibacterial or antiviral properties. It might be possible to use a blend of three essential oils which addressed the three problems, or alternatively to use one essential oil which would affect all three areas.

Case study 1

Mrs Brown is a 41-year-old woman with a cholecystectomy incision (8 days post-surgery). The incision is not healing well, and there is continual purulent drainage. The nursing care consists of the following:

- inspecting and cleaning the wound site and the surrounding area three times a day;
- applying a stomadhesive and a drainage pouch to contain the discharge and to protect the skin;
- promoting optimal nutrition and hydration.

The immediate problem would be the skin adjacent to the wound breaking down.

Aromatherapy in nursing plan
The nurse prescribes intervention using 2% essential oil of *Lavandula angustifolia* (true lavender) in a carrier oil to prevent the skin breaking down further and to promote healing. Lavender was used for wound cleaning in World War I and was approved by the French Academy of Medicine. As well as an antiseptic action, true lavender has cicatrisant and analgesic properties. Lavender was found to be a mood elevator by Rovesti, and any nurse who has cared for a post-cholecystectomy patient with a wound infection knows that such a patient is likely to be a little depressed. Lavender also has an attractive aroma which may mask the aroma of the wound infection.

The nursing diagnosis is therefore *high risk for impaired skin integrity related to draining purulent wound*.

Gordon developed a system for organizing the assessment of the functional health pattern of a patient.[7] This system lists 11 areas: health management, nutrition/metabolism, elimination, activity/exercise, sleep/rest, perception, self-perception, relationships, sexuality, coping/stress, values/beliefs. It is easy to see that aromatherapy could fit fairly readily into most of these categories. This kind of data enables nurses to make judgements on which the nursing diagnosis will be based. As the care plan will be based on the nursing diagnosis, careful analysis of the assessments is necessary.

Care plans are blueprints to enable a continuous, consistent quality of care. They will contain a diagnostic statement, desired nursing outcome criteria, nursing interventions and an evaluation.

Case study 2

A 45-year-old mother has insomnia due to anxiety about her daughter who is about to sit major examinations. The nursing diagnosis is sleep pattern disturbance.

Nursing care plan
Encourage the patient to verbalize her fears with her partner. Suggest a gentle physical exercise programme. Propose that aromatherapy might aid the patient's ability to relax mentally before bedtime. Discover if the patient

Roman Cham-omile

has a history of allergies. Introduce two essential oils, such as *Chamomelum nobile* and *Lavandula angustifolia*, and discuss how these essential oils make the patient feel. Allow the patient to choose one of the essential oils. If she is comfortable with the idea of touch, introduce the idea of a gentle hand massage using 2 per cent essential oil in a carrier oil, just before bedtime, with an additional single drop of the essential oil on a tissue to inhale immediately before sleep.

The above care plan would be evaluated as follows:

■ Was the diagnosis correct?
■ Was the goal of improving sleep achieved?
■ Was aromatherapy acceptable to the patient?
■ Should aromatherapy be continued, and if so for how long?

Take the difficult procedure of extubation (i.e. removing an endotracheal tube when a patient is capable of breathing without artificial help), which often falls within the remit of an intensive-care nurse. Textbooks state there is no one method of weaning which has clear superiority.[8] However, it is accepted that weaning readiness involves both physical and psychological preparedness.[9] Extubation is a tricky manoeuvre because the patient must be alert enough to breathe on his or her own, but not so alert that the endotracheal tube is causing distress and they are fighting the ventilator. There are reported instances of nurses using aromatherapy who have found that offering the patient a hand massage using dilute lavender (*Lavandula angustifolia*) 20 minutes prior to extubation has enabled the patient to relax and not fight the process, without being so relaxed that they are unable to breathe on their own.

Nursing diagnosis of dysfunctional ventilatory weaning response

The outcome criteria would be as follows:

■ achieve weaning goals;
■ remain extubated;
■ not be exhausted by the process of weaning.

The nursing intervention would consist of the following:

■ determine readiness for weaning;
■ ask if the patient likes the smell of lavender;
■ ask for permission to touch the patient;
■ explain the weaning process whilst giving hand massage using lavender;
■ explain the patient's role in the process of weaning;
■ enhance the patient's feelings of self-esteem through encouragement;
■ promote trust through conversation and touch;

- reduce the negative effects of anxiety and fatigue through the use of lavender;
- create a positive environment with pleasant aroma and gentle touch;
- optimize comfort status through the position of the patient, pleasant aroma and touch.

Case study 3

A 25-year-old man has just been told that his leukaemia is not responding to treatment. For the first time, he has to think about his own death and try to prepare for it.

Nursing diagnosis of spiritual distress

The outcome criteria would be as follows:

- continue spiritual practices as the patient knows them;
- express decreasing feelings of guilt and anxiety;
- express satisfaction with one's spiritual condition.

The nursing intervention would consist of the following:

- provide privacy and quiet;
- be open to the patient's needs for spiritual peace;
- contact the patient's spiritual leader where required;
- suggest that aromatherapy might enhance the patient's ability to meditate, pray or induce a state of peacefulness;
- introduce the essential oils *Boswellia carteri* (frankincense) and *Cananga odorata* var. *genuina* (ylang ylang);
- discuss the effects of both aromas.

All people have a spiritual dimension, whether they choose to accept it or not.[10] Spirituality is often at the core of a person's distress, yet most people find spirituality the most difficult subject to communicate. During acute and chronic disease, many patients may turn to their faith, lose their faith, or seek a faith where there has been none previously. Despite this, nurses commonly avoid addressing the spiritual dimension of a patient. Research suggests that the spiritual part of nursing involves *being with* the patient rather than *doing to* the patient.[11]

Aromatherapy allows us to *be with* our patient even while we may be *doing to*, in an intimate but controlled way which nurtures the relationship between the nurse and the patient. This often allows a window of inner reflection in which spiritual feelings (or needs) are verbalized. During my training as a nurse, and subsequent to it, few patients brought up the subject of spiritual matters. Yet since I have been using aromatherapy, this sensitive area has arisen time and time again, almost as though the aromas themselves provide an atmosphere of acceptance.

Larry Dossey writes about the need for thought to be accepted as being as genuine as any drug or surgical procedure.[2] The thoughts generated by gentle touch and pleasing smell have a powerful effect on our psyche and on our spirituality. It is not only what we *do* for patients, but also our good intentions to *be* with them which can aid their healing process. Nursing has a 'curative' potential. Despite the fact that 15 per cent of nurses feel that they are not prepared to provide spiritual care,[12] they can provide spiritual support just by *being* there. The use of aromatherapy gives us permission to *be* there.

Case study 4

A young mother of an 8-month-old baby. Both the mother and her baby have AIDS.

Nursing diagnosis of high risk of infection

This describes a patient whose host defences are compromised. Nursing interventions for such a patient should be centred on reducing the potential risk of infection to that individual. Because the skin is the first line of defence, it is logical to protect it from infection using anti-infectious agents. Many essential oils have proven anti-infectious properties (see section on infection in Chapter 7) and can be used diluted on the skin (1–5 per cent) with no detrimental side-effects.

Some infections are airborne. Despite the defence systems in the nasal mucous membranes, which contain immunoglobulin A and lysosomes, the inhalation of infections is common. It is very difficult to prevent infection from entering a patient's room unless they are in an isolation unit.

With regard to the nursing intervention, as well as the usual practices of preventing cross-infection, the use of aromatherapy can provide a beneficial enhancement of nursing care. Touch and smell can reduce the patient's anxiety about the possibility of infection. At the same time, specific essential oils can add additional support to the orthodox antisepsis programme in progress. The use of atomizers containing 5 per cent essential oils with known antiseptic properties would not only give a pleasant smell to the room but also provide added defence against pathogenic micro-organisms. Examples of such essential oils could include: *Eucalyptus globulus, Eucalyptus smithi, Melaleuca alternifolia* chemotype (CT) terpineole and *Lavandula intermedia* CT super. One or two of the essential oils should be used, and interchanged with the other two essential oils every 3 weeks. The atomizer needs to be sprayed in the room four times daily. At this concentration there is little likelihood of sensitivity, although if there is any concern about this, a patch test can be taken first (see section on patch testing).

CONCLUSIONS

A few case studies have been presented above – a brief argument to support the use of aromatherapy to enhance nursing care. We use many over-the-counter products which are not prescribed by a physician. We use soaps and hair-spray which are perfumed with essential oils on our patients. We use synthetic sprays to mask human smells. It is time to think what aromatherapy could mean to our nursing and how it could enhance what we do – how it could enhance who we are, in every aspect of our lives.

One of my students said that 'aromatherapy has changed my life – now I notice what smells good and what doesn't'. She went on to say 'So much in life smells bad, doesn't it? I wonder if that is because we have made a nonsense of nature'. We are making a nonsense of nursing if we are 'not allowed' to make our patients feel better through gentle touch and the use of scents which are already part of everyday life. Before palliative care became an accepted specialty within nursing, it was unknown, but nurses still did carry out palliative care. Then it became recognized as a distinctive and very caring form of health care. Before the first heart transplant, people thought that heart transplants were not possible. Now there are countless books on surgery and the nursing of these patients. Nursing is evolving as world perceptions change. Nurses are using aromatherapy in many parts of the world. They are using it *now* because it has validity whether one's view of nursing is intuitive or derived through nursing diagnosis.

How aromatherapy could be used in hospitals

There are many potential uses for aromatherapy in hospitals, ranging from the simple mood-enhancing antidepressant effects of smelling something pleasant and uplifting to the specific application of the antiseptic properties of the essential oils used in aromatherapy to combat cross-infections. At present our hospitals do not smell nice.

Medical science is now aware that how we feel affects how we are. If it is possible to manipulate our environment to be supportive in times of need, i.e. in an emergency or stress situation, surely this is something to be taken very seriously.

John Steele was responsible for some of the first important research on how aromatherapy could affect the mind, when he tested volunteers using a

John Steele how aromatherapy affects mind

Mind Mirror to demonstrate changes in electroencephalogram (EEG) following the smelling of certain essential oils. He discovered that changes in brain rhythms occurred within 15 seconds, and that a change in mood took approximately the same length of time.[13]

Patients undergoing radiotherapy or computer-assisted tomography (CAT) scans are isolated in a room during treatment and have to lie absolutely still for lengthy periods of time. Many find this experience very stressful. A soothing, relaxing essential oil such as lavender (*Lavandula vera*), vetiver (*Vetiveria zizanoides*) or bergamot (*Citrus bergamia*) in the air-vent might help them. In New York, research has shown that 60 per cent of patients exposed to a sweet vanilla-like fragrance (heliotropin) experienced less anxiety than the control group.[14]

Accident and Emergency wards are recipients of the results of catastrophes such as road traffic accidents, burns and poisoning. Immediate action is needed, and frequently, in the heat of the moment, relatives find it difficult to stay calm enough to explain exactly what happened. Medical professionals find it hard to maintain patience, knowing that every second is vital but needing precise information. By combining an antiseptic essential oil with a calming one, the environment is immediately made more reassuring and more hospitable.

Wards for care of the elderly often have a depressing smell – stale urine from incontinent patients, lingering smells of hospital food, and over-use of lavatory cleaner. Helen Passant, a nurse, managed to change that situation in Oxford when she introduced the use of aromatherapy massage. Her elderly patients responded to the use of touch and massage, becoming 'alive' again – a situation reminiscent of the film, *Beginnings*. The aromas evoked memories, and the patients began to talk about their lives and to communicate their feelings. No longer isolated men and women waiting to die, they became an active group – singing, dancing and creating. Their drug bill was reduced by one-third.

Many operating theatres have closed air-conditioning. This means that the same air is ventilated consistently. It is much less expensive than open air-conditioning, which sucks in a constant stream of new air, warms and filters it and then vents it back into the outside environment. Research has been carried out on airborne infections such as those caused by *Staphylococcus aureus*, and on the prevalence of post-operative wound infections. The incidence of such wound infections is not high, but one could argue that any post-operative wound infection should be avoided. There is sufficient data to indicate that post-operative wound infections (from pre-operatively clean wounds) are directly correlated with the length of operating time.[15] By adding an essential oil with strong antibacterial and antiviral properties, it may be possible to reduce the cost of the additional

touch
+5
oils

days incurred as in-patients for those with inatropic (hospital-acquired) wound infections.

Indeed, certain enlightened hospitals are already experimenting with the controlled use of specific antibacterial essential oils in the air-conducting vents of operating theatres, an added bonus being the prevention of cross-infection among medical personnel as well as among patients. As it is possible for each operating suite to conduct its own research into which bacteria and viruses are most prevalent, a customized cocktail of several essential oils could be employed. In addition, it is arguable that the additional use of a stimulant essential oil, such as pine (*Pinus sylvestris*) or lemon (*Citrus limonum*), after 10 p.m. at night, might also improve the concentration of operating personnel during night-shifts.

The use of aromatherapy in hospitals in England, South Africa, Switzerland and, more recently, in the USA shows a progressive trend towards supporting patients on a more holistic basis. Physicians and hospital managers are much more aware of how their patients' feelings can acutely affect the way in which they respond to treatment, and therefore how quickly they recover.

Touch is known to have a dramatic effect on patients. A consultant anaesthetist conducted a survey among his own patients, holding the hands of some while he gave them their pre-operation 'pep talk', and not holding the hands of others. The patients who had had their hands held needed significantly less sedation and analgesic post-operatively. Babies who are denied touch fail to thrive. Patients lying in a hospital bed are rarely touched, except for procedural reasons (e.g. dressing, blood pressure recording) or diagnostic one's (e.g. palpation). Aromatherapy massage quickly acknowledges their worth as an individual. A foot massage or hand massage takes only 10 minutes, but in that time can totally change how a patient perceives the environment around him or her. Touch has been shown to reduce blood pressure, reduce lower back pain, relieve anxiety and alleviate depression. This being so, not only would patients benefit from aromatherapy in hospitals, but so also would staff and visitors.

Aromas have also been shown to enhance the output of the work-force, raise feelings of job satisfaction and reduce sick-leave.[16] Specific aromas have shown specific effects. Melissa has been used for grief, lemongrass to mask *specifics* offensive smells, marjoram and lavender to aid insomnia in the elderly, and geranium and mandarin to enhance memory recall in patients with Alzheimer's disease.

Aromatherapy using touch and smell could be a complete hospital stress management package, producing a happier and more content work force, with more secure and less anxious patients. The implications of the level of interest shown by patients and nurses are sufficient to suggest an overwhelming need for a coherent investigation into such an integration.

The economics of using fragrance in hospitals to accelerate patient turnover is one analysis which few holistic therapists would care to use, but as hospitals become more and more like businesses there is an urgent need to examine the cost benefits of using essential oils to promote healing.

Some say that there is a need to address the subjects of consent and ethics in aromatherapy. Is it ethical to manipulate mood, even if not subliminally? What about those patients who do not like the aromas? The utilization of air-conditioning vents raises issues which need to be clarified, as does the use of essential oils in a ward setting where, even if they wish to do so, patients are unable to remove themselves from the aroma.

One answer could be in the form of a questionnaire for staff prior to starting to use aromatherapy, and a signed consent form for patients. This might appear to be pedantic, but it is the democratic right of a patient to seek the treatment he or she wishes, and therefore to refuse a treatment. Yet how many patients or members of staff sign a consent form approving the smell of antiseptics or air-fresheners? How many nurses enter their place of work wearing perfume or deodorant? What are the ethics involved if a patient actively dislikes that perfume or deodorant? It is difficult to have one set of rules for aromatherapy if there are no rules governing other types of aroma. What about those patients who may be allergic or sensitive to specific essential oils? What about their visitors, relatives, and doctors? There are many issues surrounding safety and ethics which will be addressed in the section on safety.

Another area of serious concern is the potential use of synthetic/adulterated essential oils, resulting in poor or negative results. It cannot be emphasized strongly enough that it is the quality of the essential oil which will determine the final result. Just as a good wine depends on the soil, sun and rain, so do the plants which produce essential oils. This means that essential oils are not all identical – different years will produce slightly different essential oils. Different areas of the world will also produce different essential oils, so there is no exact standard, but only a general template. Essential oils need to be judged like good wine. Good wine is expensive, and so are the best essential oils.

Perhaps one of the greatest concerns about the use of aromatherapy in hospitals is the possibility of incorrect use due to ignorance. Contrary to media hype, aromatherapy is not the panacea for everything, a kind of 'comfort-blanket' smell. Of equal importance is the quality of the touch. A heavy, compressing, rapid stroke will not produce the same effect as a light, slow, gentle one. The techniques used in aromatherapy cannot be learnt solely from a book or video – they need to be experienced.

lavender

There is an urgent need for adequate training, and one weekend or one week is not enough. As well as learning how to touch correctly, the specific use of the essential oils used in aromatherapy requires knowledge and experience. A simple name like lavender covers three completely different species, each with entirely different therapeutic effects, one being a sedative, one being a stimulant and one being useful in the treatment of *Pseudomonas*, but neurotoxic except in small doses.[17]

REFERENCES

1. **Leddy, S. and Pepper, J.M.** 1993: *Conceptual bases of professional nursing.* Mickleton, NJ: J.B. Lippincott Co.

2. **Dossey, L.** 1993: *Healing words.* San Francisco: Harper Collins.

3. **Carpenito, L.J.** 1993: *Nursing diagnosis: applications to clinical practice,* 5th edn. Mickleton, NJ: J.B. Lippincott Co.

4. **Bulechek, G. and McCloskey, J.** 1985: *Nursing interventions: treatment for nursing diagnosis.* Philadelphia: W.B. Saunders.

5. **Gordon, M.** 1982: *Nursing diagnosis: process and application.* New York: McGraw-Hill.

6. **Abdellah, F.G. and Levine, E.** 1965: *Better patient care through nursing research.* New York: Macmillan.

7. **Gordon, M.** 1990: Towards theory-based diagnostic categories. *Nursing Diagnosis* **1**, 5–11.

8. **Yang, K.L. and Tobin, M.J.** 1991: A prospective study of indexes predicting outcomes of trials of weaning from mechanical ventilation. *New England Journal of Medicine* **324**, 1445–51.

9. **Logan, J. and Jenny, J.** 1990: Deriving a new nursing diagnosis through qualitative research: dysfunctional ventilatory response. *Nursing Diagnosis* **1**, 37–43.

10. **Dickinson, C.** 1975: The search for spiritual meaning. *American Journal of Nursing* **75**, 1789–93.

11. **Martin, C., Burrow, C. and Pomilio, J.** 1978: Spiritual needs of patients' surveys. In Fish, S. and Shelly, J.A. (eds), *Spiritual care: the nurse's role.* Downers Grove, IL: Intervarsity Press.

12. **Stiles, M.K.** 1990: The shining stranger: nurse-family spiritual relationship. *Cancer Nursing* **13**, 235–56.

13. **Steele, J.** 1993: The fragrant hospital. In *Aroma 93 Conference Proceedings.* Brighton: Aromatherapy Publications, 22–9.

14. **Balacs, T.** 1991: Fragrance relaxes. In Research Reports. *International Journal of Aromatherapy* **33**, 8.

15. **Cruse, P.J.E.** 1980: The epidemiology of wound infection: a 10-year prospective study of 69 939 wounds. *Surgical Clinics of North America* **60**, 27–40.

16. **Lawless, J.** 1994: *Aromatherapy and the mind*. London: Thorsons.

17. **Franchomme, P. and Peneol, D.** 1990: *L'aromatherapie exactement*. Limoge: Roger Jollios.

3

THE NATURE OF AROMATHERAPY

Aromatherapy is the use of essential oils for therapeutic or medical purposes. Franchome calls it 'a powerful and reliable therapeutic method ... the treatment of illnesses by vegetal aromas, and in particular, by essential oils'.[1] Herbalist Jeanne Rose classifies it as 'the healing of essential oils through the sense of smell by inhalation, and through application of these therapeutic volatile substances.'[2] The Institute of Classical Aromatherapy defines aromatherapy as 'a natural treatment which uses the concentrated herbal energies in essential oils from plants in association with massage, friction, inhalation, compresses and baths'.[3] In Gattefosse's book, the grandfather of aromatherapy, it is called 'a therapy or cure using aromas, aromatics, scents'.[4]

According to Anne Gilt, there are four different types of aromatherapy: clinical aromatherapy, stress management aromatherapy, beauty therapy aromatherapy and smell aromatherapy.[5] Tisserand agrees that there are varying types, but classifies them slightly differently, as psycho-aromatherapy, aesthetic aromatherapy, holistic aromatherapy, nursing aromatherapy and medical aromatherapy.[6]

Without doubt, 'nice smells' added to a massage in a beauty salon are something akin to flowers on the table at a restaurant; they are not specific ingredients of the meal, but they certainly enhance it. This is a form of aesthetic aromatherapy. Beauty therapists do not usually treat disease. However, at the other end of the aromatherapy spectrum, medical aromatherapy suggests that specific medical conditions *can* be treated with essential oils. Franchomme and Peneol, Gattefosse and Belaiche have written books dedicated to this end. So these two different types of aromatherapy – aesthetic and medical – are very distinct. The misunderstandings that arise concern the others in between, including nursing aromatherapy and what it entails.

Holistic aromatherapy suggests that the therapist is involved with all parts of the patient, in other words, with mind, body and spirit. To me, and this is consistent with Tisserand's diagrammatic outlines, holistic aromatherapy involves 'supporting' a patient. It is a procedure often carried out by body workers who may or may not know much about the chemistry of the essential oils or the pathology to which they are appropriate. They are not 'treating' the patient so much as supporting other treatments that the patient may be receiving, which can be either orthodox or alternative.

Aesthetic aromatherapy is about pleasure. To choose a smell because it is pleasing is similar to studying a beautiful picture. The picture is treasured for the pleasure it gives, not for its intrinsic molecular structure. To put it another way, the use of perfume, scented bath soaps and incense sticks is the use of aesthetic aromatherapy, and the world would be a sadder place without it. When patients are nearing the end of their lives, we as nurses are more concerned with keeping them comfortable than with prolonging their life. At that stage, aesthetic aromatherapy can give pleasure and comfort.

Psychoaromatherapy concerns the ways in which smells or odours affect our brains, and can encourage the production of endorphins and noradrenaline. Whether we realize it or not, our entire lives are affected by smell. We even choose our partners through smells called pheromones. These chemicals are given off involuntarily, attracting or repelling others. Although we may not be aware of someone's smell (and this is not the same as body odour), it is this smell which really attracts us to that person.

Couples going through marriage breakdown often say that their partner 'no longer smells the same'. This is much truer than they realize: the chemical attraction between them *has* changed. It has changed from attracting mode into repelling mode, just as their emotions have changed. Pheromones work in a subliminal way, so we are unaware of them, although we still know 'something' is different.

Everyone's body odour is unique – a 'smellprint'. Recently, an electronic device known as 'The Bloodhound' was built at Cambridge University. This man-made sniffer dog can identify a person's 'smellprint', and by recording a particular person's unique body odour, the machine can recognize that same smellprint anywhere in the world.

It is also possible, using psychoaromatherapy, to manipulate mood or to change perception through the use of *subliminal* smell. A certain amount of research has been conducted on this, and the results show that we can encourage or manipulate people in a particular way using this method of aromatherapy. For example, we can encourage them to purchase an item, in preference to another identical item, by impregnating it with a pleasant subliminal smell.

Companies can 'persuade' customers to pay bills on time by impregnating invoices with subliminal offensive odours. The concept is disturbing, and the possible repercussions arguably unethical, but when has big business been overconcerned about morality? Perhaps, in time, there will be a subliminal smell which can pervade stadiums towards the end of a football match to make hooligans travel home in an orderly fashion from a match!

Psychoaromatherapy is not just about subliminal smell. The perfume industry is very concerned with how our choice of scent affects us. Millions of pounds and dollars of potential profit each year is channelled into olfaction research. Incidentally, the perfume you wear could enhance your immunity if it actually contains essential oils. However, due to their very high cost, few perfumes contain real essential oils; they are now mostly composed of synthetic derivatives.

All forms of aromatherapy have been around for many hundreds of years. They are definitely not 'New Age'. Despite the explosion of products currently on the market which include the word 'aromatherapy' on the label, the use of essential oils in products is not new, unlike the use of many of the synthetic copies.

HISTORY OF AROMATHERAPY: AN OUTLINE

Ancient history

The use of herbal medicine dates back thousands of years and is not confined to any one geographical area. Almost every part of the world has some history of the use of aromatics in its health care system.

Iraq

Perhaps the earliest use of aromatics was discovered only recently. In 1975, during investigation of a dig in Iraq, concentrated extracts of yarrow, knapweed, grape hyacinth, mallow and other plants were found near a Neanderthal skeleton dating back 60 000 years.[7] Of the eight species of herbs, seven are still being used today in medicine.[8]

France

One of the earliest records of aromatic medicine is in the form of paintings drawn on the walls of caves in Lascaux, Dordogne in France.[9] These drawings tell of the use of medicinal plants and date back to 18 000BC.

Mesopotamia

The Sumerians, who lived in Mesopotamia from 5500BC, became sophisticated in herbal medicine. In this matriarchal society, the women were the healers, either as shamans called Ashipu, or as herbalists called Asu.[10] They left as their legacy clay tablets containing prescriptions, names of plants, methods of preparation and dosages.[7] Aromatic medicine featured strongly in this early culture, and pots have been found which could have been used in plant distillation dating back to this time.

Egypt

The ancient Egyptians used aromatics in their embalming process, removing most of the internal body parts and replacing them with fragrant preparations such as cedar and myrrh. In the seventeenth century some of these 'mummies' were sold and distilled to be used in medicines themselves![11] One of the most famous manuscripts listing aromatic medicines is the Egyptian Papyrus Ebers manuscript, found near Thebes in 1872. This document, written during the reign of Khufu, around 2800BC, was closely followed by another document, written about 2000BC which speaks of 'fine oils and choice perfumes'.These manuscripts, written when the Great Pyramid was still being built, show that during the time of Moses, frankincense, myrtle, galbanum and eaglewood were some of the many aromatic herbs used. There is also mention of myrrh being used to treat hay fever.

When Tutankhamun's tomb was opened in 1922, the boy-king was wearing floral collars that were still faintly aromatic. A total of 35 alabaster jars of perfume were found in his burial chamber, all of them broken or empty as they had contained frankincense and myrrh, highly valued commodities and therefore the first items to be stolen from the tomb.[12]

China

The earliest known text of written instructions on how to use herbs as medicines was written by the Chinese. This *Great Herbal* or *Pen Ts'ao* was written by Shen Nung. In the herbal he lists some 350 plants, many of which are still being used today. One of them is the herb *Ephedra sinica*, found in the Neanderthal grave. The great Herbal dates back to about 2800BC. Another emperor, Huang Ti, sometimes called the Yellow Emperor, wrote the *Huang Ti Nei Ching Su Wen*. The English translation is called *The Yellow Emperor's Classic of Internal Medicine*.[13]

India

Vedic medicine, the precursor to Ayervedic medicine, which has been used for 5000 years, has at its core the *Vedas*, which lists 700 different items, many of them herbs and aromatics such as ginger, coriander, myrrh, cinnamon and sandalwood.

Tibet

Tibetan medicine has traditionally used aromatic herbs, many in inhalations. These herbs are usually prescribed in complex remedies, such as 'Aquilaria A', which contains aromatics including clove, cardamom, sandalwood and myrrh.[14]

Traditional Indian shamans known as *perfumeros* were healers who used the scents of aromatic plants.[12]

Greece

The ancient Greeks used aromatics. Dioskurides suggested that one of them, *Artemesia dracunculus* (tarragon) was useful in the treatment of cancer, as a cure for gangrene, as an abortifacient, and as protection against viper bites. Tarragon was later used by the Native Americans during difficult labours and to induce menstruation. It was thought to be such an important herb that it was classified as a 'chief medicine', so it was necessary for the collector to pull it (pick it) and not dig it up, out of respect for its power.

Helen of Troy was famed for her use of aromatics in mood-enhancing potions. In 300BC, Theophrastus wrote his *Enquiry into Plants*, in which he described specific uses of aromatics. At that time there was a special name for doctors who used aromatic unctions – they were called *latralyptes*. One formula of aromatics that they used, containing 16 different ingredients, was called *Kyphi*. It was used as an antiseptic and an antidote to poison, was soothing to the skin and 'would lull one to sleep, allay anxiety and brighten dreams'. It was Theophrastus, later to be called the 'father of botany'[9] who discovered that the perfume of jasmine was stronger at night, and to this day the highest quality jasmine blossoms are picked at night.

The legendary Greek Pedanios Dioskurides (frequently misspelt Dioscorides) lived in AD100. He wrote the famous *De Materia Medica*. This foundation stone of Western herbal medicine listed over 700 plants which were in use at the time.[15] Easily recognizable were aromatics such as basil, verbena, cardamom, rose, rosemary and garlic. Each section of the *De Materia Medica* begins with a drawing and description, and the contraindications are carefully listed.[8]

Army doctors travelled with large supplies of herbal remedies, but in a manual written for the Emperor Claudius in AD43, detailed instructions were found which gave advice on how to recognize plants abroad, and how to pick and pack them. Everyone seemed to be receiving herbal medicine in some form. Even audiences watching the competitive sports in the stadium in Daphne were sprinkled with rose-water to keep up their spirits and urge the games on.

Hippocrates (460BC) is recognized as being the father of medicine as we know it today – just think of the Hippocratic oath. He wrote that 'aromatic baths are useful in the treatment of female disorders, and would often be useful for the other conditions too.'[16] He understood the principles of psychosomatic disorders, and his was possibly the first statement on holism: 'in order to cure the human body it is necessary to have knowledge of the whole'.[10] However, he was also aware that aromatics had important antibacterial properties, and when an epidemic of plague broke out he urged the people to use aromatic plants to protect themselves and stop the spread of the disease.

During the immediate pre-Christian era, Jewish women would spike with myrrh the wine given to those being tortured, to enable them to go into a trance-like state, and they sometimes also added frankincense for its anaesthetic effects.

When Claudios Galenos (in English known as Galen) was appointed personal physician to Emperor Marcus (AD130–200) he continued the use of fragrant oils, and called the fragrance of narcissus the 'food of the soul'. By regimenting the whole process of classification in his massive *Peri krateos kai dunaneos ton naplon pharmakon*, he set the tone for all further identification of plants.[8]

In *Peri* he listed not only different herbs but different grades of herbs such as cinnamon.[15] Unfortunately, many of the 500 works he compiled were destroyed when his clinic was burned down in Rome. However, the system introduced in his largest work, which consisted of 11 books, survived. Galen's approach to herbs involved describing the plants' energetic profiles as well as their pharmacology, and is similar to the Chinese and Ayervedic approaches.

By describing a disease process in terms of temperature and moisture, he laid the cornerstone of modern physiology.[10] This complicated but fascinating approach to aromatics, which includes the energetic approach, has recently been covered in Peter Holmes' analysis, *The Energetics of Western Herbs, Volumes 1 and 2.*[15]

Persia

A Persian doctor living in Arabia produced a further encyclopaedia called *Collection of Simple Remedies and Foods*, in which he listed 2325 botanics. He

banned by Church

was elevated to the rank of Chief of Botanists by Sultan Al-Kamil in 1220 when he moved to Egypt.

During the early Christian era, aromatics were considered to be pagan by the Church, as they could heighten sensual pleasure, and in AD529, Pope Gregory the Great passed a law banning *Materia Medica*. The School of Philosophy at Athens closed and the works of Galen and Hippocrates were smuggled to Syria.

Arabia

Arab doctors began to play an important part in the development of aromatic medicine. By the third century, Alexandria had become a centre continuing the Greek tradition of the science of aromatics. In AD980, Avicenna invented a new kind of apparatus for distilling essential oils, called an alembic. Avicenna was also responsible for the *Canon of Medicine*, which remained a standard medical textbook until the sixteenth century.[10]

Europe

By the thirteenth century, 'the perfumes of Arabia' mentioned by Shakespeare had spread to Europe. Being surrounded by pleasant odours was supposed to give protection against disease, especially the plague. Glove-makers in London became licensed to impregnate their wares with essential oils, and many survived the Great Plague. Pomanders containing solid perfumes, which originated in the East, as well as scent boxes became popular among the aristocracy. During this time, the Abbess of Bingen, St Hildegarde, wrote four books on medicinal plants.

By the sixteenth century, many Europeans had formed their own collective works on herbs and aromatics. Among them, Walther Ryff from Strassburg produced a *Materia Medica* together with a therapeutic manual. This German herbal turned out to be much more popular among its fellow men than Culpepper's own herbal ever was. (Perhaps this is the reason why, from 1993, all German medical students have been required to study herbal medicine and to pass an examination in phytotherapy. The German people have been much more open to tisanes and tinctures – herbal teas being freely available in restaurants and coffee shops well before the 'new age era' of healthy living and vegetarianism arrived.)

With the Renaissance and subsequent world exploration, many spices were added to Europe's knowledge of herbs. Explorers such as Captain Cooke were involved who, legend has it, discovered tea tree as well as Australia. Coco leaves (resulting in the many popular chocolate houses which sprang up in Europe) were brought in from South America and balsam from Peru. Both herbs became listed in the Pharmacopoeia. During one such exploration a British man named Cartier discovered a cure for scurvy from the North American Indians, whilst he was wintering in Quebec. Most of his fellow travellers had fallen ill, but his friend, Dom Agaya, suddenly appeared to be completely cured.

Intrigued, Cartier investigated and discovered that Dom Agaya had drunk a concoction from the branch of a tree that the Native Americans called Annedda, which was probably what is now known as spruce. This was the first documentation of scurvy treatment. The Native Americans were also adept at treating wounds with tree gum such as that of *Abies balsamea.* They treated dysentery with cedar leaves, and they used sweat lodges to promote healing.

They also used narcotic plants, such as water hemlock, in topical applications, viciously scratching the skin until it bled before applying the herb. Many Native American herbs and principles are still in use, but it is only now that the medical knowledge of these people is beginning to be respected for its depth, history and sophistication.[7]

Paracelsus, a Swiss-German doctor, was watching the emergence of a plethora of 'herbals.' He poured scorn on what he felt were 'reconstituted manuals', wanting to experience something innovative and new. He subsequently became one of the first alchemists in medicine, using minerals such as mercury and antimony, as well as herbs. Paracelsus also held the belief, common at the time, that a little of like would cure like. This was a philosophy that would be reintroduced as homeopathy in later years.[8]

Paracelsus was also a firm believer in the doctrine of signatures – that plants indicated the organ that they could treat either by their shape or by the place where they grew. However, by the time of his death, Paracelsus was firmly associated with the revolution supporting mineral preparations, and he questioned many of Galen's principles. He felt that isolating an active ingredient from a plant would enhance its strength and increase its safeness.

We now know to our cost that this is not always the case. Plants have their own synergistic action which is irreplaceable. In the plant world, the sum of the parts really does add up to more than the total.[17] If the most active constituent is removed and applied in isolation, it will often have a different effect. The effect of the whole plant, as opposed to the effect of the isolated compound, is known as quenching.[18] To explain this further, in the case of citral (found in lemongrass) the isolated compound citral produces a more severe sensitization reaction at a lower concentration than the complete essential oil, which contains a higher percentage of citral.

This demonstrates that isolating all of the active ingredients and then recombining them will not necessarily produce the same effect as the complete essential oil. However, this is how drug companies usually view research into herbs – isolate and synthesize. To this day Paracelsus is regarded as the first medical pharmacologist – the patron saint of drug companies.

In 1596, Descartes declared that man was a machine with a soul based in his pineal gland. He went on to say that mind and body bore no relationship to one another and the concept of soul faded. The idea that an aromatic compound could have an effect on the body via the brain began to fall into disrepute. Not until the eighteenth century was it suggested by a physician named Gaub that 'bodily diseases may often be more readily alleviated or cured by the mind, that is by the emotions, than by corporeal remedies'.[10]

Gaub suggested that doctors should search for substances which would affect the mind. This gave Charles Fourier exactly the task that he had been waiting for. He had an idea that there *was* a cosmic olfactory foundation to life. Two hundred years later this was the task of the Arome research carried out by the French National Centre for Scientific Research.

England

William Turner (1520–1568) was one of the earliest English herbalists. A Cambridge graduate, he also believed in the doctrine of signature, and named many plants, such as lungwort and liverwort, to indicate their use. Unfortunately, at this time, qualifying as a doctor took up to 20 years. The apothecaries from whom physicians purchased their medicines were also 'prescribing' 'on the side'. In order to control this situation, in 1512 Parliament introduced the first in a series of laws to try to regulate the prescription and sale of medicines. Six years later, the College of Physicians was established.

However, the seventeenth century is mainly remembered as the golden era for herbal medicine. Culpepper, who posthumously became one of the more famous herbalists, published his *Complete Herbal* in 1660. He was closely followed by Salmon, who published first a *Dispensatory* (Pharmacopoeia) in 1696, and then, in 1710, his own *Herbal*. During the 1700s, essential oils were widely used in 'mainstream' medicine. In Salmon's *Dispensary* of 1696, he lists oils of cinnamon, lavender, lemon, clove, rue and others in a recipe to 'cheer and comfort all the spirits, natural, vital and animal'.[19]

The nineteenth century saw the first scientific evaluation of essential oils, many of the results being published in William Whitla's *Materia Medica* in 1882. The industrial and scientific revolution followed, and during the next two centuries scores of essential oils were analysed. It was thought important to identify and isolate therapeutic components of plants. In the late 1890s, specific components such as geraniol and citronellol were identified, and in 1868 William Henry Perkin announced the synthesis of coumarin. Synthetic copies of perfumes and aromatics began to be made, and the era of modern drug development dawned. Willow bark became aspirin, and foxglove became digitalis.

However, in isolating parts of plants, the pharmaceutical industry has tended to ignore synergy – a vital part of aromatherapy. Despite important research on the therapeutic effects of many essential oils by Cadeac and Meunier in France and Gatti and Cajola in Italy, essential oils and herbal medicine lost in popularity to synthetic drugs. As a result, the pharmaceutical industry has grown to become a major economic and political force. Until recently the drug companies have appeared to be disinterested in ethnobotanical research. However, this situation is beginning to change.

One example of this change leading to co-operation is a company called Shaman Pharmaceuticals Inc. Founded in 1989, Shaman works with Merck and Co., Ono Pharmaceuticals, Bayer and Eli Lily, looking at a range of plants and plant extracts. A 1996 report sponsored by the *Financial Times* suggests that this kind of collaboration will increase.

From the rest of the world we have the following records.

- Australian aborigines have used eucalyptus as an antiseptic for hundreds of years.
- North African tribes have used saffron, musk and orris throughout their history.
- In Asia, basil has been regarded as holy and its roots made into sacred beads.
- In Tahiti, women protect their hair with coconut oil scented with sandalwood.
- The Aztecs had special rooms built next to their temples to allow steam combined with flowers and herbs to treat their ailments.

Modern history

Gradually, herbal remedies were replaced with synthetic compounds, such as salicin, derived from the willow, later to be developed as aspirin. It was becoming difficult to supply sufficient herbs to meet demand, and this spurred on the early chemists to find other remedies. Non-herbal remedies began to be introduced, e.g. mercury, which rapidly became the common treatment for syphilis.

The modern renaissance of aromatherapy began in France with the work of Gattefosse, Valnet and Maury. Maurice Gattefosse, a chemist, lived in

France from 1881 to 1950. Although he was known as a pragmatist, he also had a fascination for metaphysics, and was interested in both the psychological and physiological effects of aromatics using topical application of essential oils. A meticulous chemist, his pioneering vision set the foundations for research into many of the effects of aromas which is still being conducted today.

It was through an accident that Gattefosse was first drawn to researching aromatherapy. Whilst he was working in his laboratory, an explosion occurred and he plunged his burnt arm into a vat which contained essential oil of lavender (*Lavandula angustifolia*). Impressed by the way in which his arm healed and how rapidly the pain disappeared, he dedicated his life to researching essential oils. Many of his patients were soldiers wounded in the trenches of World War I. Among the essential oils he used were thyme, chamomile, clove and lemon and, up until World War II, those essential oils were used both as 'natural' disinfectants, and to sterilize surgical instruments.[9]

Gattefosse was the first person to use the word 'aromatherapy'. In his research he discovered that essential oils take from between 30 minutes and 12 hours to be absorbed completely by the body after being applied topically. His work *Aromatherapie* giving detailed case studies, was published in France in 1937, but until recently a copy of the manuscript proved elusive. Finally, after 20 years of searching, it was discovered by well-known American herbalist Jeanne Rose. She was the first person to see the famous document, in 1990.[2] The manuscript was then translated into English by Robert Tisserand, and the book *Gateffosse's Aromatherapy*[4] was published in English in 1993.

Throughout the war, French doctors used essential oils on a multiplicity of wound infections and as a treatment for gangrene. Perhaps the course of aromatic medicine would have been different if Alexander Fleming had not discovered a piece of mouldy bread which led to the manufacture of penicillin. With the emergence of manufactured antibiotics, full of promise, profit and easy availability, the demise of aromatherapy seemed certain.

Dr Jean Valnet was born in the early 1900s, and is still alive at the time of writing this book. An army doctor, he spent much of his life researching aromatherapy, and was interviewed in 1993 by Christine Scott for the *International Journal of Aromatherapy*.[20] His publication *Aromatherapie*[21] was the first 'medical' publication on aromatherapy, full of examples of case studies and numerous references to research. He wrote that it 'is not necessary to be a doctor to use aromatherapy. But one has to know the power of essential oils in order to avoid accidents and incidents.'[20]

During his time in Indo-China, where he was commander of an Advanced Surgical Unit, Valnet practised aromatic medicine with the approval of his superiors. However, despite impressive results, when he returned to France, orthodox medical practitioners, unhappy with his use of unconventional medicine, tried to strike him off the general medical list. Fortunately for aromatherapy, some of his patients were high-ranking government officials, including the Minister of Health, so this did not happen.[20] His book, *The Practice of Aromatherapy*, possibly *the* classic on aromatherapy, has been translated into German, Italian, Spanish and Japanese as well as English.

Marguerite Maury's life was initially one of tragedy. Born in Austria, she married very early and had her first child whilst still a teenager. Sadly, her son died from meningitis, aged only two years. Shortly afterwards, her husband was killed in action, and his death was closely followed by her father's suicide. Keen to make a new start, Marguerite decided to move to France. Whilst she was working there as a surgical assistant she met and married Dr Maury. He shared her love of the arts and her fascination with alternative approaches to medicine, and together they formed a cohesive and inspirational team.

As chairman of the Comité International d'Esthétique et de Cosmétologie (CIDESCO), Marguerite won two international prizes for her research on essential oils and cosmetology. Her book, *Le Capital Jeunesse*, was published in 1961 and was translated into English 3 years later. She leaves a dedicated and now famous pupil to continue her work – Daniele Ryman.[22]

Gattefosse, Valnet and Maury may have been the first pioneers of modern aromatherapy, but there were plenty of famous names waiting in the wings. Other researchers of note included Rovesti, who demonstrated clinically the benefit of essential oils in the treatment of depression and anxiety.[23]

These pioneers were followed by Gildemeister in Germany, Guenther and Lawrence in the USA, Leclerc and Belaiche in France, and Dodd, Deans and Svoboda in the UK. For the dedicated detective there is a wealth of information and research on essential oils. Much of it is not in English, and much of it has not been published in medical or nursing journals. However, there *is* sufficient evidence to suggest that the medicine of the future could be a sweet-smelling one. Perhaps an integrated medicine which included aromatherapy might pay more than lip-service to biodiversity. It might also improve the Third World Debt, as it is in these countries that many of the most precious and costly essential oils are harvested. The use of essential oils in health care raises ecological, economic and political issues.

Clinical aromatherapy needs to be learned – it is not enough just to read a book. The practical application of aromatherapy using touch is a delicate balance which needs to be taught and learned. Not every nurse knows the chemistry of the drugs that she administers, but if a nurse is to be competent in clinical aromatherapy, she needs to have a grasp of chemistry in order to be able to choose the correct essential oils.

The following are a few more examples of how aromatherapy has been used throughout the world.

- 1930 – An American study conducted by Collier and Nitta found bergamot to be effective against gonococcus at a dilution of 1:600.
- 1958 – An American study by Maruzella *et al.* showed *in vitro* antibacterial activity of 35 essential oils.
- – A Hungarian study showed that certain essential oils reduced athero-sclerosis.
- 1963 – An English study by Ashford *et al.* showed that thymol basic ethers had a depressing effect on the central nervous system.
- 1966 – An American study showed melissa to be an effective viricide.
- 1969 – An Italian study by Jori *et al.* showed that certain essential oils increased the metabolism of pentobarbitol.
- 1973 – A Russian study showed that one of the eucalyptus oils was effective against influenza viruses A2 and A.

The above studies were all cited in *The Practice of Aromatherapy* by Valnet.

How essential oils work

The study of where essential oils go when they are absorbed by the body and how the body eliminates them is termed pharmacokinetics.[17] No one really knows how aromatherapy works. Indeed, it is a heavily debated issue. However, we do know that essential oils may be absorbed into the body through one of the three orifices (mouth, vagina and anus), by olfaction (to the lungs and limbic system) and through the skin.[24]

There is also fairly heated debate as to how aromatherapy should be used. There are those who feel that only inhalation is important, preferring the instant effect, and those who feel that slow absorption via the skin coupled with soothing touch or warmth enhances and prolongs the therapeutic effects. There is a considerable body of information to indicate that inhaled essential oils affect our brains, and almost as much research has been conducted on the effect of ingested oils, much of which has been carried out by the food and drinks industry.

There is a substantial body of knowledge about the absorption of essential oils through the shaved skin of animals or by injection into their peritoneal cavities, but published research on the absorption of essential oils through the human skin is limited. The use of aromatherapy within nursing is still in its infancy. We think aromatherapy works because we see it working in our patients, and because our patients tell us that it works, and the whole movement of aromatherapy in nursing appears to be as much patient-led as nurse-led. However, we need a great deal more than anecdotal information.

Using aromatherapy in nursing makes us pioneers, just like Florence Nightingale before us. It is impossible to provide evidence of efficacy if we do not carry out research, but before any research can be conducted, there needs to be some 'evidence' that what we wish to do will be effective. We have reached that critical point now. We think, and our patients think, that we have anecdotal evidence that what we do is effective. What is needed next is a major research movement to prove (or disprove) what this 'evidence' shows. This may take some achieving, but it is possible.

ROUTES OF ABSORPTION OF ESSENTIAL OILS

There are three methods by which essential oils can be absorbed into our bodies:

- topically, through touch, compress or bath;
- internally, by means of douches, pessaries, suppositories or capsules;
- by inhalation, with or without steam.

Each method of application has its own physiological process.

Topical application

For many years it was thought that drugs were not absorbed through the skin. Women were ridiculed for putting creams and lotions on their faces in an effort to preserve their youthfulness. Now, with the advent of patch therapy, many drugs, such as nitroglycerine, oestradiol, nicotine and scopolamine are administered on a continuous basis through the skin. Tests are currently in progress to establish whether it will be possible to add beta-blockers, antihistamines and testosterone to the list.[25]

Two processes are involved in topical absorption: penetration and permeation.[26] Penetration involves the actual entry of a substance into the skin, whereas permeation involves the subsequent passage of substances through the body. Obviously the former is more important if it is the skin which is being treated, and the latter if it is systemic treatment which is being sought.

It is thought that permeation is governed by Fick's laws, which consist of a series of mathematical descriptions of diffusion through membranes. More important than the actual concentration of the substance, in this case the essential oil, is its chemical potential. In other words, if an essential oil contains a small amount of a potent component, the chemical potential of that essential oil is greater than that of another essential oil which contains a larger amount of a less potent chemical.

If the essential oil is diluted in a substance of lower permeability, its progress, or pharmacokinetics, will be adversely influenced. In other words, applications of essential oils diluted in a fixed oil (carrier oil) will be absorbed more slowly than applications of neat essential oils.

The actual carrier medium can also affect (and to a certain extent inhibit) the concentration of the active ingredients of essential oils. For example, in one study, the germicidal effects of phenol (a common constituent of essential oils with germicidal properties) could not be exerted when it was applied to the skin in a fatty base.[27] Another factor which affects Fick's laws is whether the substance is dissolved in water, which speeds up its absorption.

Essential oils are lipid soluble, so can be absorbed through the skin within 20–40 minutes, the exact time being dependent on the weight of the molecule and certain physico-chemical properties, such as polarity and optical activity.[24] In the case of lavender, most of the two main constituents, linalol and linalyl acetate, are eliminated within 90 minutes. The disadvantage is that not all of the essential oil is absorbed, much of it evaporating due to its high volatility.

It is obvious that the greater the percentage of skin covered, the greater will be the penetration by an essential oil.[28] The friction of stroking or massage encourages dilation of blood vessels under the skin, increasing their ability to absorb essential oils.[29] Because the stratum corneum (the outer layer of the epithelium) is partly hydrophilic and partly lipophilic, some water-based and some oil-based components can pass through it.[30]

Because essential oils are mainly lipid soluble, they gain rapid access to lipid-rich areas of the body[31] such as the myelin covering of medullated nerve fibres. This lipid solubility also enables the relatively small molecules of essential oils to cross the so-called blood–brain barrier – the separation of neurones from capillary walls by astrocytes.[32]

Studies have shown that penetration of the dermis is increased 100-fold if the essential oils are dispersed in a bath.[33] Even though the palms of the hands have much thicker skin than the rest of the body, the most permeable areas of the skin are in fact the palms of the hands, the soles of the feet, the forehead, armpits and scalp.[28] Clearly this indicates that it is not necessary, or sometimes even advisable, to give a patient a full-body treatment. Patients' feet are usually easily accessible, they rarely have intravenous infusions attached to them, and are possibly the least embarrassing body part to be touched (except for the hands). Treatment of feet requires no removal of clothes apart from shoes and socks. Feet can be massaged in full view of visitors, and while they are not areas of low innervation, neither are they highly innervative areas like the face or back.[34]

Damaged or old skin will absorb substances to a lesser extent. Damaged skin includes diseased skin due to systemic disease, dermatology problems, dehydration caused by excessive exposure to sunlight, or dietary insufficiency. It is known that stress (either physical or emotional) results in peripheral shut-down, which produces cold hands and feet, making absorption less effective. Equally, when a patient is sweating, the body is trying to excrete and not absorb, and again essential oils will be poorly absorbed. Some drugs, such as steroids, affect the ability of the skin to absorb substances.

Whilst it might not be aesthetically pleasing, if the sole purpose of topical application is to allow essential oils access to body systems (e.g. in the case of antibacterial/antifungal action), potential vaporization can be reduced by using clingfilm and a towel. Covering the skin will also increase its temperature. By covering the skin with a non-permeable membrane such as clingfilm, it is possible to increase the proportion of essential oil absorbed by about 18 per cent.

The disadvantage of applying essential oils topically is that some of them, e.g. those containing phenols, can be dermacostic. Furthermore, absorption is still not fully understood, pharmacokinetics being a relatively new field. Added to this, certain components (e.g. some ketones) can be neurotoxic, and others (e.g. furocoumarins) can cause photosensitivity. However, to balance this it should be noted that for many years the most commonly used hospital bactericide was hexachlorophane, which was later found to be neurotoxic, but not before several babies had died as a result of hexachlorophane in baby powder.[35] One of the advantages of topically applied essential oils is that they do not go through the digestive process (first pass).[17] This indicates that they do not, therefore, have to be metabolized by the liver.

Finally, it is accepted that many essential oils are grown with pesticides. Whilst gas chromatography might indicate this, concentrated nitrates are not going to be beneficial to human skin, and they could also cause a reaction which has nothing to do with the essential oil itself.

Topical application of essential oils can be used for the following:

- relieving localized trauma such as bruising, sprains, stings or burns;
- relaxing and warming specific muscles;
- relieving neuralgic conditions;
- as an anti-inflammatory;
- as an anti-spasmodic;
- as a specific antiviral/antifungal/antibacterial agent for skin infections;

- systemic treatments, including hormonal imbalance;
- as a general body relaxant.

Topical applications can be given as follows:

- in a carrier oil (see section on carrier oils);
- in an ointment;
- in a gel;
- neat (see section on contraindications);
- in a bath (sitz, hand, foot or full);
- as a compress;
- in a wound irrigation.

It must be emphasized that, although essential oils *are* absorbed through the skin, a large percentage evaporates into the room and is inhaled by the patient. It is arguable whether it is, in fact, the inhaled essential oils which are the more beneficial during topical application. Perhaps it is the synergy of topically applied and inhaled essential oil, together with the fact that the patient relaxes through touch sufficiently to breathe deeply! However, it is difficult to separate the two means of entry, and it is suggested that they could work in tandem when essential oils are applied topically.

Currently there is no body of comparative knowledge on the gastrointestinal and cutaneous absorption of the same test material.[35]

Internal administration and safety issues

Apart from giving the essential oils orally in a gelule capsule or disperse (with medical supervision), they can be used in a mouthwash. It is important to remember to tell your patient to spit out the mouthwash, and not to swallow it. Essential oils can also be used diluted in douches and, for certain fungal infections, mixed in carrier oils and applied per vagina on a tampon. Both rectal and vaginal pessaries have a distinct advantage in the treatment of reproductive or urinary conditions, as they are absorbed directly into the surrounding tissue. Recurrent cystitis and vaginal thrush can respond well to this type of treatment.

It is not the purpose of this book to advise nurses on the internal uses of essential oils for their patients. This is a highly specialized and potentially dangerous field and needs training. Despite the fact that many essential oils are used as flavouring agents in our food, essential oils are concentrated and not to be experimented with casually. Just as a bottle of paracetamol can be lethal (although this drug is still sold over the counter because the public is expected to take one or two tablets at a time), so some essential oils are potentially lethal. The usual external dose is between one and five drops only.

The oral route for essential oils is important, but I personally feel that it is for medicine to prescribe this use. Taking essential oils by mouth can be an excellent way to treat gastrointestinal problems (most other problems can be helped using another method). However, I do not consider that it is part of our nursing brief to advise patients to take essential oils by mouth – this is aromatic medicine. Aromatic medicine can produce miraculous results, especially with resistant infections (see Chapter 7 on infections). Training in aromatic medicine is open to nurses as well as to doctors and herbalists in the UK, but at the time of writing is a hotly debated subject. Aromatic medicine is not the subject of this book.

Several people have written books and articles on the subject of aromatic medicine. However, I consider that a much safer option for nurses is to offer patients herbal teas. These are much gentler and, as they are sold over the counter, have already been researched, passed as safe, and should not produce side-effects. Common tissanes or teas are chamomile, peppermint, rosehip, fennel and lime blossom.

Warning
Encouraging your patients to take essential oils by mouth is not advised unless those oils are prescribed by, or through, the doctor responsible for the patient.

Inhalation: olfactory system

Of all the methods for introducing essential oils into the human body, this is the simplest and fastest. It is also the oldest, the use of aromatics in rituals being well documented. Indeed the very word, *'perfume'* comes from the Latin *'fumare'*, meaning to cleanse with smoke. This is similar to fumigation, which means to disinfect with fume or perfume.[36]

Smell produces an instant reaction, both physiologically (until very recently smelling salts were the standard method for reviving someone who had fainted) and psychologically. We know immediately if the smell is pleasant or unpleasant, and what memories it evokes.

Smell is a chemical reaction, receptors in the brain responding to chemicals within the essential oil. As we breathe in, these chemicals move up to behind the bridge of the nose, just beneath the brain, where they attach themselves to millions of hair-like receptors which are connected to the olfactory bulb. These receptors are extremely sensitive and can be stimulated by very subtle scents. Because olfactory receptors are so sensitive, they are easily fatigued, which explains why smells seem less obvious as the body adapts to them, or tires.[32] Odours breathed through one or the other nostril produce different effects. However, there are no differences with regard to the electrical changes in the brain between the left and right nostrils.[37]

An electrical phenomenon discovered by Grey in 1964, and called contingent negative variation (CNV), showed that sedative effects caused by nitrazepam decreased CNV, and the stimulant effect produced by caffeine increased CNV. When fragrances were tested, these too caused different effects. Lavender produced a similar reaction to nitrazepam, decreasing CNV, and jasmine had 'the reverse effect and increased CNV.[38] Recent research has shown that olfactory receptors are also affected by non-volatile molecules in aerosols.[23]

From the olfactory bulb, the smell is conducted via the olfactory tract to the olfactory centre of the brain. There it is connected to the limbic system, beginning a series of chain reactions which affect every part of our body. The limbic system (LS) is the oldest part of the human brain, supposedly having evolved first. In lower vertebrates it is called the 'smell brain', these animals being dependent on their sense of smell for survival. The main structures in the limbic system are the amygdala, septum, hippocampus, anterior thalamus and hypothalamus. These structures are connected by a number of complicated pathways.[32]

As well as influencing how we express our emotions, instinctive behaviours, drives and motivations, the limbic system plays an essential role in learning and memory.[39] Buchbauer stated that the limbic system is responsible for our sexual desires, and feelings of wellness and harmony. It also receives most of our sensory input and passes it on to the voluntary and involuntary motor centres. Gatti and Cayola noted that odour produced an immediate effect on respiration, pulse and blood pressure, and therefore concluded that odour had, by a reflex action, produced a dramatic effect on the functioning of the central nervous system.[40]

Essential oils are a complex mixture of molecules, each conveying a chemical message. When the essential oil reaches the limbic system, the 'message' is relayed to the hippocampus and amygdala, where it is analysed. It is this part of the brain which is directly involved with memory.[41] Maybe this is why Kipling wrote that 'smells are surer than sounds or sights to make your heartstrings crack'.[42] (It has been suggested that an animal's response to smell is all learned.) This belief would explain why some smells upset some people and not others. The message is then passed on to the hypothalamus. This gland works as a regulator, that alleviates anxiety, depression and hormonal imbalances.[43] It is interesting to note at this point that certain benzodiazepines have specific binding sites on olfactory cells.

The hypothalamus now has the option of relaying the sense impulse in one of four directions.

- The impulse could go to the *thalamus*, which secretes the neurochemical encephalin – a painkiller, mood elevator and antidepressant.
- The impulse could go to the *locus ceruleus* to trigger *noradrenaline* to work against lethargy, tiredness and immune deficiency problems.
- The impulse could go to the *pituitary gland* to stimulate the follicle-stimulating hormone, luteinizing hormone, or adrenocorticotrophin (ACTH). ACTH controls growth hormones, the production of cortisol and thyrotrophin (thyroid-stimulating hormone).
- The impulse could go to the *raphe nucleus* to release *serotonin*, a sedative that relieves insomnia, anxiety and hypertension.

It is not known exactly how the limbic system determines to which organ the 'smell' should be sent.

On a psychological level, as early as 1690 Sir William Temple wrote in his *Essay on Health and Long Life* that 'The use of scents is not practised in modern physic but might be carried out with advantage seeing that some smells are so depressing and others so inspiring and reviving'. Professor Dodds of Warwick University has pointed out that stimulation of olfactory responses by odorants is a branch of molecular pharmacology.[44] It is similar to mood changes brought about by some psychotropic drugs. Responses to pleasant odours are conducted unconsciously, although both olfactory nerve connections and measured physiological changes indicate that the response is of an emotional and hormonal nature.

Smell is also a language of communication. We communicate, without being able to control this, through our pheromones. We talk about 'smelling danger', or that someone or something 'smelt wrong'. The French have a saying 'je ne peux pas le sentir' which means 'I don't trust him', although the literal translation is 'I can't smell him'.

Unconsciously we choose our friends and partners by smell. This kind of smell is called subliminal smell, i.e. it can affect us without our knowing it. Research has shown that subliminal smell on a waiting-room chair attracted a statistically significant proportion of patients entering that waiting-room. Other research, conducted in America, has shown that the sale of training shoes can be enhanced by using a subliminal smell.

Learned memory is the reaction to a smell which has been learned through experience, e.g. a bad trauma linked with a smell. When that odour is smelled again, fear, or the emotion originally experienced, is triggered. This should be remembered when lavender is used. For many elderly people, lavender is associated with linen bags, and for some the odour is closely linked with care of the dying.

Lavender has undergone a tremendous revival with aromatherapy, and although it appears to be universally enjoyed by those under 60 years of age, those in their seventies or older are sometimes not quite so enthusiastic. Kirk-Smith relates the story of a 55-year-old man who had been terrified of a female teacher who wore a particular perfume. In later life, that same perfume still evoked a sense of anxiety.[39] Learned memory of smell is hard to undo.

The functioning of the human body is greatly affected by the mind. Fortunately, medicine is now beginning to accept the mind/body connections. The immune system has receptors for endorphins, proving that our immune system is strongly affected by our sense of well-being. This continual conversation between brain and immune system is affected by bereavement, anxiety and stress.[45] By combining two external communicators, smell and touch, we are enhancing our patients' abilities to communicate internally.

Smell is closely linked to taste (although it is 10 000 times more sensitive) which is why, when we have a cold, food does not smell appetizing. As well as tasting pleasant (otherwise we would not eat it), food has a molecular structure which our bodies break down into atoms which have both physiological and psychological effects. Smells can give us similar pleasure, but they also affect us physiologically and psychologically.

Methods of administration via the olfactory system

- Diffusers and nebulizers. The 'burner'-type, which consist of tiny pots of water heated over a candle are unsuitable for hospital use due to safety regulations.

Warning
Do not burn essential oils; not only is the smell very unpleasant, but burning actually changes the chemistry of the oil (would you really burn a bunch of flowers?).

- One to five drops in a hot bowl of water with a towel over the head and the eyes kept closed. This method is useful for sinusitis, heavy colds or dry coughs. The nurse should stay with the patient for the 5 to 10 minutes necessary for the essential oils to take effect.
- In an atomizer spray, such as a plant spray. It is important to shake the container vigorously as essential oils are not soluble in water. This is an ideal method to use in damp dusting to combat cross-infection.
- Applied neat on a tissue – breathe naturally through the tissue for up to 15 minutes or put under a pillowcase. Again, this is a perfectly acceptable method for patient use.

■ Added to a bowl of hot water on a ward radiator. This method is acceptable for use in a ward, provided that the bowl cannot be tipped accidentally.

Inhaled essential oils can be particularly useful for the following:

■ for upper and lower respiratory tract infections;
■ for hay fever, sinusitis and headache;
■ for asthma – they have antispasmodic and relaxing effects;
■ for people who cannot be touched, for physical reasons (e.g. burns) or psychological reasons (e.g. rape);
■ for the prevention of cross-infection;

Finally, the nose, as well as governing our smell system, contains a touch system, which is often (wrongly) thought to be part of the smell system. This touch system is the trigeminal system, and forms part of the fifth cranial nerve. It can detect aggressive odours such as acetic acid and ammonia, and causes the head-swivelling reflex.[46]

REFERENCES

1. **Franchomme P**. 1980: *Phytoguide: aromatherapy advanced therapy for infectious illnesses*. International Phytomedical Foundation, France. Limoges: Jollois.

2. **Rose, J.** 1992: *The aromatherapy book*. San Francisco: North Atlantic Books.

3. **Kusmerik, J.** 1992: *Aromatherapy for the family*. Institute of Classical Aromatherapy. London: Wigmore Publications.

4. **Gattefosse, R.** 1993: *Gatefosse's aromatherapy*. Saffron Walden: CW Daniel.

5. **Gilt, A.** 1992: Aromatherapy 2000 and beyond. *Journal of Alternative and Complementary Medicine* **9**, 19–20.

6. **Tisserand, R.** 1993: Aspects of aromatherapy. In *Aroma 93 Conference Proceedings*. Brighton: Aromatherapy Publications, 1–9.

7. **Erichsen-Brown, C.** 1979: *Medicinal and other uses of North American plants*. New York: Dover Publications Inc.

8. **Griggs, B.** 1981: *Green pharmacy*. London: Jill Norman & Hobhouse.

9. **Ryman, D.** 1991: *Aromatherapy*. London: Piatkus.

10. **Lawless, J.** 1994: *Aromatherapy and the mind*. London: Thorsons.

11. **Levabre, M.** 1990: *Aromatherapy workbook*. Vermont: Healing Arts Press.

12. **Steele, J.** 1991: Anthropology of smell and scent in fragrance. In Van Toller, S. and Dood, G. (eds), *The Psychology and biology of perfume*. London: Elsevier Applied Science, 287–302.

13. **Rose, J.** 1992: A history of herbs and herbalism. In Tierra. M. (ed.), *American herbalism*. Freedom, CA: Crossing Press, 3–32.

14. **Lawless, J.** 1992: *The encyclopedia of essential oils*. Shaftesbury: Element Books.

15. **Holmes, P.** 1989: *The energetics of western herbs, Vols 1 and 2*. Berkeley: Nat Trop.

16. **Chadwick, J. and Mann, W.N.** 1983: Aphorism 28. In *Hippocratic writings*. Harmondsworth: Penguin Books, 24.

17. **Mills, S.** 1991: *Out of the earth*. London: Viking Arkana.

18. **Watt, M.** 1991: *Plant aromatics*. Witham: Watt.

19. **Tisserand, R.** 1979: *The art of aromatherapy*. Saffron Walden: CW Daniel.

20. **Scott, C.** 1993/1994: In profile with Valnet. *International Journal of Aromatherapy* **5**, 10–13.

21. **Valnet, J.** 1937: *Aromatherapie: Les huiles essentielles hormones vegetales*. Paris: Girardot (translated by R. Tisserand as **Gattefosse, B.** 1993: *Aromatherapy*. Saffron Walden: CW Daniel).

22. **Maury, M.** 1964: *Le Capital Jeunesse* (translated by D. Ryman as *The secrets of life and youth*). London: Macdonald.

23. **Rovesti, P. and Columbo, E.** 1973: Aromatherapy and aerosols. *Soaps, Perfumery and Cosmetics* **46**, 475–7.

24. **Jager, W., Buchbauer, G., Jirovetz, L. and Fritzer, M.** 1992: Percutaneous absorption of lavender oil from a massage oil. *Journal of the Society of Cosmetic Chemists* **43**, 49–54.

25. **Cleary, G.** 1993: Transdermal drug delivery. In Zatz, J.L. (ed.), *Skin permeation: fundamentals and applications*. Wheaton, IL: Allured Publishing 207–37.

26. **Reiger, M.** 1993: Factors affecting sorption of topically applied substances. In Zatz, J.L. (ed.), *Skin permeation: fundamentals and applications*. Wheaton, IL: Allured Publishing, 37–61.

27. **Zatz, J.** 1993: Modification of skin permeation by solvents. In Zatz, J.L. (ed.), *Skin permeation: fundamentals and applications*. Wheaton, IL: Allured Publishing, 127–62.

28. **Balacs, T.** 1993: Essential oils in the body. In *Aroma 93 Conference Proceedings*. Brighton: Aromatherapy Publications, 12–20.

29. **Pratt, J. and Mason, A.** 1981: *The caring touch*. London: Heyden.

30. **Riviere, J.E.** 1993: Biological factors in absorption and permeation. In Zatz, J.L. (ed.), *Skin permeation: fundamentals and applications*. Wheaton, IL: Allured Publishing, 113–25.

31. **Buchbauer, G.** 1993: Molecular interaction. *International Journal of Aromatherapy* **5**, 11–14.

32. **Anthony, C.P. and Thibodeau, G.A.** 1983: *Nervous system cells in anatomy and physiology*. St Louis, MO: Mosby.

33. **Buchbauer, G.** 1993: Biological effects of fragrances and essential oils. *Perfumer and Flavorist* **18**, 19–24.

34. **Weiss, S.** 1979: The language of touch. *Nursing Research* **28**, 76–9.

35. **Jackson, E.** 1993: Toxicological aspects of percutaneous absorption. In Zatz, J.L. (ed.), *Skin permeation: fundamentals and applications*. Wheaton, IL. Allured Publishing, 177–93.

36. **Oxford Dictionaries** 1964: *Concise English dictionary*. Oxford: Oxford University Press.

37. **Walter, R.G., Cooper, R., Aldridge, V.J., McCullum, W.C. and Winter, A.L.** 1964: Contingent negative variation: an electric sign of sensorimotor association and expectancy in the human brain. *Nature (London)* **203**, 380–4.

38. **Torii, S., Fukada, H., Kanemoto, H., Miyanchi, R., Hamauzu, Y. and Kawasaki, M.** 1991: Contingent negative variation (CNV) and the psychological effects of odour. In Van Toller, S. and Dodds, G. (eds), *Perfumery: the psychology and biology of fragrance*. London: Chapman and Hall, 107–18.

39. **Kirk-Smith, M.** 1993: Human olfactory communication. In *Aroma 93 Conference Proceedings*. Brighton: Aromatherapy Publications, 86–103.

40. **Gatti, G. and Cayola, R.** 1923: L'Azione delle essenze sul sistema nervosa. *Rivista Italiana delle Essenze e Profumi* **5**, 133–5.

41. **Engen, T.** 1977: Odor memory. *Perfumer and Flavorist* **2**, 8–11.

42. **Birchall, A.** 1990: A whiff of happiness. *New Scientist* **25 August**, 44–7.

43. **Sidebottom, B.** 1991: The gentle art and science of aromatherapy. *Caduceus* **Autumn**, 5–7.

44. **Dodds, G.H.** 1991: The molecular dimension in perfumery. In Van Toller, S. and Dodds, G. (eds), *Perfumery: the psychology and biology of fragrance*. London: Chapman and Hall, 19–46.

45. **Quinn, J. and Strelkauskas.** 1993: Psychoimmunologic effects of therapeutic touch on practitioners and recently bereaved recipients: a pilot study. *Advances in Nursing Science* **15**, 13–26.

46. **Van Toller, S. and Dodd, G.H.** 1991: Preface. In Van Toller, S. and Dodds, G. (eds), *Perfumery: the psychology and biology of fragrance*. London: Chapman and Hall, xii–xv.

4

ESSENTIAL OILS

EXTRACTION OF ESSENTIAL OILS

Essential oils are steam distilled from aromatic plants. David Williams describes them as 'odorous volatile products obtained by a physical process from a natural source of a single species, which corresponds to the source in both name and odour.'[1] He further states that it is impossible to obtain an essential oil by a physical process without to some extent changing its composition. Essential oils are described by the International School of Aromatherapy Safety Guide as 'the pure volatile portion of aromatic plant products normally extracted by distillation ... the main exceptions to the distillation method of extraction are the citrus essential oils.'[2]

Tisserand and Balacs describe essential oils as 'volatile, organic constituents of fragrant plant matter.'[3] The Essential Oil Trade Association Ltd suggests that they should be described 'as the exclusive product of the extraction of the aromatic principles contained in the substances of vegetable origin of which they bear the name.'[4] Most aromatherapy schools will describe true essential oils as being obtained by steam distillation or by expression (from the peel of citrus fruit only).

In order to clarify the situation it should be explained that there are several other ways of obtaining extracts from plants. It is this diversity which can produce different odorous compounds which are *not* classified as essential oils. Traditionally, distillation has always been the method of choice for therapists. It involves a still, usually of copper, but now more often of stainless steel. The plant material is placed in the still and steam is passed through it.

The steam, mixed with volatile oils, is passed through a condenser which cools it. The result is two-layered: an aqueous mixture which is mostly water with a very small percentage of essential oil dispersed in it (known as floral water or hydrolats), and a layer of essential oil floating on top of the floral water (see Figure 4.1). The essential oil can then be tapped off. It floats on the top because the majority of essential oils are *non-soluble* in water.

To give some idea of quantity, 200 kg of *Lavandula angustifolia* flowers will produce 1 kg of essential oil. However, between 2 and 5 metric tons of rose petals will be needed to produce the same quantity of rose oil,[5] giving a clear indication which of these oils will be the more costly to buy.

Some plants are more volatile than others. The perfume industry refers to this volatility as *notes,* and divides it into top, middle and base notes.[6] These divisions indicate how rapidly the essential oil will lose its vitality. A top note might last, in an unstoppered bottle, for a few hours before losing its odour, a middle note might last a couple of days, and a base note, such as frankincense, might last for 2000 years, as the opening of Tutankhamun's tomb showed. However, the term 'notes' is generally deployed by perfumers, not by therapists, and was first used by Septimus Piesle in the nineteenth century.[1] Sometimes middle notes are referred to as body notes and base notes as dry-out notes.[7]

The odour of an essential oil deteriorates as a result of oxidation. This is explained by David Williams in his comparison of the volatility of essential oils. He writes about the speed at which an essential oil evaporates, stating

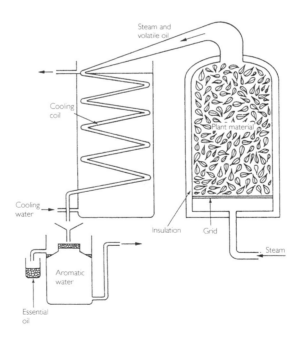

FIGURE 4.1 Steam distillation. Reproduced from Price, S. (1983) *Practical Aromatherapy,* with the kind permission of Harper Collins, London.

that no 'essential oil is highly volatile, but that some evaporate more quickly than others'. For example, citrus oils such as bergamot or grapefruit will evaporate faster than flower oils such as rose. The least volatile oils are the resins and the woods. Oxidation, which can be speeded up by heat and light, not only affects the odour of an essential oil, but also affects its therapeutic potential.[3]

Modern extraction of essential oils uses liquid carbon dioxide (hypercritical). The advantages of this method are that extraction occurs in a few moments and, because the solvent is inert, there are no chemical reactions.[8] However, it is arguable whether this method of extraction does produce exactly the same chemical formula as steam distillation.[9] In steam distillation, which can last up to 24 hours, the amount of time (and magnitude of the heat) is a vital part of the process, as it is known that some components of plants are very sensitive to heat. Essential oils are composed of volatile, liquid and solid compounds which have widely varying boiling points.[5] Furthermore, the actual duration of the distillation process is directly related to the resulting chemical formula of the essential oil.

There are other methods of extraction which produce compounds mainly used by the fragrance and cosmetics industry. One such compound is called an absolute. Mistakenly, some people think absolute stands for the 'absolute best'. In the world of essential oils this is not so. An absolute is not a true essential oil but an extract obtained by chemical extraction using petrol-based chemicals. Initially this method produces a waxy concrete, which is often solid. Further extraction with alcohol produces the absolute. It is impossible to remove all of the chemical solvent.

In 1989 the International Fragrance Association (IFRA) issued guidelines on the recommended level of benzene in an absolute, stating that it should not exceed 10 parts per million (ppm).[2] However, these types of compounds are best avoided in therapeutic use, as the solvent could provoke adverse reactions.

More recently, the solvent gas hexane has been used to extract absolutes. Hexane is believed to be safe, and is used in several food extraction processes. However, it is impossible to remove all of the solvent following extraction.

A new chemical process called phytonics has been developed in England by rose-grower and scientist Peter Wilde. This method involves extracting essential oil by means of new solvents. The unique character of these solvents is that their boiling points are around −30°C. The extraction of the plant material can be carried out at room temperature and the solvent removed without boiling. This ensures that the plant material is not damaged by high temperature, and although the extracts do have a residual solvent residue, its levels are very low. The extract is neither acid nor alkaline. (When using liquid carbon dioxide, some CO_2 dissolves, lowering the pH and producing an acidic product. The phytonics process is being patented and is one to be watched with interest.[10] Of particular note is the fact that these products do not produce concretes which require further refining with alcohol.[11]

Resinoids are obtained from resins such as amber and mastic, balsams such as benzoin, or gum-like substances such as frankincense and myrrh. Frequently the method used is extraction by hydrocarbon solvents. Frankincense and myrrh can also be obtained by straight steam distillation. Resins are soluble in alcohol but not in water; gums are soluble in water but not in alcohol.[2]

Essential oils can also be obtained via *expression*, a process in which the skin of a citrus fruit is compressed, by machine or by hand, releasing the 'zest' (the essential oil) and a little juice, which is then steam distilled.

Enfleurage is another method, which used to be traditional in France. It is described in Jeanne Rose's book.[12] Flowers are laid in vats of fat, or as stated by Jeanne Rose, on ridged panes of glass which have been 'painted' with jojoba oil. These are left for a couple of days for the fat to absorb the essential oils. Pure alcohol is then added to the mixture and left for several weeks. Finally, the concoction is separated and the alcohol filtered. Enfleurage is labour-intensive but interesting to try.

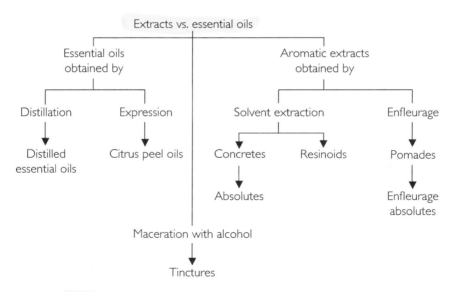

FIGURE 4.2 Extracts vs. essential oils. Adapted from Williams, D. (1989) *Lecture Notes on Essential Oils*, with the kind permission of Eve Taylor, London.

Because commercial enfleurage is so expensive, it was until recently restricted to jasmine, tuberose and a few other oils, but has now been almost completely replaced by solvent extraction. However, the resulting essence will still not be a true essential oil as it will be alcohol-based. See Figure 4.2 for a comparison of the extraction procedures used for aromatic extracts and essential oils.

FUNCTIONS OF ESSENTIAL OILS IN LIVING PLANTS

Essential oils are derived from living plants, a great many being found in the Lamiaceae family. The plant uses its essential oils to attract (or repel) animals and to defend itself against parasitic or bacterial invasion.[13] Possibly it is this inherent property which leads the American wormseed plant to produce ascaridole, an anthelmintic, which Indian tribes have used in the treatment of roundworms, hookworms and intestinal amoebas for hundreds of years.[14]

Some scientists consider that essential oils can help a plant to maintain an equable temperature, the vaporization of the oils absorbing excess heat, some consider that essential oils are merely waste products of the plant, while others think that they play a vital role in sealing plant wounds, or acting as an emergency food reserve.[13]

The amount of essential oil contained in a plant varies tremendously. *Ruta graveolens* is so saturated with essential oil and normal paraffins that the oil can be ignited whilst it is still in the plant. However, it is not just the *amount* of essential oil that is relevant, but also what the essential oil *contains*. Sometimes the smallest quantity of a chemical in an essential oil has a major part to play. For example, the smell of a rose (*Rosa damascena*) originates from 0.1 parts per million. The most poisonous plant in the world, Himalayan monkshood (*Aconitum ferox*) is so toxic because it contains 0.2 per cent nepaline, a poisonous alkaloid. This concentration is sufficient to kill someone who merely smells it.[2] Death occurs within an hour, and is caused by circulatory and respiratory failure.

The chemical make-up of all living plants alters depending on climate, including rainfall, sunlight, soil acidity, altitude and pollution.[13] The chemistry of a rose grown in Bulgaria will not be the same as that of one grown in England. Similarly, *Lavandula angustifolia* grown high up a mountain will contain more esters, which are thought to have a greater antispasmodic effect, than *Lavandula angustifolia* grown further down the mountain, where more linalol (alcohol) will be produced.

The chemistry of a plant affects the essential oil which is distilled from it. So many factors can affect a plant that the only way to be certain of the composition of the essential oil is to determine its biological fingerprint. This is done by a process called gas-liquid chromatography(GLC). A very small amount of essential oil is injected into a finely coiled tubular column, and the time taken for each chemical component of the essential oils to appear at the far end of the temperature-controlled column is recorded on a trace, which is printed out on paper. Each batch of oil will vary slightly, one being the standard to compare with another. This is why it is so useful to have a batch number on a bottle of essential oil.

There are hundreds of aromatic plants, but not all of them produce essential oils in sufficient quantity for distillation to be viable. For example, hyacinth is usually obtained by solvent extraction and the solvent distilled.[15] The same is true for lily of the valley and lilac.[2] Some plants produce essential oils which are poisonous, and some produce oils which can be toxic, e.g. thuja, wintergreen,[16] arnica and narcissus.[15] (Arnica is traditionally used in very small amounts in homeopathic treatments.) Some essential oils are not safe for use in pregnancy or on young children, and some are contraindicated for patients with cancer (see section on contraindications).

It is important to remember that essential oils are highly concentrated – often 99 times more concentrated than the essential oil normally found in a living plant.[17]

There are countless plants world-wide which man has not yet examined. Each newly discovered essential oil will probably contain several new compounds. There is an urgent need to ensure the conservation of biological diversity and to explore the role of ethnobotany in pharmaceutical prospecting. The future of aromatic medicine depends on intellectual property rights and biodiversity conservation. These are far-reaching issues and are covered very well in Timothy Swanson's book.[18]

USE OF ESSENTIAL OILS

Of the hundreds of essential oils which *are* produced, there are classics which are used regularly, on a daily basis, by therapists all over the world. These are essential oils which have research-based therapeutic properties and/or a long history of use. However, apart from aromatherapy, essential oils play an important part in our lives. Some of the uses of essential oils might be surprising. For example, they are used in the following products and processes: adhesives; animal feed; automobile industry; prepared food industry, including meats and baked goods; canning industry; chewing gum and confectionery business; dentist's and dental preparations; insecticides; household goods such as furniture polish and washing powder; ice-cream industry; meat-packing industry; paint, paper and printing works; perfume manufacturers; pharmaceutical industry; alcohol manufacturers; rubber industry; soap industry; soft drinks manufacture; textile industry; tobacco industry; veterinary suppliers; candle-making; ceramics; contact lens manufacture.[13]

Essential oils are derived from different parts of plants but they all come from parts that contain the essential oil sacs or glands. These include the following:

- whole herb, e.g. thyme, rosemary, dill;
- flower, e.g. ylang ylang, melissa, rose;
- resin, e.g. frankincense, myrrh;
- wood, e.g. rosewood, cedarwood;
- seed, e.g. black pepper, cumin;
- root, e.g. ginger.

Many herbs are used in cooking, e.g. basil, thyme, coriander, rosemary, dill, oregano, bay. Some are drunk in tisanes, e.g. peppermint, lime flower, chamomile. Several of the names of plants which produce essential oil will already be familiar. Some of them have been used in orthodox medicines for centuries, e.g. peppermint in gripe water, eucalyptus in Vicks vapour rub and other 'cold remedies'.

Different parts of a plant can be used in the extraction, e.g. root in ginger, bark in cinnamon, fruit in nutmeg, flowering heads in chamomile. Some contemporary aromatherapists, such as Dietrich Gumbel, consider that there is a correlation between the metabolism of flowers, shoots and roots and human skin layers. He writes that the various parts of plants are closely related to the head, sense and nerve functions of the human body.[19] This is particularly interesting in view of the fact that distilling different parts of the same plant can sometimes produce entirely different essential oils.

Perhaps what is not so commonly known is how many different species of the same plant exist, and how confusing this can be for the beginner. For example, consider one of the most popular of essential oils, namely lavender. There are three different species of lavender as well as a whole array of hybrids.[20] Lavender belongs to a family of herbs called the Lamiaceae (Labiatae) which includes many plants used in herbal medicine. The genus *Lavandula* denotes all lavenders, rather like a surname. The species (like a Christian name) denotes exactly which type of lavender is being referred to.

In botanical language there are three different types of lavender: *Lavandula angustifolia*, *Lavandula latifolia* and *Lavandula stoechas*. However, as frequently happens in the plant family, two of the species have other names. *Lavandula angustifolia* is sometimes called *L. vera* or *L. officinalis*, although the correct name is *L. angustifolia*.[21] It is also called English lavender, French lavender and true lavender. Latifolia is often called spike lavender, which is completely different to spikenard (*Nardostachys jatamansi*), which is closely related to valerian and belongs to a completely different family (Valerianaceae).

Until recently, *Lavandula angustifolia* and *Lavandula latifolia* were listed in the *British Pharmacopoeia* and supplied to hospitals in vats labelled 'lavender'. However, whilst *L. angustifolia* has sedative, relaxant and hypotensive properties, *L. latifolia* is a stimulant and expectorant.

Chamomile can cause confusion to the newcomer, too. There are three different types of chamomile: German, Roman and Moroccan. They are completely different in chemistry, each has a different genus, but they all belong to the same family (Asteraceae, which used to be called Compositae).

German chamomile, *Matricaria recutita*, is a lovely smokey-smelling deep blue oil which contains chamazulene, a powerful anti-inflammatory with a history of use in the treatment of skin problems.[22] It also contains alpha-bisabolol, which produces the most anti-inflammatory effect.[23] As well as having hormone-like properties, this chamomile is a powerful antibiotic, effective against *Staphylococcus aureus,* haemolytic *Streptococcus* and *Proteus vulgaris* in very low dilutions. Wound infections bathed with a solution of 1 part in 100 000 of German chamomile have been healed.[24] Jeanne Rose states that German chamomile 'will stimulate liver regeneration and subcutaneous treatments will initiate formation of new tissue'.[12] It should be noted that chamazulene is not present in the fresh flower but is produced during distillation.[15]

Roman chamomile (*Anthemis nobilis* or *Chamaemelum nobile*) is a pale blue oil which turns yellow with storage. Listed in the *British Herbal Pharmacopoeia*, it contains up to 80 per cent esters. Esters have antispasmodic properties, and Roman chamomile is traditionally used as an antispasmodic and relaxant. It does also have some anti-inflammatory properties,[25] particularly if the oil is collected from white-headed flowers instead of the classic yellow-headed flowers.[26]

Moroccan chamomile (*Ormenis multicaulis*) is a relative newcomer used by the perfume industry. Little is known about its therapeutic effect. In all respects, it is different to the other chamomiles and cannot be regarded as a substitute for them.

As mentioned previously, specific parts of plants are used in the distillation process. Sometimes a plant can produce different essential oils. In the case of the bitter orange plant (*Citrus aurantium* subsp. *amara*), two different types of essential oils can be obtained: a petitgrain from the woody stem and twigs, and a neroli from the petals. Bergamot is obtained from the skin of the fruit, thought to be a subspecies of this plant. The shorthand for *Citrus aurantium* subsp. *bergamia* (bergamot) is *Citrus bergamia*.[27] Bergamot, neroli and petitgrain are also generic names for types of essential oils which are obtained from the peel, flowers and stems, respectively, of citrus fruit.

There are many citrus fruits, e.g. grapefruit, lemon and lime, which can produce their own bergamot, neroli and petitgrain type of essential oil, which is why it is so important to know the complete botanical name of the plant.

Sometimes a plant produces essential oils which have the same name, but with the specific part of the plant named, e.g. cinnamon bark, cinnamon leaf. Cinnamon bark contains about 50 per cent cinnamaldehyde, which is dermacostic but can inhibit bacterial growth on food for 30 days.[28] Cinnamon leaf has a higher eugenol content (80 to 96 per cent) and can corrode metal.[9] Small amounts of both cinnamon bark and leaf are used by the fragrance and pharmaceutical industries. Cinnamon is one of the flavours in Coca-Cola.[15]

To complicate the situation still further, it is possible, by growing a plant in different climates (and using slower or higher-temperature distillation techniques) to produce different chemotypes (CTs) of the same essential oil. This means that the essential oil has a specific chemical profile which could make it more suitable for treating a particular ailment, or might make it safer to use. *Thymus vulgaris* has several chemotypes, the most common being CT thymol, CT linalol, CT thujanol and CT geraniol. CT geraniol and CT linalol both have a high alcohol content. These are safe to use (diluted) on the skin. However, CT thujanol and CT thymol contain high levels of phenol. Phenols can cause skin irritation, but have potent antimicrobial activity (see section on infection in Chapter 7).

Tea tree, eucalyptus, rosemary and German chamomile are other essential oils with specialized chemotypes. The tea tree which we probably hope to have is *Melaleuca alternifolia* CT terpineol – a chemotype with a high alcohol content. However, there is another CT called cineole, which is an oxide and therefore harsher on the skin. The all-important alpha-bisabolol found in German chamomile is only found in one of the chemotypes.[23] This is further discussed by Franz in his chapter on plant genetics in *Volatile Oil Crops*.[29]

CHEMISTRY OF ESSENTIAL OILS

Essential oils contain two main types of molecules: hydrocarbons (terpenes) and oxygenated compounds (terpenoids). The hydrocarbon section is composed entirely of terpenes. The oxygenated group is much more diverse, and includes alcohols, aldehydes, esters, ketones, phenols, lactones and oxides.[3] A description of some of the main characteristic therapeutic effects of each of the above will follow.

The terpene section can be subdivided into monoterpenes (molecules with 10 carbon atoms), sesquiterpenes (which have 15 carbon atoms) and diterpenes (which have 20 carbon atoms).

Living organisms contain organic (carbon-containing) and inorganic (non-carbon-containing) compounds. Organic compounds always contain hydrogen, and usually oxygen, as well as carbon. Many of them also contain nitrogen and/or sulphur. The structure of an organic compound is of great importance, as the physical positioning (spatial positioning) of some of the atoms can alter the overall properties of the compound.

- The structural formula of a large number of compounds found in plants can be divided up into branched chains of carbon atoms.
- Although these usually occur in a chain-like formation, there are exceptions which occur most frequently in the sesqui-, di- and triterpenes (compounds containing 15, 20 or 30 carbon atoms, respectively).
- Benzene (aromatic) rings can easily be formed from aliphatic (non-benzene rings) but the reverse reaction rarely occurs.
- Oxidation, reduction, shifting of double bonds and polymerization (changes in the spatial position of atoms within the molecule) take place readily.
- The branched C_5 unit is distinguishable in the formulae of a number of non-terpenes coupled with non-branched structures.
- The terpenes are often accompanied by propylbenzene derivatives and straight-chain hydrocarbons.[13]

Terpenes

Monoterpenes occur in most essential oils. They all have antiseptic properties and many of them end in '-ene'. They include camphene, caryophyllene, phellandrene, pinene, myrcene and limonene. Limonene is thought to be antitumoural,[30] and occurs in most citrus oils, as well as in dill (*Anethum graveolens*). Myrcene in *Cymbopogon citratus* (lemongrass) has been found to have analgesic properties.[31]

Monoterpenes have a generally stimulating effect, and are often skin irritants. Because they are insoluble in water, the perfume industry frequently removes terpenes from an essential oil during distillation so that the oil can be used in toilet water. In this case the essential oil is said to be 'terpeneless'. This process is described by Guenther in Volume 1 of *The Essential Oils*.[13]

Sesquiterpenes have much stronger odours, are strongly anti-inflammatory and have bactericidal properties. Several sesquiterpenes have recently been discovered to have antitumour activity.[32] Chamazulene and farnesol are found in German chamomile, bisabolene is found in black pepper and caryophyllene is found in *Cananga odorata* (ylang ylang).

Very few diterpenes are found in essential oils, as their molecular weight is too high for them to be distilled. However, they may occur in solvent extracts.

Terpenoids

Alcohols

Alcohols are found in many essential oils. They are thought to be good antiseptics, and some are antiviral and uplifting. Usually essential oils with a high percentage of alcohols are safe to use in the correct dilution and have few side-effects. Examples include geraniol in *Cymbopogon martini* (Palmarosa), linalol in *Lavandula angustifolia* and citronellol in *Eucalyptus citriodora*.[33]

Phenols

Phenols need to be treated with caution as many of them are skin irritants. Most have very strong antibacterial properties and can have a stimulatory effect on both the nervous system and the immune system. Thymol (from *Thymus vulgaris*) also has anthelmintic properties. Eugenol is a powerful anti-inflammatory,[34] decreases gut motility in diarrhoea and inhibits prostaglandin synthesis.[35] Examples of phenols include cavacrol in oregano, eugenol in clove and nutmeg, thymol in thyme, anethole in star anise, and methyleugenol in cinnamon.

Aldehydes

Aldehydes often have a sedative, calming effect, as well as being important in the aroma of the plant. Examples include citral in lemon balm (*Melissa officinalis*), citronellal in lemongrass (*Cymbopogon citratus*) and citronellal in *Cymbopogon nardus*, geranial in *Eucalyptus citriadora* and neral in lemon verbena (*Aloysia triphylla*). Citral has strong antiseptic and antibacterial properties.[36] Citronellal possesses antifungal properties.[37]

Esters

Esters have very useful antispasmodic properties, and are calming and antifungal. They often smell very fruity. Examples include linalyl acetate found in lavender (*Lavandula angustifolia*), clary sage (*Salvia sclarea*) and bergamot (*Citrus aurantium* subsp. *bergamia*) and genaryl acetate found in sweet marjoram (*Origanum majorana*). An essential oil with a very high ester content (85 per cent) is Roman chamomile (*Chamaemelum/Anthemis nobilis*), which includes angelic and tiglic esters.[38]

Ketones

Although ketones can sometimes be difficult to use due to their potential toxicity, this mainly relates to situations where they are taken internally. However, some ketones should always be treated with caution. Definitely toxic ketones include *d*-pulegone (found in pennyroyal), which caused the death of a 23-year-old woman in 1897. It must be stressed that this lady did drink a tablespoonful (15 ml) of undiluted essential oil.[39]

There are some non-toxic ketones, and these are useful as mucolytics.[12] Franchomme states that ketones are traditionally good for the skin, a view which is supported by Lavabre.[8] Safe ketones include jasmone in jasmine[2] fenchone in fennel (*Foeniculum vulgare*) and menthone in geranium (*Pelargonium graveolens*). Although beta-damascerone is only present at a concentration of 0.05 per cent, it is this ketone which gives roses their wonderful smell. 'Safe' means when used in reasonable amounts – even water can prove lethal in excess.

Oxides

The most common oxide in *Eucalyptus* is cineole – a strong expectorant. Both forms, 1,4-cineole and 1,8-cineole occur in essential oils.[3] Cineole is found in *Eucalyptus globulus* (blue gum), *Rosmarinus officinalis* CT cineol (rosemary) and *Lauris nobilis* (bay laurel). Other oxides are ascaridole, found in wormseed (*Chenopodium ambrosiodies* var. *anthelminticum*). The freshly baked smell that is wafted around bread counters in supermarkets is often due to an oxide called 2-furaldehyde.[38]

Lactones

Lactones are present in most expressed oils. The percentage of lactones present may be low, but lactones play an important role as expectorants and mucolytics. Alantolactone is present in *Inula helnium*, used to treat purulent bronchitis.[40] A bicyclic lactone (a phthalide) is responsible for the odour in celery root. One of the main lactones is called coumarin.[38]

Coumarins

Coumarins may be present in small amounts, but they are very potent. Franchomme states that coumarins augment the antispasmodic effect of esters. However, the fermentation of coumarin itself yields a chemical called dicoumarol which is the basis of warfarin, an anticoagulant.[32] It is the furanocoumarin bergapten, in bergamot, which is responsible for the phototoxic effect observed when skin treated with bergamot is exposed to ultraviolet light. The skin discolours and the resulting pigmentation can remain for life. Other coumarins include khellin and visnagin, strong vasodilators found in *Ammi visnaga*.[33] Khellin is also a bronchodilator.[41] It was the reconstituted compounds from this plant that formed the ingredients of the pharmaceutical product, Intal.[12]

Peneol states that the 'energy facet of essential oils is revealed through the biophysical approach, for example through the determination of the bioelectronigram (pH, rH_2 and resistivity)'.[42] Franchomme, in his lectures, states that bacteria and viruses need an alkaline medium in which to grow. He goes on to say that essential oils have a high pH, which is not favourable for pathogenic micro-organisms, but is favourable for a healthy human body.

Franchomme and Peneol believe that the electrical charge of an aromatic molecule plays a vital part in its therapeutic property. They say that this is the ability of molecules to 'give' protons or electrons. Franchomme and Peneol consider that by 'giving' electrons, the patient will become negatively charged, resulting in a calming effect. By 'giving' protons, the patient will be stimulated and energized. Protonization results in a reduction in pH.[25]

Furthermore, Peneol and Franchomme discuss molecules as having yin- and yang-like qualities. The yang-like qualities are thought to tone the whole body, stimulate immune growth, support the metabolic response, raise the internal temperature and stimulate the nervous system. The yin-like oils are thought to reduce the temperature, decrease activity in the nervous system and have a calming effect. This approach of attributing yin- and yang-like properties to essential oils is carried through in Peter Holme's work[43] and Gabriel Mojay's book.[44]

BUYING ESSENTIAL OILS

In the last few years there has been an explosion in the number of essential oil companies. Many operate by direct mail. The listings sections of magazines such as *Aromatherapy Quarterly*, the *International Journal of Aromatherapy* and the *International Society of Aromatherapy Journal* carry several pages of mail-order advertisements. Most health-food shops, some chemists and certain department stores also carry a range of essential oils, and of course there is the ubiquitous Body Shop. A great many essential oil mail-order companies have been set up specifically to milk the new market and to make a quick profit.

Although many companies appear to provide true essential oils, often this is not the case. Some honest dealers openly state in their literature or on the bottle that their oils are diluted. Other companies are not so honest, and the public is led to believe that the bottle they are purchasing contains pure 100 per cent strength essential oil.

Essential oils are extremely easy to dilute or to adulterate.[13] The most common method of dilution is the addition of a vegetable oil. When this occurs, the 'essential oil' will leave a ring on evaporation. If alcohol is added, it is sometimes discernible in the aroma. Adulteration by adding a cheaper substitute, e.g. putting geranium oil in rose oil, or petitgrain/bergamot in neroli, is commonplace. Real melissa is extremely difficult to find, as it is frequently adulterated with lemongrass or citral. Sometimes particular components are added, such as citronella, geraniol or linalol.[45] Some of the best melissa is actually grown very close to home – in Ireland.

First and foremost, one should only buy an essential oil which is correctly labelled. *Much* more is needed than just the generic name. Product lists and bottle labels should bear the complete botanical name. Product lists should include the country of origin, the part of the plant, and whether it has been grown wild or grown without pesticides. Also mentioned on the product list should be the type of extraction, and whether the batch number is known. Organically grown plants used for essential oil production are certified by the Organic Farmers and Growers Ltd, UK. The chemotype, where relevant, also needs to be specified. Some distributors are members of the Essential Oils Trade Association (EOTA), and some are members of the trade arm of the Aromatherapy Organisation Council (AOT).

Labelling provides a good indication of how scrupulous the supplier is. Bottles should contain integral droppers, and should be of coloured glass. 'Pure 100 per cent essential oil' should be clearly marked. Basic safety precautions such as 'do not take by mouth', 'keep away from children' and 'avoid contact with eyes' should appear on the label. Apart from the label and the price, the only reliable indicators are an experienced nose and a reputable company that would lose too much by compromising itself. It is best to ask around. Qualified and registered aromatherapists tend to buy from the same suppliers, who usually operate by mail order.

Some of the best suppliers will tell the buyer whether the whole flowering plant was used, or just the flowering heads. Reputable suppliers are keen to supply the very best, and can provide gas-chromatography data. However, they are *not* in business to answer questions about which essential oil to use.

There is a list in Appendix 3 at the back of this book of essential oil suppliers I have personally bought from in the past. I make no secret of the fact that I buy from Fragrant Earth, Saffron Oils, Essentially Oils, Butterbar and Sage, Rosa Medica and Quintessence in the USA, and feel that they represent some of the very best. However, I am biased, as I have used them for a long time and have built up a relationship of mutual trust. I am sure that there are new companies which may be as good. It is important to remember that you get what you pay for, and that aromatherapy is only as good as the essential oils used.

ESSENTIAL OIL TOXICITY

There are several ways in which essential oil toxicity can be measured. One of them is by oral dosage. This is usually tested on mice or rats, and when 50 per cent of the animals die the strength of the essential oil is deemed to be toxic.[2] Another method is by skin tests, used on a shaved area of the skin of animals, and again when 50 per cent of them die the oil is assumed to be toxic. There have been very few clinical tests on humans. Those that have been carried out are ones in which volunteers experience a patch test over a 24-hour period.[17] The largest study was conducted by the Japanese. It spanned 8 years and involved testing 200 human volunteers using 270 000 patch tests. However, it is recognized that oriental skin is more sensitive than Caucasian skin.[2]

In skin tests, adverse reactions can be divided into cutaneous irritation, allergic sensitivity reaction and phototoxic reaction[17] (sensitivity and safety will be covered in the section on sensitivity and safety). It should be borne in mind that essential oils naturally occurring in the living plant are about 0.1 to 1 per cent concentrated. When essential oils have been distilled and are purchased in a bottle, they are up to 100 per cent concentrated. At this concentration, their potency is up to 1000 times stronger than it is in their naturally occurring state.[2] This is why they must always be diluted before use. In general, a 2 per cent dilution is acceptable, although up to 5 per cent and down to 0.05 per cent is not uncommon.

Those therapists with a leaning towards homeopathy, such as myself, strongly contest that a lower dilution is more powerful, as well as being safer.

There was considerable media hype about sage a few years ago. It was suggested that sage stuffing mix could cause pregnant women to miscarry. This was based on research conducted on rats who were forced to ingest vast quantities of sage. However, the liver metabolism of a rat is different to that of humans. Moreover, humans rarely sit down and consume plate after plate of sage, even when they are pregnant. Most qualified aromatherapists consider that sage is safe to use although, because of its high thujone content (ketones), the need for special care *is* emphasized. Thujone can exist as any of four different isomers (alpha, beta, etc.), each of which has different effects.[46]

Sage contains estragole. When estragole was given to rats in doses of 0.5 g/kg/day it caused hepatocellular cancer. However, estragole is eaten regularly by humans in a normal diet at a level of around 1 mg/kg/day;

1 mg is equivalent to 20 drops. The World Health Organization/Food and Agriculture Organization (WHO/FAO) joint expert committee on food additives stated that 'we do not know how much estragole is absorbed through the skin. ... At low doses a compound may be safely disposed of metabolically.'[3] Sometimes essential oils or herbs are classified as unsafe even when they could be used with caution.

Perhaps this would be a good opportunity to explain that the effects of the essential oil from a plant, and the effects of the plant itself as used in herbal medicine, are often different. Herbal remedies are made up from the dried herb, which is macerated in alcohol – the 'mother tincture'. This 'mother tincture' is then added to water, and the diluted tincture is taken by mouth. Essential oils are steam distilled, concentrated and (for the most part) inhaled or applied to the skin.

HERBAL OILS AND FLORAL WATERS

There are three different kinds of 'oils' used in aromatherapy:

- essential oils;
- carrier oils;
- herbal oils.

In this book there is no A to Z of essential oils listing their properties, as is common in many aromatherapy books, but there is a list of potentially safe essential oils which might be incorporated into a nursing protocol in the summary.

Carrier oils

Essential oils need to be diluted when applied to the skin, as they are too concentrated to use on their own except in specific situations, involving specific essential oils. Because essential oils are often diluted in a carrier oil, it might be relevant at this point to mention some of these carrier oils (sometimes called base oils). Carrier oils are fatty oils, many of them have their own therapeutic properties, and all of them are vegetable based. Although this book is about aromatherapy, it could be relevant to use some specialized carrier oils on their own in certain cases when essential oils might be contraindicated (see section on contraindications and precautions).

All carrier oils should be cold-pressed. This rules out cooking oils, which are intended to be ingested, not applied to the skin, and which for the food and drinks industry need to be 'purified' at very high temperatures. Heating a vegetable oil to 212°F radically changes its chemistry, so the vegetable oil ends up increasing the risk of peroxidation – a process which encourages free radical cell damage. Free radicals are formed when the double bonds in the chemical structure of a vegetable oil are attacked by oxygen molecules, producing highly unstable hydroperoxides which are thought to cause premature ageing.[47]

Most vegetable carrier oils are odourless, their main purpose in aromatherapy massage being to serve as a carrier for the essential oil. However, carrier oils contain linoleic acid, which the body can convert into gamma-linolenic acid (GLA). GLA is an essential component of the membranes surrounding every skin cell, and is required to strengthen the protective lipid barrier which lies beneath the surface of the skin and guards against moisture loss.[48] A lack of linoleic acid affects the ability of collagen to support the skin.

Warning
Many carrier oils are extracted from nuts. Nut allergies appear to be increasing, so it is important to ask your patients first whether they have a nut allergy. Before using any essential oil, carrier oil or phytol it is essential to take detailed case notes.

The most common carrier oils are grapeseed and sweet almond. Grapeseed has a thin, almost non-greasy feel and is the cheapest emollient. It is also quickly absorbed. Sweet almond oil is more luxurious, has a higher linoleic acid content, and takes longer to absorb. It is also used by the pharmaceutical trade as a base for mild laxatives and some ointments.

Other carrier oils which are more expensive and have specific therapeutic effects can be added to grapeseed or sweet almond oil, or used on their own. A brief description of some of these now follows.

Apricot kernel
This is used for mature or dry skins. It is an expensive oil containing vitamin A.

Avocado
Only a small quantity of this oil is required as it is a sticky green viscous oil with a slight aroma. The green colour is caused by chlorophyll. Avocado is very effective for deep penetration into adipose tissue and, as it contains proteins, vitamins, lecithin and fatty acids, is useful for treating itchy dry skin problems such as psoriasis, as well as for protecting the skin against degeneration. It is a natural sunscreen. The cosmetic industry uses avocado oil in a wide selection of products, including lipstick, hair conditioner and cleansing cream.

Camellia

This carrier oil is thought to be excellent for the nerve tissue in the skin. It has none of the bronchodilating properties of the tea that is made from the plant.

Evening primrose

This is the only carrier oil that contains gamma linolenic acid (GLA), the precursor of linoleic acid. It is excellent for the dry flaking skin which frequently accompanies viral conditions, alcoholism, smoking and most chronic diseases. This naturally occurring polyunsaturated fatty acid has been used to good effect in the treatment of a range of inflammatory diseases, including rheumatoid conditions and eczema.[49]

Jojoba

This carrier oil is rich in vitamin E and, because it has a very fine texture, it is excellent for treatment of acne or greasy skins as it penetrates the skin easily. It was employed as the natural alternative to sperm whale oil when this mammal became an endangered species in 1970.[47]

Kiwi seed

This carrier oil contains very high levels of compounds essential for the synthesis of prostaglandins and cell membranes. As well as linoleic acid, it contains alpha-linolenic fatty acid, which is excellent for promoting the cellular growth of skin. Patients with multiple sclerosis have been found to have low levels of this particular fatty acid.

Palm kernel (Tamanu) (Calophyllum inophyllum)

This is a thick dark green viscous sticky oil with exceptional properties. It is anti-inflammatory and analgesic, and often used in pessaries. It should be used sparingly with another carrier oil. Tamanu, which comes from the South Sea Islands, has been used for generations as an analgesic medicine to treat sciatica, rheumatism and to help ulcers and wounds heal. It is useful for promoting the healing of burns. It also has antibiotic-like properties, and is a wonderful healing carrier oil with anti-inflammatory properties. It is recommended for use in all mucous membrane lesions, including wounds and ulcers, and in the treatment of burns (both chemical and physical). Care should be taken not to confuse it with enriched cocoa butter masquerading as the real thing.

Passionflower

This carrier oil is good for maintaining skin elasticity. It does not have any of the anti-inflammatory or narcotic properties of the extract from the flower.

Rosa rubignosa – Rosehip

This a fairly new carrier oil. It has a high content of unsaturated fatty acids and is called a biological balancer. It is thought to decrease old scarring (especially keloid) and pigmentation.

This vegetable oil is the only one that contains 21 per cent palmitoleic acid. With 61 per cent oleic acid it closely resembles human sebum, and thus is contraindicated for individuals with acne or greasy skin. It is thought to be excellent for slowing down lipid peroxidation (free radicals which create autocatalytic chain reactions resulting in damage to membrane permeability and decreasing the functioning of enzymes).[50] It is because of this effect that rosehip carrier oil may well have cell protection functions.

Wheatgerm

This carrier oil is thought to be a good anti-scarring agent, being rich in vitamin E. Because it is dark and aromatic, with a distinctive nutty smell, it should be used sparingly. It is contraindicated for patients with coeliac disease or gluten intolerance. It is a natural anti-oxidant, and if added to other carrier oils will increase their shelf-life.

All carrier oils should be supplied in coloured glass bottles or metal containers, to protect them from light, which will turn them rancid. Usually they will keep for 9 months. However, every time the bottle or container is opened, oxygen will attack the contents, so small bottles are best. The carrier oils should be kept cool. This may lead to some clouding, which is merely an indication that the oil has not been refined (heated). The clouding is caused by the saturated part of the oil sinking to the bottom. The sell-by date should always be checked.

Herbal oils

Herbal oils, sometimes called phytols are infused oils. They usually have a basis of either olive oil or sunflower oil. A selected herb is macerated in the oil over a period of time. This maceration or infusion can be hot, cold or, in a commercial setting, under a vacuum.

Today aromatherapists add a few drops of an essential oil to a carrier oil in order to obtain an 'aromatherapy mix'. However, some plants are reluctant to yield their essential oils. Herbal oils provide one means of obtaining a ready-to-use aromatherapy-type oil for topical application. Phytols can be a useful adjunct to other carrier oils when a more specialized approach is indicated. The majority of phytols contain herbs which have a long history of use in traditional herbal medicine.

Arnica (*Arnica montana*)

This species is indigenous to Central Europe, growing in mountain pastures from 800 to 2400 metres. It has aso been found in the UK and the USA. The scented daisy-like flowers appear in the second summer, and the plant flowers all season. The roots, leaves and flowers are used. The active ingredients contain 0.3 per cent volatile oil, 50 per cent of which is found in the flowers. Arnica has stimulatory properties, it is a uterotonic, and has antiphlogistic properties, making it highly suitable for its classic use, namely the treatment of sprains and bruising. Repeated use can cause inflammation of the skin. It provides some relief from chilblains and rheumatic pain. Essential oil of arnica is highly toxic and therefore contraindicated. The phytol is safe to use because it contains about the same amount of arnica as a homeopathic remedy. (Tincture and ointments contain very small amounts of arnica – often in homeopathic dosages).

Calendula (*Calendula officinalis*)

This species is an annual herbaceous plant 30–50 cm high with oblong hairy leaves and stems. The daisy-like flowers have many petals and an orange centre. The plant flowers throughout the summer. It is believed to have originated in India, but is now native to Southern Europe and Asia. Only the flower parts are used. It is traditionally used by the pharmaceutical industry for healing skin cracks and sores. It is useful in the treatment of impetigo, acne, burns and chilblains. It can be used on cracked nipples and is non-toxic to the baby. Its classic uses are as an anti-inflammatory and in the treatment of burns.

Calendula essential oil is extremely difficult to obtain and very expensive, but the phytol is easy to prepare and very inexpensive. Calendula (sometimes called marigold) is often confused with Mexican marigold (*Tagetes minuta*), but the oil from the latter is completely different and is used mainly to treat fungal infections.

Centella (*Centella asiatica*)

This species mainly grows in tropical areas. It is a perennial plant with a ground-hugging, creeping appearance. Because it is very adaptable it can be found at low as well as high altitudes, and in both marshy and arid climates. The small clusters of flowers are white or pale pink and appear from June to September. The parts used are the leaves. Because of its supposedly effective action in the treatment of leprosy and skin tuberculosis it is currently being researched by various interested parties. Centella appears to break down leprosy nodules by dissolving the waxy coating of the leprosy bacillus. It also seems to stimulate collagen synthesis and enhance the development of connective tissue. Its classical uses are for anti-inflammatory, anti-scarring and wound-healing purposes.

Comfrey (*Symphytum officinalis*)

This species is a common rough, hairy perennial growing up to 1 m in height. Its large leaves are tongue-shaped. It thrives in moist fields but is very adaptable. Two to five crops of comfrey can be produced per year, depending on the climate. The leaves of this plant contain more protein in their structure than the leaves of any other known member of the vegetable kingdom. The roots are used. Allantoin at a concentration of 0.75 to 2.5 per cent is found in comfrey root. Allantoin stimulates tissue regeneration. The recent discovery of specific alkaloids in Russian comfrey (*Symphytum × uplandicum*) has cast doubt on the desirability of using comfrey internally, although the danger of carcinogenesis has not yet been proven. Comfrey is extremely useful in the treatment of fractures, sprains, strains, wounds and ulcers. Its classic use is in the reduction of swelling and the treatment of fractures.

Devil's claw (*Harbagophytum procumbens*)

This is a perennial plant that grows in the swamps of the Kalahari desert. It has secondary tuberous roots and violet or red trumpet-shaped flowers which later develop into very tough barbed fruits – hence its name. These fruits have been known to ensnare wild animals. The parts used are the tuberous roots. Devil's claw has a long history of use in the treatment of rheumatoid arthritis and osteoarthritis. It has analgesic and anti-inflammatory properties, and it is also an important antispasmolytic. It is classically used as an anti-rheumatic.

Echinacea (*Echinacea purpurea*)

This perennial plant grows in North America. It is very similar to *Echinacea angustifolia*, which was used by the Native Americans and early settlers. It grows in clumps and has edible roots. The large flowers have dark pink petals with a brownish-red centre. The parts used are the rhizome and root. Echinacea has a long history of use for antifungal, antibacterial and possibly antiviral purposes. Currently it is being researched for the treatment of AIDS. Its external use is very specific and effective in wound infections, inhibiting the production of hyaluronidase, increasing capillary permeability and stimulating phagocytosis. It has been used effectively on boils, abscesses, infected burns and snake bites. It is also thought to decrease wrinkles and stretch marks. Its classical use is in the treatment of wound infections.

Fenugreek (*Trigonella foenum-graecum*)

Sometimes erect and sometimes growing horizontally, this annual plant produces pale lemon pea-like flowers in the summer. The fruits subsequently produce seeds with a distinctive smell a little like that of celery. The seeds take 4 months to mature. Fenugreek was used by the Egyptians in the embalming process. The seeds are the parts used. Fenugreek has been shown to have a hypoglycaemic effect on animals. However, its effect on human diabetes has been inconclusive (internal use only). Fenugreek seeds contain 0.6 to 1.7 per cent steroid aponogenins which could potentially provide a useful source of steroid drugs in the future. It is used to treat mouth ulcers, chronic cough, swollen glands and digestive problems, and is also used in the production of mock maple syrup. Its classic uses are in the treatment of fevers and mouth ulcers.

Lime blossom (*Tilia* × *europaea*)

Lime trees grow to a height of about 40 metres or more. The small fragrant flowers are yellowish-white and hang down in bunches. The tree is frequently grown in suburban streets. The flowers are the parts used. The macerated oil has an emollient action and is also soothing and antispasmodic. It is useful in the treatment of skin diseases, especially those involving scaling. It can also be used for headache. Its classic use is for soothing the skin.

Meadowsweet (*Filipendula ulmaria*)

This is a perennial plant which grows in North America and Europe, especially in moist areas. The upright clusters of small fragrant cream-coloured flowers appear from June to August. The parts used are the flowers. Meadowsweet has been used since the Middle Ages to treat joint pain and arthritis and to regulate the bladder. Recent research has shown that meadowsweet is effective in the treatment of dysentery, diarrhoea and most digestive problems. It has a mildly sedative action and is useful in the treatment of toothache. Its classic uses are in pain relief and as a sedative.

St John's wort (*Hypericum perforatum*)

This is a hairless perennial plant which grows in North America and Europe. The bright yellow flowers, which are covered in tiny black dots, appear from July to September. The flowers are the parts used. The plant is much disliked by farmers, as cattle that have eaten the plant become sensitive to sunlight and start to scratch themselves continually. Used externally, St John's wort has remarkable soothing and healing properties. It is extremely effective on painful joints, gout or lumbago, and works by increasing the blood supply to the affected area. It is very effective when used in a compress applied to bruises and sprains, to which it brings almost instant relief. The use of St

John's wort on the hands is thought to prevent the development of age spots. It is also used in many antiwrinkle preparations. Its classic uses are in the treatment of bruised skin, ulcers and varicose veins.[51]

REFERENCES

1. **Williams, D.** 1989: *Lecture notes on essential oils*. London: Eve Taylor.

2. **International School of Aromatherapy** 1993: *A safety guide on the use of essential oils*. London: Nature by Nature Oils Ltd.

3. **Tisserand, R. and Balacs, T.** 1995: *Essential oil safety*. London: Churchill Livingstone.

4. **Van Moppes** 1995: *Information pamphlet*. St Leonards: Essential Oil Trade Association.

5. **Guenther, E.** 1976: *The essential oils. Volume V*. Malabar, FL: Krieger.

6. **Price, S.** 1983: *Practical aromatherapy*. London: Thorsons.

7. **Arctander, S.** 1961: *Perfume and flavor materials of natural origin*. Carol Stream, IL: Allured Publishing.

8. **Lavabre, M.** 1990: *Aromatherapy workbook*. Vermont: Healing Arts Press.

9. **Ryman, D.** 1991: *Aromatherapy*. London: Piatkus.

10. **Tisserand, R.** 1994: Profile: Peter Wilde. *International Journal of Aromatherapy* 6, 3–7.

11. **Wilde, P.** 1995: Flavour, fragrances and essential oils. In *13th International Congress Proceedings, Istanbul*. Eskisehir, Turkey: Anadolu University Press, 351–7.

12. **Rose, J.** 1992: *The aromatherapy book*. San Francisco: North Atlantic Books.

13. **Guenther, E.** 1972: *The essential oils. Volume 1*. Malabar, FL: Krieger.

14. **Erichsen-Brown, C.** 1979: *Medicinal and other uses of North American plants*. New York: Dover Publications Inc.

15. **Lawless, J.** 1992: *Encyclopedia of essential oils*. Shaftesbury: Element.

16. **Tisserand, R.** 1988: *The essential oil safety data manual*. Brighton: Tisserand.

17. **Watt, M.** 1991: *Plant aromatics*. Witham: Watts.

18. **Swanson, T.** 1995: *Intellectual rights and biodiversity conservation*. Cambridge: Cambridge University Press.

19. **Gumbel, D.** 1986: *The principles of holistic skin therapy with herbal essences*. Heidelberg: Haug.

20. **Blackwell, R.** 1991: An insight into aromatic oils: lavender and teatree. *British Journal of Phytotherapy* 2, 25–30.

21. **Lawrence, B.** 1989: *Essential oils: 1981–1987*. Carol Stream, IL: Allured Publishing.

22. **Jakovlev, V.** *et al.* 1983: Pharmacological investigations with compounds of chamomile. VI. Investigations on the antiphlogistic effects of chamazulene and matricin. *Planta Medica* **49**, 67–73.

23. **Carle, R. and Gomaa, K.** 1992: The medicinal use of *Matricaria flos*. *British Journal of Phytotherapy* **2**, 147–53.

24. **Valnet, J.** 1990: *The practice of aromatherapy*. Saffron Walden: C.W. Daniel Co. Ltd.

25. **Franchomme, P. and Peneol, D.** 1990: *L'aromatherapie exactement*. Limoges: Jollois.

26. **Rossi, T., Melegari, M., Bianchi, A., Albasini, A. and Vampa, G.** 1988: Sedative, anti-inflammatory and anti-diuretic effects induced in rats by essential oils of varieties of *Anthemis nobilis*: a comparative study. *Pharmacological Research Communications* **20** (Suppl. 5), 71–4.

27. **Guenther, E.** 1976: *The essential oils. Volume III*. Malabar, FL: Krieger.

28. **Moleyar, V. and Narasimham, P.** 1992: Antibacterial activity of essential oil components. *International Journal of Food Microbiology* **16**, 337–42.

29. **Franz, C.** 1993: Genetics. In Hay, R.K.M. and Waterman, P.G. (eds), *Volatile oil crops: their biology, biochemistry and production*. Harlow: Longman Scientific and Technical, 63–96.

30. **Zheng, G.-Q., Kenney, P.M. and Luke, T.L.** 1992: Anethofuran, carvone and limonene: potential cancer chemopreventive agents from dill weed oil and caraway oil. *Planta Medica* **58**, 338–41.

31. **Lorenzetti, B.B., Souza, G.E., Sarti, S.J., Santox Filho, D. and Ferreira, S.H.** 1991: Myrcene mimics the peripheral analgesic activity of lemongrass tea. *Journal of Ethnopharmacology* **34**, 43–8.

32. **Mills, S.** 1991: *Out of the Earth*. London: Viking Arkana. p. 295.

33. **Lewis Walter, H. and Elvin-Lewis Memory, R.F.** 1977. *Medical botany*. New York: John Wiley.

34. **Sharma, J.N., Srivastava, K.C. and Gan, E.K.** 1994: Suppressive effects of eugenol and ginger oil on arthritic rats. *Pharmacology* **49**, 314–18.

35. **Bennett, A., Stamford, P. and Tavares, I.A.** 1988: The biological activity of eugenol, a major constituent of nutmeg (*Myristica fragrans*): studies on prostaglandins, the intestine and other tissues. *Phytotherapy Research* **2**, 124–30.

36. **Onawunmi, G.O. and Oguniana, E.O.** 1981: Antibacterial constituents in the essential oil of *Cymbopogon citratus. Ethnopharmacology* **24**, 64–8.

37. **Hmamouchi, M., Tantaoui-Elaraki, A. and Es-Safu, N.** 1990: Illustration of antibacterial and antifungal properties of *Eucalyptus* essential oils. *Plantes Medicale Phytotherapie* **24**, 278–9.

38. **Bauer, K., Garbe, D. and Surburg, H.** 1990: *Common fragrance and flavor materials*. Weinheim: VCH Verlagsgesellschaft.

39. **Allen, W.T.** 1897: Note on a case of supposed poisoning by pennyroyal. *Lancet* **1**, 1022–3.

40. **Rose, J.** 1994: *Guide to essential oils.* San Francisco: Jeanne Rose Aromatherapy.

41. **Budavari, S. et al.** (ed). 1996: *The Merck index,* 12th edn. Whitehouse Station, NJ: Merck & Co. Inc.

42. **Peneol, D.** 1991: This is also aromatherapy. *International Journal of Aromatherapy* **3**, 14–16.

43. **Holmes, P.** 1989: *The energetics of Western herbs.* Berkley: NatTrop Publishing.

44. **Mojay, G.** 1996: *Aromatherapy for healing the spirit.* London: Gaia.

45. **Wagner, H., Bladt, S. and Zgainski, E.M.** 1984: *Plant drug analysis.* Berlin: Springer-Verlag.

46. **Price, S.** 1993: *Aromatherapy workbook.* London: Thorsons.

47. **Earle, L.** 1991: *Vital oils.* London: Vermilion Press.

48. **Egbaria, K. and Weiner, N.** 1993: Topical application of liposomal preparations. In Zatz, J.L. (ed.), *Skin permeation.* Wheaton, IL: Allured Publishing, 193–206.

49. **Hansen, T.M. et al.** 1983: Treatment of rheumatoid arthritis with prostaglandin E, and precursors *cis*-linoleic acid and γ-linolenic acid. *Scandinavian Journal of Rheumatology* **12**, 85–8.

50. **Lackie, J.M. and More, I.A.R.** 1992: Cells and tissues in health and disease. In MacSween, N.M. and Whaley, K. (eds), *Muir's textbook of pathology.* London: Edward Arnold, 1–35.

51. **Kusmirek, J.** 1993: *Essential herbal oils.* Taunton, Devon: Fragrant Earth.

5

CONTRAINDICATIONS

Just because essential oils are natural or pure, this does not mean that they will never produce an adverse reaction. Many such reactions can be avoided if essential oils and not extracts are used. Essential oils are steam distilled, and therefore the potential for adverse reactions to something other than the essential oils (e.g. a solvent) is eradicated. Equally, it is logical to assume that essential oils which have been adulterated or extended are more likely to cause a problem, although this would be difficult to prove. However, the possibility of adverse reactions using pure, unadulterated essential oils cannot be ruled out, especially among patients who are already receiving medication, or who are allergy prone. Patch testing can do much to avoid these reactions, although a few essential oils are toxic, and some essential oils cause dermal irritation.

POSSIBLE SKIN REACTIONS

These include the following:

- irritation;
- sensitivity;
- phototoxicity.

Irritation

This is produced by a component within the essential oil, and occurs immediately, producing contact dermatitis. Contact dermatitis from a 2 to 5 per cent dilution of a true essential oil is a rare event. More often, the irritation is due to a chemical used in the extraction method, indicating that an extract and not an essential oil has been used. Possible skin-irritating oils include cinnamon and clove. There have been incidences of erythema following the use of topical benzoin.[1,2] Benzoin is often used in a proprietary spray prior to elastoplast dressing.

Cinnamon has been reported to be responsible for an adverse reaction to trichlorophenol (TCP)[3] (cinnamon is no longer used in this product). Even tea tree, so often recommended for its gentleness, has produced contact dermatitis when used undiluted on the skin. In this particular case, the actual oil used was found to have a high eucalyptol content. Another name for eucalyptol is 1,8-cineol (an oxide).[4] However, true tea tree oil is supposed to have a high content of 1-terpinen-4-ol (an alcohol), not 1,8-cineole. This highlights the importance of knowing exactly what is in the bottle. The user has to rely entirely on the integrity of the supplier.

Chemical burns

These have been reported from *neat* peppermint oil which was inadvertently spilt on skin which had already been traumatized by skin grafts. The area necrosed and required excision and further surgery.[5]

Sensitivity

Sensitization to an essential oil is an allergic reaction which occurs over time. On the first occasion nothing much may happen. However, in a similar manner to some drug sensitivities (such as that to penicillin), subsequent exposure will produce stronger reactions. These reactions can occur in the form of inflammation, or as a rash. Sensitivity is not very common, and usually occurs after long-term habitual use. However, allergic reactions are not unknown in patients who are sensitized. Juniper took 25 years to produce sensitivity in the case of a lady who sold food smoked and spiced in juniper oils. She developed a dry cough and asthma. Skin tests showed a sensitivity to juniper, although it was not established whether it was the wood resin that was to blame, or the berries.[6]

It is thought that patients who are already on medication are more sensitive to essential oils than those who are not taking medication. Obviously those patients who are already suffering from an allergy-like illness such as asthma, eczema or hay fever are also more likely to be sensitive. A florist who presented with an allergic reaction to Roman chamomile (*Chamaemelum nobile*) was found to have a prior sensitivity to chamomile tisanes and ointments.[7] Another florist, who had had dermatitis of the face for 1 year, was found to be allergic to the sesquiterpenes in German chamomile (*Matricaria recutita*).[8] Lavender, which is supposed to be the safest of all essential oils, caused an allergy in a hairdresser who habitually used lavender shampoo. It is thought that the allergen involved was linalol or linalyl acetate.[9] However, almost anything can be an allergen, even water.

Sometimes a mixture of another chemical and an essential oil can trigger an allergic reaction. This was the case when an aromatherapist sprayed her roses with an insecticide, and 24 hours later developed an acute bilateral hand eczema. She had been using French marigold (*Tagetes patula*) on a patient. The French marigold had been obtained by solvent extraction (so was not a true essential oil). Tests showed that the allergic reaction was caused by a cross-reaction between the synthetic pyrethoid in the insecticide and the acetone-soluble extract of the marigold leaves and flowers.[10] French marigold is an unusual choice in aromatherapy – it smells unpleasant and always needs to be used with caution due to the high percentage of tagetone, which can cause skin reactions. Its main use is in the treatment of fungal infections, but even in this respect it has been mainly replaced by tea tree. One wonders if the aromatherapist believed that she was using common marigold (*Calendula officinalis*), which is non-irritant and used for its powerful skin-healing properties.

Although it is accepted that citral is a potential sensitizer, lemongrass, melissa and verbena rarely produce sensitivity reactions in aromatherapy, although they each contain citral. It is thought that the presence of *d*-limonene produces a quenching effect. This means that there is something else within the plant which balances it. If that is taken away by isolating what is thought to be the active ingredient, then the effect of the chemical becomes much stronger, even though the actual concentration might be lower. For lists of potential sensitizers please refer to *Essential Oil Safety* by R. Tisserand and T. Balacs.[14]

The most common skin reaction is a stinging, painful weal with occasional generalized urticaria. It is sometimes accompanied by bronchial inflammation producing asthma-like symptoms.[11]

Phototoxicity

Phototoxicity results from a reaction between a component in the essential oil, the skin, and ultraviolet light. This means that exposure to either sunbed radiation or natural sunlight can produce a skin reaction. Such reactions can vary from pigmentation of the skin to severe full-thickness burns. The most common components causing phototoxicity are furanocoumarins. Lemon oil contains oxypeucedanin and bergapten (both of which are furanocoumarins), which produce phototoxic reactions. Lime and bitter orange oil also contain these components, but in smaller quantities.[12] Angelica root oil can produce phototoxicity.

Bergamot was used in fake sun-tan preparations until recently, when 12 cases were reported of a skin reaction following the use of this type of product.

In two cases (in which skin had been exposed to the sun immediately after application of the tanning cream) symptoms of erythema as well as pigmentation were presented.[13] Bergamot oil can be obtained without the furanocoumarins which produce the pigmentation. This oil is then classified as bergaptene-free or furanocoumarin-free (FCF). Many therapists will not use FCF essential oils, and some distributors will not supply them, saying that they will only use 'whole' oils. Deterpenated citrus oils will contain higher concentrations of furanocoumarins, and are best avoided.

Patch tests can be used to avoid skin reactions, and are suggested for all potential risk patients.

- Irritation – the essential oil is mixed with a carrier oil at double the concentration to be used. Two drops of the mixture are applied to a Band Aid, which is left on the skin for 48 hours.
- Sensitivity – the procedure is as described above, but repeated a second time. It is important to look for itching, redness or blistering. If an adverse skin reaction occurs, the patient's skin should be washed with an unperfumed soap and left exposed to the air. Tisserand and Balacs suggest that the application of a limonene-rich oil such as lemon might reduce the severity of such a reaction.[14]

CHRONIC TOXICITY

This is defined as a toxic reaction caused by repeated low-level doses over a period of time resulting in organ tissue damage, most commonly in the liver or kidneys. Death may eventually occur, but it is the preceding slow tissue damage which is the main problem. Although chronic toxicity is a term usually used in relation to oral use of essential oils, it is thought that some essential oils could cause similar problems if used over extended periods of time. For this reason extended use of a single essential oil or blend is not advised. An extended period refers to a span of more than 14 days. It is extremely unlikely that chronic toxicity can occur at the low dosages used in aromatherapy, particularly when the application is topical. Please consult one of the specialist books listed at the end of this book.

REACTIONS WITH ORTHODOX DRUGS

Drug combinations and pharmacokinetics

A working definition of an interacting drug combination is 'one that has the potential, documented in humans, to produce a clinically significant change in the pharmacological response to its constituent drugs that is larger or smaller than the sum of the effects when the drugs are administered separately'.[15]

It has been assessed that 7.4 per cent of all hospitalized patients receive an interacting drug combination during their hospital stay.[16] Compounding this problem is the knowledge that individual patients will respond in varying ways to the same dose of the same drug. This variation is thought to be directly related to the pharmacokinetics, i.e. the mathematical description of the rate and extent of absorption, distribution and elimination of drugs in the body.[17] These three processes determine the movements of drugs within the body. However, despite advances in understanding, a great deal is not yet known about drug combinations and pharmacokinetics.

As there are documented differences between individuals with regard to the absorption of several orthodox drugs, e.g. phenytoin and digoxin, it is expected that the absorption of essential oils will also vary. Absorption is dependent on the mode of delivery, the transdermal route being thought to be slower and more controlled. It is considered that this reduces the difference between the maximum and minimum drug concentrations attained during a dosing interval.[15] The distribution of any drug is controlled by blood flow to the tissue or organ, as well as by the drug's ability to bind to plasma proteins. It is also related to whether the molecule is lipid-soluble or water-soluble.

Elimination takes place at the same time as distribution, and occurs primarily through the liver and kidneys. However, some lipid-soluble non-ionized drugs can be completely reabsorbed and metabolized in the liver. This metabolism includes chemical conversion to allow the drug (or essential oil) to become more water-soluble, and therefore easier to excrete in the urine. Metabolism is the mechanism whereby drug action is terminated or, in the case of some drugs, such as aspirin, activated.[18] Essential oils that are inhaled or applied topically do not go through the first stage of metabolism by the liver.[19]

Because they are lipid-soluble, essential oils gain easy access to the brain. When they are being transported by the bloodstream they travel readily to the adrenal glands and kidneys.[14] The rate of elimination of a drug from the body is proportional to the concentration of that drug in the bloodstream. In most instances the biological half-life ($t_{1/2}$), rather than the elimination rate, is documented. The half-life is the time taken for the drug concentration in the blood to decrease to one-half of its initial value. It is dependent on both the volume of distribution of the drug and the rate at which that drug is eliminated from the body (clearance).[17]

Drugs and essential oils are excreted via the kidneys, lungs and skin. In addition, many nursing mothers will also excrete drugs, and therefore, essential oils, in their breast milk.[20]

Theoretically, essential oils could interact with orthodox drugs in several ways: by combining with a cellular receptor (and thereby competing with the drug), by combining with plasma protein, or by combining with and somehow altering the chemistry of the drug to produce a different compound with different effects.[14]

Essential oils and drug metabolism

Cellular receptors

Most drugs combine with a molecular structure, found on the surface of cells, which is called a receptor. This produces a molecular change in the receptor and leads to a chain of events called a *response*. The same situation occurs with naturally formed neurotransmitters and hormones secreted by the body itself. Some drugs produce the same effect as naturally occurring substances because they combine with the same receptors at a cellular level. An example of this is morphine mimicking the effects of endorphins.[21]

It is known that receptors will only react with a limited number of substances which have a similar molecular structure. Therefore, an essential oil that has a molecular structure similar to that of a drug known to bind to a particular receptor may also combine with that receptor. An example of this is anethole and its polymers, dianethole and photoanethole, which bear a striking resemblance to the catecholamine dopamines, adrenaline and noradrenaline.[22] Also worthy of mention are the non-steroidal compounds with oestrogenic activity, found in plants, which mimic the A-ring of steroids.[23]

Combining at the plasma level

Most drugs found in the vascular compartment will bind with one of the macromolecules in the plasma (compartmental modelling is used as a theoretical vehicle for assessing the distribution of drugs).[15] This binding is reversible, as only an unbound drug can diffuse through the capillary wall, produce systemic effects, be metabolized and then be excreted. As the macromolecule circulates within the bloodstream, so the vascular system works as a human drug distributor.

There is no reason to suppose that an essential oil could not also bind with plasma protein. It could bind with one of the most important plasma proteins, albumin, as most albumin-bound drugs are only slightly soluble in water. Drug binding at this level is non-specific, and displacements frequently occur when a newer drug with a higher affinity comes along. This means that the previous drug is suddenly freed to become distributed to another part of the body. In some diseases, such as uraemia, plasma protein binding is reduced.

Changing the action of a drug through potentizing or opposing physiological effects

It is known that undiluted essential oils aid the penetration of drugs through the skin of animals.[24] Therefore it is possible that the topical application of diluted essential oils could increase the level of drug being received by a patient on patch therapy, e.g. hormone replacement therapy (HRT). However, no documented information is available to confirm whether this is so.

In a study conducted in 1993, it was found that *b*-myrcene affected the metabolism of barbiturates in rats. The rats were given *b*-myrcene orally 1 hour before an intraperitoneal injection of pentobarbital. This potentized the sleeping time and was attributed to pentobarbital-biotransforming enzymes. However, when myrcene was given 1 day before the barbiturate, the sleeping time was reduced by 50 per cent.[25] Sheppard-Hangar states that *b*-myrcene is found in lemongrass, rosemary (CT camphor and verbenone), clary sage, juniper berry and bay.[26]

Wintergreen and sweet birch are essential oils that are not in common use because they contain high levels of methyl salicylate (closely related to acetylsalicylic acid, or aspirin), and in safety data manuals are marked 'hazardous'.[14,27] However, it is still possible to buy them – they are on sale in health-food shops in the USA and through mail-order firms. Aspirin is known to affect the blood-clotting mechanism. A combination of an aspirin-like substance and warfarin could lead to haemorrhage. Several proprietary brands of creams for arthritis contain similar acetylsalicylic acid-like components.

Essential oils containing *b*-asarone or *d*-pulegone may potentize the toxic effects of a drug, as they both induce the detoxifying enzyme, cytochrome P450. Drugs which induce this enzyme include progestogens (found in the contraceptive pill), diphenhydramine (antihistamine), pethidine, nitrazepam, phenobarbitone and phenytoin, the last four being frequently used hospital drugs.[14] Fortunately, very few essential oils contain *b*-asarone or *d*-pulegone, and few are in regular use. They include wintergreen, cultivated carrot seed and calamus, which contain *b*-asarone, and pennyroyal, cornmint, peppermint, sweetmint and applemint, which contain *d*-pulegone[26] (although peppermint contains less than 1 per cent).[19] Tisserand and Balacs stated that the amounts used in aromatherapy would be insufficient to induce changes in cytochrome P450 activity.[14]

Peppermint was shown to enhance the effect of pentobarbitone in rats in a study published in 1990. Both *Mentha rotundifolia* and *Mentha longifolia* significantly potentized sodium-pentobarbital-induced sleep.[28]

Lavender was also shown to potentiate pentobarbitol-induced sleep in rats, although the effect ceased if treatment lasted for longer than 5 days.[29] Another study also demonstrated the potentizing effect of lavender (*Lavandula angustifolia*), although this may only show that the essential oil was sedative.[30]

In a paper dating back to 1969, several components of essential oils were studied in order to establish whether they affected the metabolism of drugs in rats. The components were eucalyptol (cineol), guaiacol, menthol and essential oil of *Pinus pumilio* (which contained *a*-pinene, phellandrene, dipentene, sylestrene and bornyl acetate). In this study, eucalyptol was shown to increase the activity of the microsomal enzymatic reaction. This altered the metabolism of drugs and appeared to result in increased tolerance of barbiturates.[31]

However, Tisserand and Balacs state that essential oils are used in such small amounts compared to orthodox drugs that, unless they are given orally, they are unlikely to affect the therapeutic action of most orthodox pharmacology.[14]

Specific essential oils or specific components of essential oils and other drugs

Certain essential oils may react with other medication. In some instances they may potentize the effects of orthodox drugs, while in other cases they may interfere at a cellular level, reducing the effect of medication. *Cananga odorata* (ylang ylang) enhances the dermal absorption of 5-fluorouracil (5-FU) sevenfold.[24] *Eucalyptus globulus* enhances the activity of streptomycin, isoniazid and sulfetrone in *Mycobacterium* tuberculosis.[32] Eucalyptol (found in *Eucaplytus smithii*, *E. globulus* and *E. fruticetorum*) produced a significant decrease in pentabarbitol effects, and dose-related effects on the liver enzyme activity of rats could also be measured.[31] The reduction in sedative effect occurred even when the eucalyptus had been administered 36 hours previously.

Chamaemelum nobile (Roman chamomile) was found to be incompatible with the administration of products containing Peruvian bark, tannin or silver salts.[33] These are often present in certain old-fashioned preparations that are still used for pressure area care.

Paracetamol is a commonly used household drug. It reduces the level of glutathione in the liver. Glutathione is responsible for absorbing free radicals, and when the level of glutathione falls, reactive molecules such as free radicals can attack the liver cells, with potentially fatal consequences.

It is extremely unlikely that the small amounts of essential oils used in aromatherapy could adversely affect glutathione production. However, in a patient using the maximum recommended dosage of paracetamol, it might be advisable to avoid essential oils which have a potential for liver toxicity, such as those containing *trans*-anethole, estragole and eugenol.[14] This would mean avoiding the following essential oils: fennel (*Foeniculum vulgare*), coriander (*Coriandrum sativum*) and aniseed (*Pimpinella anisum*).

Terpineol is thought to enhance prednisolone absorption through the skin.[24] Terpineol is found in many essential oils, including niaouli, ravensara, sweet marjoram and geranium.[26]

Limonene is thought to affect indomethacin absorption.[14] Indomethacin is a drug commonly used in arthritis. Limonene is a monoterpene and it occurs in many essential oils.

Cedrus atlantica (cedarwood) was found to reduce the effect of barbiturate-induced sleep.[34] This study also showed that cedarwood reduced the amount of dicoumerol in the blood. Dicoumerol is an anticoagulant that can be obtained from sweet clover.[35] Eugenol has been shown to have anti-platelet activity,[36] and should be avoided in patients receiving anticoagulant therapy. It occurs in clove and cinnamon.

Finally, some patients with particular enzyme deficits or specific conditions may be affected by certain essential oils. Babies of Chinese, West African, Mediterranean and Middle Eastern origin are more likely to have a deficiency of an enzyme called glucose-6-phosphate dehydrogenase (G6PD). This enzyme is responsible for liver detoxification of menthol. When the enzyme is missing, toxic build-up of menthol can occur in the body.[37]

Cardiac patients may be affected by rosemary, which has been shown to interfere with calcium influx into the myocardial cells.[14]

Patients with glaucoma should avoid citral-rich essential oils, although the risk is greater with an oral dose than with a topical or inhaled dose.[38] More information can be found in an essential oil safety manual.

Hormone replacement therapy (HRT) is not thought to be adversely affected by aromatherapy.[14]

ESSENTIAL OILS AND HOMEOPATHY

Although Hippocrates may have been the first to say that 'like cures like', it is accepted that homeopathy dates back to 1810 when Samuel Hahnmann, a German physician, introduced the idea. He had discovered that chinchona bark taken by a healthy person produced the symptoms of malaria. At that time, chinchona bark was administered as a herbal remedy to cure malaria. (It would later be discovered that chinchona bark has an ingredient called quinine which would become a classic drug against malaria.) Hahnmann thought that giving a minute dose of what could have caused symptoms of the disease might stimulate the body to fight and overcome that disease.

He tested this hypothesis on himself and his family, compiling a huge encyclopaedia of knowledge which now forms the foundation of homeopathic literature. The first homeopathic hospital opened its doors to the public in 1850. Apart from 'like cures like', homeopaths consider that the more dilute the dose the more potent it may be. Often the medicines are so dilute that there are no molecules of medicine left in them. This has caused much derision among the medical profession, who feel that leaving the 'curing' of the patient to the 'learned memory of water' is something of a joke. However, rigorous scientific studies are now showing that homeopathy is indeed a valid and useful form of medicine.[39]

There is some controversy concerning the use of essential oils in patients who are receiving homeopathy. The traditional view has always been that they do not mix, and certainly during my training in aromatherapy, I was taught not to mix the two. They are indeed very different therapies. Homeopathic preparations are highly diluted, and essential oils are highly concentrated. In particular, it is thought that peppermint, eucalyptus and thyme and those essential oils which have pungent and strong aromas are best avoided by patients who are using homeopathy.

However, in a paper given at the Aroma '95 conference, Caroline Stevensen, who works on a daily basis with both homeopathy and essential oils, stated that 'I would find it difficult to envisage a clash of effects between homeopathy and aromatherapy'.[40] Certainly as a clinician she would be in a very good position to judge whether aromatherapy adversely affects homeopathy. I consider that it would be sensible to suggest using only the gentle floral aromas such as rose, lavender, geranium and neroli, and the softer herbs, such as Roman chamomile.

CONTRAINDICATIONS

Some essential oils are contraindicated in certain aromatherapy situations, or contraindicated altogether, even though they may be used as food flavourings or in perfumery. The amount used in flavouring is often very tiny. For example, mustard, a well-known flavouring, is contraindicated in aromatherapy as extremely toxic. Tisserand comments on the dose used by the food industry – one-hundredth of a drop of mustard to 50 grams of pickle. It would be impossible to measure one-hundredth of a drop in aromatherapy. However, if just one drop was used (1 per cent), the resulting dilution would be 1000 times higher than that in pickle![41]

There are several safety data manuals available which go into detail as to why some essential oils are contraindicated. Tisserand and Balacs's *Essential Oil Safety* is particularly recommended.[14] If wards are to become involved in the use of essential oils, it is suggested that they have a safety data manual to hand. The most hazardous oils are almost impossible to buy in the UK, although they are on sale in many health-food shops elsewhere in the world, especially in the USA. It is interesting to note that some essential oils, such as croton, savin and wormseed oil, whilst not being common, are illegal unless obtained on prescription.[42]

Some fairly common essential oils are generally contraindicated for all therapeutic uses. These include boldo leaf, calamus, cassia, bitter fennel, mugwort, mustard, dwarf pine, rue, sassafras, tansy, wintergreen and wormwood. All of these essential oils contain toxic constituents (refer to an essential oils safety manual for further information). The essential oils that are contraindicated for topical application include oregano, clove, cinnamon bark, camphor and red thyme. Essential oils that are contraindicated in hypertension include rosemary, spike lavender, hyssop, juniper, thyme and clove. Contraindicated in epilepsy are hyssop, fennel, peppermint, rosemary and thyme (all chemotypes).

Contraindications in oncology

As it is recognized that many malignant growths are oestrogen dependent, the use of essential oils that are either oestrogen-stimulating or oestrogen-like is contraindicated. According to Franchomme, the specific chemical components which are associated with oestrogen stimulation or oestrogen-like properties are sesquiterpenic alcohols such as sclareol and viridiflorol, phenyl methyl ethers such as anethole, and 'certain' ketones which he does not specify. Animal studies suggest the use of citrus peel oils such as bergamot should be avoided in patients who have a history or symptoms of melanoma.[43]

Contraindications in pregnancy

Whilst appreciating that midwifery is a separate field to general nursing, it might be interesting for the reader to know a little about the use of essential oils in this field.

The use of essential oils in pregnancy is a contentious area, especially during the vital first 3-month period. Many aromatherapists will not treat expectant mothers, as we know that essential oils cross the placenta and we do not know what effect they have on the unborn child. Whilst some midwives are happy to use essential oils during labour, to promote contractions, and for their analgesic properties, and some essential oils have been used in water births, it is generally agreed that for the first 24 weeks of pregnancy essential oils should be avoided.[44] Too little is known about how essential oils can affect the unborn child. An extremely good analysis of the situation has been provided by Tiran.[45]

Obviously the advice is the same for pregnant nurses or for health professionals wishing to use aromatherapy to enhance their patient care. There are specific reasons for avoiding certain essential oils during pregnancy. Some of them have an abortifacient tendency, or a possible carcinogenic action, and some have emmenagogic actions which could theoretically induce a miscarriage.[46]

SAFETY AND STORAGE

Safety

Aromatherapy requires knowledge and training. In the wrong hands, essential oils can be hazardous. Just like paracetamol and aspirin, which can be bought over the counter almost anywhere, essential oils should *always* be kept well away from children.

The lethal doses for a 3-year-old child (if taken orally) are as follows:

- basil – 8 ml (2 medicine spoonfuls);
- aniseed – 25 ml (this tastes quite sweet);
- clove – 19 ml (either leaf or stem);
- *Eucalyptus globulus* – 5 ml;
- Hyssop – 19 ml;
- *Mentha longifolia* (German spearmint) – 7 ml;
- *Mentha rotundifolia* (Egyptian) – 10 ml;
- Origano – 21 ml;
- parsley seed oil – 21 ml;
- pennyroyal – 3 ml;
- sage (*officinalis*) – 26 ml;
- savory – 19 ml;
- tansy – 5 ml;
- tarragon – 26 ml;
- thuja – 10 ml;
- wintergreen – 5 ml.

These are samples taken from *Plant Aromatics*[42] which deals with adverse reactions and toxicity in greater detail. However, many other essential oils may be lethal if taken orally in sufficient amounts.

If copious amounts of essential oils have been taken orally, encourage the patient to drink milk, and contact the nearest poisons unit (often listed in the front of a telephone directory). If essential oils get into the eyes, either diluted or not, it is important to irrigate the eyes as rapidly as possible *with milk or carrier oil followed by water*, and to seek medical help. If there is a skin reaction to an essential oil, dilute it with carrier oil and then wash the area with an unperfumed soap.

Storage

Essential oils are highly concentrated, and it is extremely important that they are stored well away from children, the confused, or those unaware of what essential oils are. It takes just 4 ml (less than a teaspoonful) of ingested *Eucalyptus globulus* to produce severe cardiovascular, respiratory and nervous symptoms necessitating emergency peritoneal dialysis, haemodialysis and mannitol infusion.[47]

Keeping concentrated essential oils on a ward is a potential hazard, and they should be stored in a locked container at all times. One possible solution could be to dilute a small selection of essential oils in a carrier base and only have 2 to 5 per cent solutions available. However, this would only be practicable if several patients were likely to require the same mix. Once diluted, essential oils lose their potency quite quickly. However, if stored under optimum conditions, undiluted essential oils can keep for several years.

To store essential oils under optimum conditions, they should be kept in coloured (blue or amber) glass bottles to protect them from ultraviolet light. The bottles should be tightly stoppered and have an integral dropper contained in the lid to prevent spillage. All bottles should be stored away from heat and sunlight (ideally in a refrigerator). (In a ward situation, this would be similar to the storage of heparin.)

All bottles should carry a firmly attached label, stating the botanical name, the supplier's name and the batch number. Most reputable companies also include a label warning that the oils should be kept away from the eyes, out of reach of children, and not be taken by mouth. Some also have a note printed on them that they are of medicinal strength. It would be useful to keep a register listing when each essential oil was purchased, the supplier's name and the price. A separate list could be kept of patients names, the name of their consultant, the dates when they received aromatherapy and any therapeutic (or adverse) results. In this way a portfolio on the use of essential oils in hospitals could be maintained, and ultimately a database could be developed.

Essential oils are highly flammable, so they *must* be stored away from naked flames such as candles, fires, matches, cigarettes and gas cookers. Sprinkling them on top of light bulbs can be dangerous.

Warning
Just a small amount of certain essential oils can seriously impair electrical components, including those of a computer keyboard.

ESSENTIAL OILS AS MEDICINES

Medicines Control Agency

In a written response to a personal letter, Dr Linda Anderson of the Medicines Control Agency wrote that 'As a rule we would not normally consider an aromatherapy product to be licensable where it was used for a cosmetic purpose and did not have any medical claims associated with it'. In situations where aromatherapy practitioners use essential oils for therapeutic purposes on individual patients, such products would be considered to be 'medicinal products'. However, these products are exempt from the requirement to hold a manufacturer's or product licence under Section 12(1) of the Medicines Act 1968, provided that they fulfil the criteria laid down in that section:

(a) that the remedy is manufactured or assembled on premises of which the person carrying on the business is the occupier and which he is able to close so as to exclude the public;

(b) that the person carrying on the business sells or supplies the remedy for administration to a particular person after being requested by or on behalf of that person and in that person's presence to use his own judgement as to the treatment required.

Essential oils used by aromatherapy practitioners as described in paragraph (b) above would be considered to be 'herbal remedies'. In the USA herbal remedies are classified as dietary supplements.

If nurses are using aromatherapy as part of their nursing care, are those aromatherapy mixtures the same as herbal remedies? Are they medicines? Consider lavender. If it is used to promote relaxation, it is not a medicine. If lavender is used to give pleasure, it is not a medicine. If it is given to enhance sleep, it is not a medicine. If it is used to help skin heal following burns, it might be seen to have medicinal properties. If it is used for its antibiotic effects, it could be seen to be a medicine. But what would the answer be if lavender was used for all of the above? Can lavender be a medicine one moment and not a medicine the next? It must be understood that essential oils are pharmacologically active substances and therefore have a physiodynamic effect which can range from an increase in parasympathetic response to an antibiotic action.

Synthetic antibiotics do not smell pleasant, give pleasure or enhance sleep – they are simply antibiotics. However, most essential oils have numerous properties which can have advantageous effects on patients, and these various effects can happen simultaneously. What makes a medicine a medicine? The dictionary defines the subject of medicine as the 'art of restoring and preserving health, especially by means of remedial substances and regulation of diet'. The word 'medicinal' is defined as something having 'healing properties'. Does this mean, now that prayer has been shown to have healing properties, that only doctors can pray? Does it mean that when a rotation diet works, it is medicine, and therefore should be prescribed? Do essential oils need a prescription? Despite the fact that essential oils are not covered by the Medicines Act, they are pharmacologically active substances.

Perhaps the words 'medicine' and 'medicinal' need to be redefined. The same dictionary defines nursing as 'to wait upon and try to cure sickness'. However, the very word 'cure' seems to cry out 'medicine'. Where is the boundary? Where does aromatherapy in nursing lie? I think that the answer lies in the intention of the giver. If nurses want to enhance their nursing care, that is clinical aromatherapy which needs training and regulation but, I would argue, not prescription. If doctors want to treat an infection using an essential oil as an antibiotic, and that essential oil is given orally, that would be perceived to be medicine – aromatic medicine which would need to be prescribed for a nurse to administer it. I feel that there are clear boundaries. I cannot envisage a scenario in which a doctor would prescribe lavender, but I can envisage a scenario in which a doctor could prescribe tea tree, even though both can be purchased over the counter by the public.

Aromatherapy and the DDAs and Poison Act

Carol Horrigan, who was instrumental in devising the aromatherapy component of the BSc Nursing course at the Royal College of Nursing, states that aromatherapy does not need a prescription. She gives the reasons for this as being 'because the oils are not standardised and, if used correctly, are non-toxic'.[48] She is right on both counts. However, with research concentrating on the therapeutic effects of essential oils, and a growing body of published work demonstrating antibacterial, antifungal, antiseptic and a whole host of other medicinal properties, it is arguable that nurses might actually lose their ability to use essential oils because of the therapeutic effects of those oils, whether they were standardized or used correctly.

There is a scenario in which aromatherapy could be limited to prescription only. This could pose awkward problems for the perfume and cosmetics industry. If essential oils were to be designated as medicinal, they would have to comply with the legislation which controls the administration of drugs. They would need to be controlled either as a poison or as a drug (it is unlikely that they would be classified with opiate drugs). Essential oils would therefore need to be kept in a locked cupboard in the treatment room of a hospital ward. This would mean that they could not be used except by boarded prescription, and a record of their administration would need to be signed and countersigned by a registered nurse.

Following written prescription by a doctor, the label of the essential oil would need to be checked by both signatories (one of whom would have to be a registered general nurse). The number of drops of each of the essential oils would then be counted out by both nursing staff, who would next go to the patient and check his or her name (with the patient and on the wristband). They would then both witness the application before signing in the book that the treatment had been given.[49] The keys to the essential oil cupboard would need to be attached to the person in charge of the unit.

All substances intended for medicinal use must conform to certain standards as specified in the *British Pharmacopoeia (BP)* or the *British Pharmaceutical Codex (BPC)*.[48] For essential oils and aromatherapy to come under exactly the same control as drugs might be perceived as an unfortunate fate for this branch of complementary therapies. Under present regulation, this would mean that essential oils would need to be 'standardized' or, in other words, rectified. This does not need to happen. By establishing an acceptable range of components within an essential oil, rectification would not be necessary. Herbal medicines are not 'standardized'.

Although essential oils have been used for thousands of years, there appear to be very few cases of sensitivity, allergy or fatality *when they are used within established guidelines*. Lovell suggests that the family Labiatae (which contains many aromatic plants used in perfumery, cooking and medicine) could produce allergic contact dermatitis.[50] He cites Canlan, who recorded six positive reactions to lavender oil patch tests in 1147 patients. The incidence of adverse reactions to essential oils during established use would appear to be lower on a percentage basis than the incidence of adverse reactions to synthetic drugs. Not only do the reactions appear to be less frequent, but also they are less severe.

REFERENCES

1. **Rademaker, M. and Kirby, J.D.T.** 1987: Contact dermatitis to a skin adhesive. *Contact Dermatitis* **6**, 297–8.

2. **Lesesne, C.B.** 1992: The postoperative use of wound adhesives. Gum mastic versus benzoin, USP. *Journal of Dermatology and Surgical Oncology* **18**, 990–91.

3. **Cainan, C.D.** 1976: Cinnamon dermatitis from an ointment. *Contact Dermatitis* **2**, 167–70.

4. **De Groot, A.C. and Weyland, J.W.** 1992: Systemic contact dermatitis from tea tree oil. *Contact Dermatitis* **27**, 279–80.

5. **Parys, BT.** 1983: Chemical burns resulting from contact with peppermint oil: a case report. *Burns Including Thermal Injury (Bristol)* **9**, 374–5.

6. **Roethe, A., Heine, A. and Rebohie, E.** 1973: Oils from juniper berries as an occupational allergen for the skin and the respiratory tract. *Berufsdermatosen* **21**, 11–16.

7. **Van Ketel, W.G.** 1982: Allergy to *Matricaria chamomilia*. *Contact Dermatitis* **8**, 143.

8. **Van Ketel, W.G.** 1987: Allergy to *Matricaria chamomilia*. *Contact Dermatitis* **16**, 50–1.

9. **Brandao, F.M.** 1986: Occupational allergy to lavender oil. *Contact Dermatitis* **15**, 249–50.

10. **Bisland, D. and Strong, A.** 1990: Allergic contact dermatitis from the essential oil of French marigold (*Tagetes patula*) in an aromatherapist. *Contact Dermatitis* **23**, 55–6.

11. **Watts, M.** 1991: *Plant aromatics*. Witham: Watts.

12. **Naganuma, M., Hirose, S., Nakayama, K. and Someya, T.** 1985: A study of the phototoxicity of lemon oil. *Archives of Dermatological Research (Berlin)* **278**, 311–6.

13. **Meyer, J.** 1970: Accidents due to tanning cosmetics with a base of bergamot oil. *Societé Francaise de Dermatologie et de Syphiligraphie* **77**, 881–4.

14. **Tisserand, R. and Balacs, T.** 1995: *Essential oil safety*. London: Churchill Livingstone.

15. **Blaschke, T.F. and Bjornsson, T.D.** 1995: Pharmacokinetics and pharmacoepidemiology. *Scientific American* **8**, 1–14.

16. **Hansten, P.D. and Horn, J.R.** 1989: *Drug interactions: clinical significance of drug–drug interactions*, 6th edn. New York: Lea and Febiger.

17. **Gwilt, R.P.R.** 1994: Pharmacokinetics. In Craig, C. and Stitzel, R.E. (eds), *Modern pharmacology*. Boston, MA: Little, Brown & Co., 55–64.

18. **Grant, T.S.** 1994: Metabolism of drugs. In Craig, C. and Stitzel, R.E. (eds), *Modern pharmacology*. Boston, MA: Little, Brown & Co., 33–46.

19. **Price, S.** 1995: *Aromatherapy for health professionals.* London: Churchill Livingstone.

20. **Berndt, W.I. and Stitzel, R.** 1994: Excretion of drugs. In Craig, C. and Stitzel, R.E. (eds), *Modern pharmacology.* Boston, MA: Little, Brown & Co., 47–53.

21. **Fleming, W.W.** 1994: Mechanisms of drug action. In Craig, C. and Stitzel, R.E. (eds), *Modern pharmacology.* Boston, MA: Little, Brown & Co., 9–18.

22. **Albert-Puleo, M.** 1980: Fennel and anise as estrogenic agents. *Journal of Ethnopharmacology* **2**, 337–44.

23. **Murad, F. and Kuret, J.A.** 1990: Estrogens and progestins. In *Goodman and Gilson's pharmacological basis of therapeutics,* 8th edn. 1384–6.

24. **Williams, A.C. and Barry, B.A.** 1989: Essential oils as novel human skin penetration enhancers. *Journal of Pharmaceutics,* **57**, R7–R9.

25. **Freitas, J.C., Presgrave, O.A.F.** *et al.* 1993: Effect of *b*-myrcene on pentobarbitol sleeping time. *Brazilian Journal of Medical and Biological Research* **26**, 519–23.

26. **Sheppard-Hangar, S.** 1995: *The aromatherapy practitioner's reference manual. Volume II.* Tampa, FL: Atlantic School of Aromatherapy.

27. **International School of Aromatherapy.** 1993: *A safety guide for the use of essential oils.* London: Nature by Nature Oils.

28. **Perez Raya, M.D., Utrilla, M.C. and Jimenez, J.** 1990: CNS activity of *Mentha rotundifolia* and *Mentha longifolia* essential oil in mice and rats. *Phytotherapy Research* **4**, 232–4.

29. **Delaveau, P., Guillemain, J., Marcisse, G. and Rousseau, A.** 1989: Neuro-depressive properties of essential oil of lavender (French). *Comptes Rendus des Séances de la Societié de Biologie et de ses Filiales* **183**, 342–8.

30. **Guillemain, J., Rousseau, R. and Delaveau, P.** 1989: Neurodepressive effects of the essential oil of *Lavandula angustifolia. Annales Pharmaceutiques Francais* **47**, 337–42.

31. **Jori, A., Bianchetti, A. and Prestinit, P.E.** 1969: Effect of essential oils on drug metabolism. *Biochemical Pharmacology* **18**, 12081–5.

32. **Kufferath, F., Mundualgo, G.M.** 1954: The activity of some preparations containing essential oils in TB. *Fitoterapia* **25**, 483–5.

33. **Chieji, R.** 1984: *The Macdonald encyclopedia of medicinal plants.* London: Macdonald.

34. **Wade, A.E.** *et al.* 1968: Alteration of drug metabolism in rats and mice by an environment of cedarwood. *Pharmacology* **1**, 317–28.

35. **Budavari, S.** (ed.) *Merck index.* 12th edn. Whitehouse Station, NJ: Merck & Co. Inc.

36. **Janssens, J., Laekeman, G.M., Pleters, L.A.** *et al.* 1990: Nutmeg oil: identification and quantification of its most active constituents as inhibitors of platelet aggregations. *Journal of Ethnopharmacology* **29**, 179–88.

37. **Owole, S.A. and Ramson-Kuto, O.** 1980: The risk of jaundice in glucose-6-phosphate dehydrogenase deficient babies exposed to menthol. *Acta Paediatrica Scandinavica* **69**, 341–5.

38. **Leach, E.H. and Lloyd, J.P.F.** 1956: Experimental ocular hypertension in animals. *Transactions of the Ophthalmological Societies of the UK* **76**, 453–60.

39. **Kleijinen, J., Knipschild, P.** *et al.* 1991: Clinical trials of homeopathy. *British Medical Journal* **301**, 316–32.

40. **Stevenson, C.** 1995: Aromatherapy and homeopathy – working together. In *Aroma 95: One Body – One Mind. Conference proceedings.* Hove: Aromatherapy Publications: 146–51.

41. **Tisserand, R.** 1988: *The essential oil safety data manual.* Brighton: Tisserand.

42. **Watts, M.** 1991: *Plant aromatics.* Witham: Watts.

43. **Elegbede, J.A., Maltzman, T.H., Verma, A.K., Tanner, M.A., Elson, C.E. and Gould, M.N.** 1986: Mouse skin tumour promoting activity of orange peel oil and di-limonene: a re-evaluation. *Carcinogenesis* **7**, 2047–9.

44. **Mason, M.** 1996: Aromatherapy and midwifery. *Aromatherapy quarterly* spring issue, 32–4.

45. **Tiran, D.** 1996: Aromatherapy in midwifery: benefits and risks. *Complementary Therapies in Nursing and Midwifery* **2**, 88–93.

46. **Balacs, T.** 1992: Safety in pregnancy. *International Journal of Aromatherapy* **4**, 12–15.

47. **Gurr, F.W. and Scroggie, J.G.** 1965: Eucalyptus oil poisoning treated by dialysis and mannitol infusion, with an appendix on the analysis of biological fluids for alcohol and eucalyptol. *Australasian Annals of Medicine.* **14**, 238–49.

48. **Horrigan, C.** 1993: Aromatherapy in patient care. In *Aroma 93. Conference proceedings.* Hove: Aromatherapy Publications, 130–35.

49. **Hector, W.** 1960: *Modern nursing.* London: Heinemann.

50. **Lovell, C.** 1993: *Plants and the skin.* Oxford: Blackwell Scientific Publications.

6

REGULATIONS AND HEALTH AND SAFETY POLICIES

Since I began writing this book in the spring of 1995, two important legislative documents have come into the public domain: The Control of Substances Hazardous to Health Regulations 1994 (COSHH) and The Chemical (Hazard Information and Packaging for Supply) Regulations 1994 (CHIP). Both will greatly benefit clinical aromatherapy in nursing because nurses will have to take aromatherapy much more seriously. Safe practice using essential oils will now mean risk assessment. This involves obtaining (or producing) safety data sheets on every essential oil to be used in nursing. It will mean identifying any hazards involved in the use of essential oils, not just to patients but also to colleagues and to nurses themselves. It will also mean creating and maintaining health and safety protocols for hospital staff to follow.

COSHH

This document is concerned with safety and risk management of potentially hazardous substances in the workplace. According to CHIP Regulations 1994, hazardous substances include essential oils, as they are all flammable, and some can be skin irritants or sensitizing. The object of COSHH in aromatherapy is to assess and evaluate risk, thereby reducing the possibility of harm for those using essential oils either directly or indirectly. Risk and safety phrases to be used are listed in the document. By standardizing them in this way, anyone looking at a COSHH document on an essential oil will immediately be able to recognize its potential risk. Although not a legal requirement, COSHH will enable nurses and hospital managers to make an informed judgement about the safety of each essential oil in a clinical setting. This will demonstrate that the nurse is trying to address the guidelines laid down by COSHH, which can only indicate how seriously she takes aromatherapy and the safe use of essential oils.

COSHH assessment means that nurses can demonstrate they are aware of the potential hazards and risks involved in clinical aromatherapy by using the language laid down in the document. To be acceptable to COSHH, this assessment must be carried out *every time a nurse uses an essential oil*. Essential oils which are defined as dangerous, i.e. corrosive, irritant or toxic, will be clearly identified. The nurse will know the maximum exposure limit (MEL) and the occupational exposure limit (OEL) of any given essential oil, as this information is detailed in the Health and Safety Executive guidelines on occupational exposure limits (EH40).[1]

By quoting the maximum exposure limit, nurses will be able to demonstrate a knowledge of the toxicity of an essential oil. Toxicity is measured by the oral dose needed to kill 50 per cent of experimental animals (LD_{50}). It is expressed in milligrams per kilogram of body weight (mg/kg). The dose needed to kill 50 per cent of experimental animals when taken other than orally is the lethal concentration (LC_{50}).

Extremely toxic	I mg or less
Highly toxic	I–50 mg
Moderately toxic	50–500 mg
Slightly toxic	0.5–5 g
Virtually non-toxic	5–15 g
Relatively harmless	15 g or less

COSHH classifies essential oils more simply, merely giving them a T (for toxic) hazard sign. An essential oil classified in this way will also have specific risk phrases such as 'toxic if inhaled, toxic if swallowed, toxic if in contact with the skin', or 'harmful if inhaled, harmful if swallowed, harmful if in contact with the skin', and specific safety phrases.

Lists of essential oil classifications/guidelines are available from CHIPS. These grade essential oils giving them hazard symbols and acceptable risk (R) and safety (S) phrases to use. Some essential oils, such as cedarwood, clary sage and geranium, have no hazard symbol or R and S number. Some, like grapefruit and lemongrass, have no hazard symbol and no safety phrase, but carry a risk phrase such as R10 (which means flammable) or R38 (which means irritating to the skin).[2] It is curious that not all essential oils are thought to be flammable, although some do have a higher flash point (risk of igniting).

Some essential oils, such as hyssop, carry a combined safety phrase (S24/25) which means 'avoid contact with skin and eyes'.[3] Keeping essential oils away from the eyes is the standard recommended safety procedure for anyone using aromatherapy. CHIPS recommends that undiluted hyssop be kept out of contact with the skin. Hyssop is classified as causing no irritation or sensitization at 4 per cent dilutions in humans.[4]

Myrrh, which is thought to be non-irritant to the skin and only mildly toxic when taken orally,[5] is listed by CHIP as a *category 3 carcinogen* and given the hazard symbol Xn, although reading through the risk category, myrrh is rated R22 (harmful if swallowed) and given the safety phrase S24/25 (keep away from eyes and skin). Thus it is difficult to assess whether the supposed carcinogen risk is from swallowing the essential oil or applying it to the skin. Price states that the lethal dose required to kill a 70-kg adult is 389 ml of myrrh.[6] Two ketones, isopinocamphone and pinocamphone, are thought to be responsible for the toxicity.[7]

Another point that is of interest to nurses using aromatherapy is safety phrase S26: 'In case of contact with eyes, rinse immediately with plenty of water and seek medical advice.' As essential oils are non-soluble in water, this safety phrase should really read: 'In case of contact with eyes, rinse immediately with plenty of *milk or carrier oil*, and then with water, and seek medical advice.'

An example of a possible COSHH document follows (Figure 6.1). Obviously computerization linked to a database on the hazardous components of essential oils would make the whole procedure much easier. A nurse would be able to key in tea tree, for example, and a COSHH safety form relevant to tea tree, listing LD_{50}, toxicity, hazard, risk and safety factor information, would immediately be printed out. Work has begun on documents linked to a database for potential use in hospitals.

CHIP

CHIP 1994 is a large document (427 pages, with its own integral package of three floppy discs) and it contains all of the information required for a supplier to understand the requirements of the Chemicals (Hazard Information and Packing for Supply) Regulations. It should be emphasized that the data required by CHIP is for the *supply and storage* of hazardous chemicals. The document is divided into seven parts, each supplied with a blue interface, and the whole document is designed to fit into a ring-binder. CHIPs is intended for the essential oil supplier. The document is arranged in the following order.

Part I   – Alphabetical listing of substances
Part II   – Mixtures of named substances or mixtures/specific isomers
Part III – Risk phrases
Part IV – Safety phrases
Part V   – Classification and labelling information
Part VI – Information for classification on pesticides
Part VII – Additional information for complex coal- and oil-derived substances

COSHH SAFETY FORM FOR ESSENTIAL OILS

Nurse's name	**Patient's name**	**Date**	**Time**
Florence Nightingale	John Doe	11/11/96	3p.m.

Essential oil
Melaleuca alternifolia CT terpineol

Number of drops
1–5

Known hazards	**Risks**
Xn: Cat 3 carcinogen	R10/22/38
LD_{50} = 190 mg/kg	Flammable, harmful if swallowed, irritating to the skin

Safety	**Other safety data**
S24/25	No sensitization[8]
Avoid contact with skin and eyes	No phototoxicity[8]
	Very mildly irritant[5] (depends on cineole level)

Emergency treatment
If swallowed, drink milk and
seek medical advice.
If in eye, irrigate with milk followed
by water, then seek medical advice

Application method	**Contraindications**	**Precautions**
Topical, inhalation	In a hot bath can cause prickly heat	Do not use undiluted on broken skin, causes intense stinging

Other information
Can be used neat on insect bites/stings/spots
Can be used in gargle and mouthwash (1–2 drops)
Can be used vaginally diluted in carrier oil
Insoluble in water: dissolve in alcohol/milk

Ensure correct chemotype = low cineole. Cineole can be a skin irritant[6]

FIGURE 6.1 Example of a possible COSHH safety document for essential oils.

So complicated is the document that a free guide entitled *Understanding CHIP 2* comes with it.

The safety data sheet which identifies hazards of particular essential oils is intended to warn people purchasing them of any risk factors and, according to COSHH 'it is incumbent on the person responsible for supplying the substance or preparation to supply information specified under these headings.'[9] Therefore we should be able to ask for a safety data sheet on every oil that we purchase. However, few distributors appear to be complying with these regulations (listed below) so far.

1 Identification of the substance/preparation and company
2 Composition/information on ingredients
3 Hazards identification
4 First aid measures
5 Firefighting measures
6 Accidental releases measures
7 Handling and storage
8 Exposure controls/personal protection
9 Physical and chemical properties
10 Stability and reactivity
11 Toxicological information
12 Ecological information
13 Disposal considerations
14 Transport information
15 Regulatory information
16 Other information

Most important for aromatherapy is the product identification. This needs to include the plant material, physical constants, registrations (usually in the form of numbers) and safety and toxicity considerations such as the flashpoint (the temperature at which an essential oil will ignite). The information should be available from the essential oil dealer, but if it is not, it is the responsibility of the nurse to formulate this document.

Below are listed some of the organizations governing registration numbers which may be named on a CHIP document.

CAS	Chemical Abstracts Service
EINECS	European Inventory of Existing Chemical Substances
FEMA	Flavour and Extracts Manufacturers Association
GRAS	Generally Recognized as Safe
IFRA	International Fragrance Association
REFM	Research Institute for Fragrance Materials
CTFA	Cosmetic Toiletry and Fragrance Association
INCI	International Nomenclature of Cosmetic Ingredients
EFFA	European Flavour and Fragrance Association
IOFI	International Organization of the Flavour Industry

FDA	Food and Drug Administration
DPD	Dangerous Preparations Directive
AIS	Association Internationale de la Savonnerie et de la Detergence
USES	Uniform System for the Evaluation of Substances

Taking tea tree as an example, a material data sheet should look similar to that shown in Figure 6.2.

SAMPLE MATERIAL DATA SHEET

Product identification

Name	Tea tree
Botanical name	*Melaleuca alternifolia*
Chemotype	Terpineol
Fema number	
CAS number	68647-73-4
Extraction	Steam distillation of the leaves

Specification

Odour	Fresh, eucalyptus type, herbaceous, antiseptic
Origin	Australia
Appearance	Clear to faintly yellow

Analytical data

(1) Physical constants	Specific gravity: 0.895–0.905 g
	Optical rotation: @ 20°C + 6.5–+9.5
	Refractive index: @ 20°C 1.476 to 1.481
	Solubility: 1 vol of oil in 0.75 vol of 85% ethanol
(2) Chemical composition	See GLC

Toxicity

Low cineole content > 6% (as used for medicinal and dental purposes) reported to be non-irritant. LD_{50} = 400 mg (moderately toxic)

Flash point

57–61°C

Legislation

FIGURE 6.2 Example of a material data sheet for tea tree oil.

This meets IFRA and RIFM guidelines. Some essential oils have many more regulatory numbers. For example mandarin (*Citrus reticulata blanco*) has the following:

REFM   250
FEMA   2657 (GRAS)
FDA   182.20
CAS   8008-31-9

Risk phrases (which are listed in the CHIP guidelines) give an indication as to how flammable an essential oil may be, if it is harmful when swallowed, if there is a risk of eye damage, if it may cause birth defects, etc. Safety phrases provide an indication of how to store the oil and dispose of it, and what it will mix with. Both phrases are expressed as numbers. Mandarin has risk phrases number R10 and safety phrase number S3.

Some essential oils are not on the CHIP list. Ravensara is one such example. When an essential oil is not listed, it should in theory be possible to evaluate the risk and safety issues from the chemical components within the essential oil. Ravensara contains compounds such as 1,8-cineole, alpha-pinene, etc. The International Organization of the Flavour Industry (IOFI) sent out a letter in 1994 informing all those involved in the essential oils trade about the new European Union (EU) regulations regarding labelling of dangerous substances. Now all labels used by member states within the European Union must conform to set standards. The regulations list classifications of chemicals, many of which are found in essential oils. Cineole and alpha-pinene are not listed. Thus for a nurse to be able to write a health and safety policy or a COSHH-acceptable safety document, she will need to consult with a phytochemical database or a reference book such as *Essential Oil Safety*.[5]

For a hospital to be confident that a nurse has thought through the whole process of using aromatherapy in a clinical setting, a health and safety policy is essential. This should be checked through with the hospital Health and Safety Officer, and amended where necessary. A sample policy is provided below.

SAMPLE HEALTH AND SAFETY POLICY

Accident procedures

- Problem – essential oil in the eye.
- Answer – irrigate the eye with milk or carrier oil, and then with water. Seek medical assistance. Keep the bottle to show which essential oil was being used.

- Problem – dermal irritant essential oil (undiluted) spilt on the skin.
- Answer – dilute with carrier oil, then wash the area with unperfumed soap and water and dry it. Seek medical assistance.

- Problem – more than 5 ml of essential oil taken by mouth.
- Answer – give milk to drink, keep the bottle and seek medical assistance. Essential oils when taken in amounts greater than 5 ml by mouth should be treated as poisons.

- Problem – bottle dropped and broken, and essential oil and glass on floor.
- Answer – use a paper towel to soak up the liquid and collect the glass. Put the mixture in more paper, and dispose of it in a secured polythene bag.

General safety

Storage

All essential oils should be stored as follows:

- locked up;
- out of reach of children;
- in a cool place;
- in tightly closed containers;
- away from food, drink or animal feed stuff;
- away from heat;
- away from naked flames.

Labelling

All bottles containing essential oils should be clearly marked with:

- labels that are indelible and stay on;
- the full botanical name;
- relevant safety phrases;
- the quantity of oil;
- the company name and address.

Packaging

All essential oils should be packaged as follows:

- in coloured glass bottles;
- with an integral dropper of UK standard (20 drops per ml).

Procedures

- Essential oils should only be used in a clinical setting by a member of staff or outside contractor who is qualified in aromatherapy and has permission to use them (see protocol).
- Whenever possible, essential oils should be used in enclosed areas to prevent the aromas from spreading.
- All essential oils used in nursing should be documented within the patient care plan.
- The positive and negative effects of essential oils should be evaluated and noted in the care plan.
- Only a 1 to 5 per cent dilution should be used, except in specific situations as recommended by safety guides.
- Essential oils that carry a high risk should be avoided. They are listed in safety guides. A suggested list of safe oils can be found at the end of this chapter.

Clothing

Essential oils leave stains, and therefore an apron or special clothing should be worn.

Disposal

Essential oils are highly flammable and carry intense aromas. They should be disposed of in a sealed polythene bag.

In addition, every hospital will need an essential oils protocol which must be followed by all nurses using aromatherapy.

SAMPLE HOSPITAL PROTOCOL

Before essential oils can be used in a clinical setting, all individuals involved (including domestic staff and visitors) need to be informed as to what aromatherapy is, what essential oils will be used, how they will be used, and their possible positive and negative effects.

(a) Consent will be needed from:
    (i)   the patient (written);
    (ii)   the patient's hospital consultant;
    (iii) support nursing staff and hospital administration.

(b) Qualification
    (i)   Nurses wishing to use essential oils to enhance nursing care need to have completed a recognizable course and be able to show that they are competent and accountable.

(ii) Documentation of each nurse's training, stating hours and place of study, should be kept on the ward.

(iii) Nurses should be aware of the potential hazards, risks and safety classifications of the essential oils that they wish to use as laid down by COSHH, as well as the potential side-effects, contraindications and possible effects on orthodox medication.

(c) Guide books

(i) A safety guide should be available.

(ii) At least one reference book should be kept on the ward.

(d) Legislation

(i) COSHH assessment should be documented for each treatment.

(e) Methods of application

Essential oils (1 to 5 drops) can be applied

(i) topically:
- by massage to the skin, diluted in a vegetable carrier oil, a cream or a lotion;
- by compress, diluted in warm water;
- by bath (hand, foot, sitz or full bath). Essential oils should be dissolved in a small amount of milk or rubbing alcohol in order to avoid possible corneal damage during splashing.

(ii) by inhalation:
- directly (over a bowl of hot water);
- indirectly with a nebulizer or vaporizer. Electrical equipment must meet the requirements of the Health and Safety at Work Act 1974 (i.e. burners with candles or ceramic rings for light bulbs cannot be used).

(f) Documentation

The full botanical name of the essential oil(s), the number of drops, method of use, time of day, reason for treatment, and positive or negative effects should be recorded in the nursing care plan.

(g) Storage

(i) Essential oils should be stored in a locked container in a cool place, preferably the ward refrigerator.

(ii) The keys to the container should be kept only by nurses trained in aromatherapy .

(h) Patch testing

All patients who have given their consent to receive aromatherapy treatment should be patch-tested for sensitivity.

(i) Apply essential oil at a 5 per cent dilution to the inner elbow or inside of the wrist. Cover the area with a Band-Aid. Remove the plaster after 12 hours. Repeat at a different site for a further 12 hours.

(i) Length of treatment
   (i)   Individual treatments should not last longer than 1 hour.
   (ii) Daily treatment should not continue for more than 3 weeks.

(j) Essential oil supply
   (i)   Essential oils should be obtained from a supplier with a CHIP data sheet.
   (ii) Gas-liquid chromatograms should be available.

(k) Continuing treatment
   (i)   Bottles containing essential oils/carrier oil blends must be labelled with:
      ■ the name of the patient;
      ■ the number of the patient;
      ■ the full botanical name of the essential oil(s) and the carrier oil;
      ■ the number of drops;
      ■ the date.
   (ii) A record sheet should be kept with the bottle, and completed after each treatment.

COSHH and CHIP have given us the baselines to enable us to use safe practice and to be seen to do so. It is in our interest and that of our patients to ensure that aromatherapy is seen to be not only efficacious but also safe.

RECOMMENDED ESSENTIAL OILS FOR USE IN A CLINICAL SETTING

Angelica archangelica (root)	Angelica
Boswellia carterii	Frankincense
Cananga odorata	Ylang ylang
Chamaemelum nobile	Roman chamomile
Citrus bergamia	Bergamot
Citrus reticulata	Mandarin
Citrus aurantium var. *amara flos*	Neroli
Citrus aurantium var. *amara fol*	Petitgrain
Commiphora myrrha	Myrrh
Cupressus sempervirens	Cypress
Cymbopogon martini var. *motia*	Palma rosa
Cymbopogon citratus	Lemongrass
Eucalyptus globulus	Blue gum

Eucalytpus smithi	Gully gum
Eucalyptus citriodora	Lemon gum
Foeniculum vulgare	Fennel
Helichrysum italicum	Everlasting flower
Juniperus communis	Juniper
Lavandula officinalis	True lavender
Lavandula latifolia	Spike lavender
Lavandula hybrida CT grosso	Lavendin
Matricaria recutita	German chamomile
Melaleuca alternifolia CT terpineol	Tea tree
Melissa officinalis	Melissa
Mentha piperita	Peppermint
Ocimum basilicum (European)	Basil
Origanum majorana	Marjoram
Pelargonium graveolens	Geranium
Piper nigrum	Black pepper
Rosa damascena	Rose
Rosmarinus officinalis CT cineole	Rosemary
Salvia sclarea	Clary sage
Santalum album	Sandalwood
Zingiber officinale	Ginger

REFERENCES

1. **Health and Safety Executive.** 1995: *The Health and Safety Executive Guidance Note (EH40). Occupational exposure limits.* Sheffield: Health and Safety Executive Books.

2. **Health and Safety Commission.** 1994: *CHIP Part III. Risk phrases.* Sheffield: Health and Safety Executive Books.

3. **Health and Safety Commission.** 1994: *CHIP Part IV. Safety phrases.* Sheffield: Health and Safety Executive Books.

4. **Opdyke, D.L.J.** 1978: Monographs on fragrance raw materials. *Food and Cosmetics Toxicology* **16**, 783–4.

5. **Tisserand, R. and Balacs, T.** 1995: *Essential oil safety.* London: Churchill Livingstone.

6. **Price, S.** 1995: *Aromatherapy for health professionals.* London: Churchill Livingstone.

7. **International School of Aromatherapy.** 1993: *A safety guide on the use of essential oils.* London: Nature by Nature Oils Ltd.

8. **Ford, R.A.** *et al.* 1988: Tea tree oil. *Food and Chemical Toxicology* **26**, 407.

9. **Health and Safety Commission.** 1994: *Safety data sheets for substances and preparations dangerous for supply.* Sheffield: Health and Safety Executive Books.

Part 2

Clinical use of aromatherapy

7

GENERAL HOSPITAL CARE

Hospital-acquired infections (HAI)

Infection, or rather infectious disease, was until recently the most common cause of death.[1] Despite an increase in the standard of living conditions among the technically advanced and so-called 'civilized' countries of the world, infections such as the common cold and upper respiratory tract infections (RTI) are major causes of working days lost. The incidence of diphtheria may have decreased, but viral infections are on the increase. Tuberculosis (TB) is also on the rise again, as are infections acquired as a result of being a patient in a hospital.[2]

Infection is caused by organisms such as bacteria, viruses, fungi, protozoa and parasites. Gascoigne[3] suggests that these organisms can be spread in the following ways:

- by droplet infection, e.g. sneezing, coughing;
- by implantation, e.g. wound infections, *Streptococcus* and *Staphylococcus* skin infections;
- by direct contact, e.g. scabies and sexually transmitted diseases;
- by food or water contamination;
- by injection by either man or insect, e.g. HIV virus, hepatitis, yellow fever and malaria.

Being a hospital patient brings with it the threat of infection. Every year almost two million American patients acquire an infection in a hospital. Of these, 80 000 patients die.[4] The situation is similar in the UK. The common forms of hospital-acquired infections (HAI) are *Campylobacter enteritis*, *Pseudomonas aeruginosa* and methicillin-resistant *Staphylococcus aureus*. Hospital-acquired infections, or nosocomial infections, can be gained in one of two ways:

- from an outside source, such as poor hygiene standards of staff, equipment, or even visitors;
- as a result of self-infection.

Meers' study showed that 9.2 per cent of all hospital patients had a hospital-acquired infection.[5] Of these patients, 30 per cent suffered from urinary tract infections, 20 per cent from chest infections and 20 per cent from wound infections (see Figure 7.1).

The implications of HAI are widespread. In the current climate of hospital trusts, each day needs carefully budgeting. Bed occupancy due to HAI affects the turnover of a hospital, and therefore influences its budget. A report by the Hospital Infections Working Group (1988) estimated that some 950 000 bed days were lost each year in the UK, causing a staggering monetary loss of £111 million per year.[6]

In England, 44 per cent of hospital patients who are (urinary) catheterized for more than 48 hours, develop bacteriuria. Between 1 and 3 per cent of these patients also develop septicaemia. It is estimated that 2 out of every 1000 hospital patients die as a result of an infection directly related to urinary catheterization.[2] However, England is not alone in this unexpected, and unnecessary, increase to the cost of the nation's health care. In a study of HAI in the USA, it was found that urinary tract infections (UTI) increased the

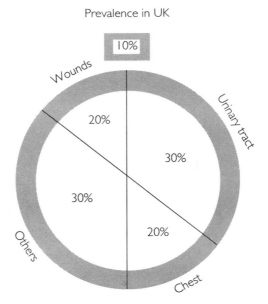

FIGURE 7.1 Prevalence of hospital-acquired infections. Reproduced with permission from Ward, K. (1993) *Nursing Practice and Health Care* (Hinchcliff, S., Norman, S. and Schober, J., eds), published by Edward Arnold, London.

duration of hospitalization by 5.1 days. A wound infection increased the period of hospitalization by 12.9 days – a heavy price to pay.[7]

A commensal is a bacterium that is symbiotic to the health of the host (e.g. *Escherichia coli* in the gut). However, when the commensal is transplanted into another part of the body, an 'infection' will ensue. A common example is *E. coli*, which when transported from the gut to the urinary tract causes cystitis.

Common forms of hospital-acquired infection

Campylobacter *enteritis*

This is now one of the commonest forms of infective diarrhoea in England.[8] This form of diarrhoea is caused by organisms that affect the digestive tract, many of which have not yet been identified, or are totally new. Following two particularly virulent outbreaks of salmonella in late 1980 in which 47 patients died, a Committee of Inquiry revoked the Crown Immunity which was until then held by all hospital kitchen premises. From 1980, hospitals could be prosecuted under the Food Hygiene Act. Before then, hospital kitchens were above the law.[2]

Pseudomonas aeruginosa

This bacillus has reared its ugly head in recent years, and is becoming increasingly common in hospitals. A strictly aerobic Gram-negative bacillus, it flourishes in water and aqueous solutions. The organism produces a pigment called pyocyanin as well as fluorescein, and these compounds together create the characteristic blue pus.[1] *Pseudomonas* is rapidly becoming resistant to antibiotics and proving very difficult to treat. It frequents surgical wards, and is the cause of extreme discomfort and embarrassment to the patient, who is often only too aware of how unpleasant he or she smells.

Methicillin-resistant Staphylococcus aureus

This has been responsible for world-wide outbreaks of infections, characterized by rapid spread. It was a mutated form of methicillin-resistant *Staphylococcus aureus* that produced the so-called 'flesh-eating bug' of 1994. *Staphylococcus* infections tend to remain localized; possibly due to the production of coagulase which clots fibronogen.[1]

The above three common causes of HAI tend not to respond to orthodox medication. However, *in-vitro* studies suggest that these infections can respond to the antibacterial action of specific essential oils (see chapter on aromatograms). Pathologists who are expert in the use of essential oils as antibacterial agents stress that 'the terrain' of the patient can affect the efficacy of the antibacterial action of an essential oil, and an

individual aromatogram is required. However, the standard aromatograms described will give a general idea as to which essential oils might
be efficacious in a patient.

Multiple resistant Serratia marcescens *and* Klebsiella

These were the cause of an epidemic involving four hospitals in the USA in the
1970s. The spread of infection was finally narrowed down to the hand-washing
of personnel who worked in all four hospitals. By the time the infection was
under control, 400 patients had been infected and 17 patients had died.[4]

Although the bacteria mentioned above are becoming more common in
hospitals, there is a whole range of pathogenic organisms which surround us
every day.

There follows a classification of bacteria and a description of some
research into the antimicrobial effects of essential oils. This research suggests
that essential oils could be used as a complement (or by a doctor as an
alternative) to an antibacterial/antifungal/antiviral synthetic drug.

Bacterial classification

Although to many nurses the following information may seem elementary, I
have found that some nurses need to have the basics reiterated so that the
information on essential oils that they require makes more sense.

Bacteria are first classified according to their shape (Figure 7.2). The two
main groups are cocci and bacilli.[9] These two groups are then subdivided
into Gram-positive and Gram-negative bacteria (Gram was the
microbiologist who devised the staining method). Gram staining uses a
mixture of violet dye and iodine to stain the magnesium ribonucleate (found
in some bacteria) deep purple. The purple stain cannot be washed out by
alcohol. Bacteria which stain purple are said to be Gram-positive. Those
bacteria which do not contain magnesium ribonucleate do not retain the
purple stain and are described as Gram-negative.[2] *Mycobacterium* (the cause
of TB and leprosy) is not revealed by the Gram stain method, and instead is
stained with an acid-fast method called the Ziehl-Nielsen method.[1]

Another subdivision is between aerobic organisms, which need air, and
anaerobic organisms, which do not require air. An increasingly common
anaerobic bacterium causes vaginitis, which conventional medicine seems
unable to help.

Coccus bacteria

The cocci bacteria include *Staphylococcus* (named after the Greek word 'staphyl',
meaning 'grapes', because under a microscope the bacteria take this
characteristic shape). *Staphylococcus* is the cause of many skin infections.

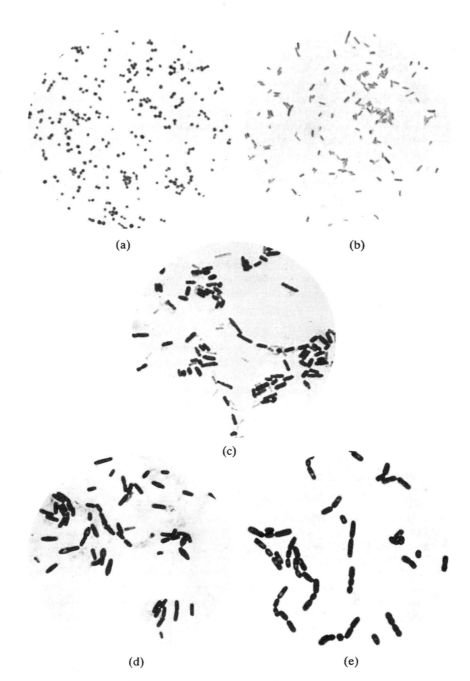

FIGURE 7.2 Types of bacteria. Reproduced with permission from Hobbs, B. and Roberts, D. (1993) *Food Poisoning and Food Hygiene*, 6th edn, published by Edward Arnold, London.

Streptococcus is named after the Greek word 'streptos', meaning 'twisted', as the bacteria resemble twisted chains. *Streptococcus* often causes throat infections. Other members of the coccus family include *Pneumococcus*, which causes pneumonia, and *Neisseria*, which causes gonorrhoea. Streptococcus can be further classified into A, B, or non-haemolytic and aerobic or anaerobic types.

Bacillus bacteria

The bacillius group includes Enterobacteriaceae such as *E. coli* and *Salmonella*, both of which can cause diarrhoea. It also includes *Proteus mirabilis* and *Bacillus anthracis*, which cause proteus and anthrax, respectively. Other bacteria in the bacillus group include *Corynebacterium diphtheriae* which causes diphtheria, *Pseudomonas aeruginosa*, and *Mycobacterium tuberculosis*, which causes TB. Anaerobic bacilli include *Clostridium tetani*, which causes tetanus, and *Clostridium difficile*, which causes pseudomembranous colitis.

In addition to the two main groups, there are the spirochaete group and a further group of organisms which are neither viruses nor bacteria, but something in between. This group includes *Rickettsia*, which causes typhus fever, and *Chlamydia trachomatis*, which causes genito-urinary infections.[9]

Bacteria divide approximately every 20 minutes in optimum conditions *in vitro*.[1]

A classification of pathogens is shown in Figure 7.3.

Antibiotics

The antibiotics industry has seen huge growth in the last 20 years, with sales increasing from $94 million in 1971 to $8 billion today.[4] Orthodox western medicine uses synthetic antibiotics to kill the bacterium which is causing an infection.

Antibiotics (which roughly translated means 'against life') are secondary metabolites of micro-organisms, and are, at high dilutions, inhibitory to other micro-organisms. They play no part in the formation of cell walls, nor do they contribute to the energy balance of the organism. An antibiotic is capable of inhibiting the growth of a micro-organism, or of destroying it.[10] Although many antibiotics are synthetic, most are natural substances. The most commonly used type of antibiotic is a broad-spectrum one which is non-selective.

Laboratory testing of a swab or blood sample will indicate which antibiotic is appropriate. This method of testing has largely been abandoned in favour of broad-spectrum antibiotics. However, these do not always succeed in killing the bacterium. A specific pathogenic organism needs a medicine that will target it specifically. There is no point throwing the

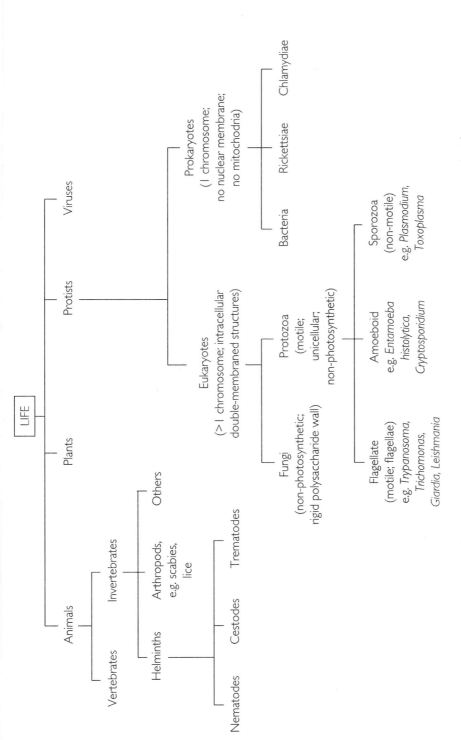

Figure 7.3 The classification of pathogens. Reproduced from Hope, R., Longmore, J., Hodgetts, T. and Ramrakha, P. (1993) *Oxford Handbook of Clinical Medicine*, by permission of Oxford University Press, Oxford.

kitchen sink at it, if the kitchen sink does not contain the specific component. Broad-spectrum antibiotics remain very popular. Testing to discover which antibiotic would be suitable is frequently considered to be old-fashioned, non cost-effective and time-consuming, particularly when doctors are under intense pressure to prescribe immediately.

Broad-spectrum antibiotics act as 'flame-throwers'. Although they may save time and, initially, money, this crude attempt to wipe out the offending bacteria also succeeds in destroying almost every other 'friendly' gut bacterium with it. As a result, there are now a great many people supporting colonies of fungi which have taken the place of the 'friendly' digestive bacteria. Nature abhors a vacuum. Candidiasis, once denied existence by the medical profession, is now thriving in millions of people who have taken broad-spectrum antibiotics and not replaced their 'friendly' bowel flora.

The majority of antibiotics are (or have been until recently) active against Gram-positive micro-organisms (which make up the huge plethora of common infectious agents such as *Staphylococcus* and *Streptococcus*). These antibiotics work either by inhibiting the synthesis of the cell wall, or protein or nucleic acid production, or by reducing the permeability of the cytoplasmic membrane. This prevents the bacteria from reproducing so rapidly, and enables the host to work towards eliminating the organism.[11]

Although man-made antibiotics are becoming ever more complex in an attempt to compete with organisms which can mutate and thereby initiate resistant colonies, they are not as complicated as most essential oils. Essential oils have a hundred or more components, so it is arguable that an organism would find it more difficult to become resistant to them. Without a doubt, synthetic antibiotics have saved lives, and will continue to do so. However, the over-use and, it might be suggested, improper use of antibiotics over the last few years has led to a growing population of resistant bacteria.[4]

Penicillin, the 'first' antibiotic, was found to be effective against *Staphylococcus* but completely ineffective against *E. coli*. As early as 1942, Fleming (who discovered penicillin) was advising the medical profession of the possibility that *Staphylococcus* could become resistant to penicillin. Today, 95 per cent of *Staphylococcus* is resistant to penicillin.

Antibiotics are also listed in the group of drugs most frequently associated with adverse reactions.[12] In addition, they are thought to be linked to the increase in food allergies and chronic fatigue syndrome (ME).[13]

Some bacteria can be killed within a few hours with direct exposure to sunlight, and most are killed at a temperature of 100°C (boiling point of water). However, some bacteria are notoriously difficult to eradicate, especially in an immune-compromised person. From Figure 7.4, it is easy to see how many bacilli and cocci have become resistant to antibiotics, resulting in the development of the so-called 'superbugs'.

FIGURE 7.4 Susceptibility of selected bacteria to certain antibacterial drugs. Reproduced from Hope, R., Longmore, J., Hodgetts, T. and Ramrakha, P. (1993) *Oxford Handbook of Clinical Medicine*, by permission of Oxford University Press, Oxford.

	Penicillin V/G	Flucloxacillin	Amp/Amoxycillin	Carbenicillin/Ticarcillin	Piperacillin/Azlocillin	Cephradine/Cephalothin/Cefazolin	Cefuroxime/Cephamandole/Cefotaxime	Ceftazidime	Imipenem	Erythromycin	Lincomycin/Clindamycin	Tetracyclines	Chloramphenicol	Trimethoprim	Aminoglycosides	Vancomycin	Metronidazole	Ciprofloxacin
Staphylococcus aureus (penicillin sensitive)	I	0	0	0	2	2	0	2	2R	2R	2R	2R	R	2	2	2	R	2
Staphylococcus aureus (penicillin resistant)	R	R	R	R	2	2	0	2	2R	2R	2R	2R	R	2R	2	2	R	2
Streptococcus (group A)	I	0	0	0	2	2	0	2	2	2R	R	R	R	R	R	0	R	R
Streptococcus pneumoniae	I	2	0	2	2	2	2	2	2	2R	2R	2R	R	R	R	0	R	R
Enterococcus faecalis	R	R	R	2	R	R	R	2	0	R	R	R	R	R	R	2R	R	R
Neisseria meningitidis	0	0	2	0	0	0	2	2	0	0	2	R	2	R	R	R	R	0
Listeria monocytogenes	2	I	0	0	0	0	R	2	2	2	0	2	2	2	R	0	R	0
Haemophilus influenzae	R	IR	R	R	R	R	2	2	2R	R	2R	R	R	0	0	R	R	2
E. coli	R	IR	R	R	R	2R	2R	2	2	R	R	R	IR	2R	2R	R	R	2
Klebsiella species	R	R	R	R	2R	2R	2R	2	2	R	R	R	IR	2R	2R	R	R	2
Serratial/Enterobacter species	R	R	R	R	2R	2R	2R	2	2	R	R	R	IR	2R	2R	R	R	2
Proteus species	R	IR	R	R	R	2R	2R	2	2	R	R	R	IR	2R	2R	R	R	2
Pseudomonas aeruginosa	R	R	R	R	R	R	R	2	2	R	R	R	R	1R	R	R	R	2
Bacteroides fragilis	R	2R	R	2	2R	R	R	2	2	2R	2R	2R	R	R	R	R	–	R
Other Bacteroides species	R	R	R	R	2R	2R	2R	2	2	2R	2R	2R	R	R	R	R	–	R

Key: I = susceptible, first choice 2 = susceptible, second choice R = resistance likely to be a problem 0 = usually inappropriate

Resistance to antibiotics – *the superbugs*

Some strains of bacteria have become resistant to antibiotics for various possible reasons.

- Patients have not completed a course of antibiotics. This means that the bacteria are not completely eradicated, and become immune to the next dose of that particular antibiotic.
- Antibiotics have been prescribed for viral illness (in the USA, some 900 000 prescriptions were for antibiotics to treat the common cold).[4]
- Antibiotics have been used prophylactically (in the USA, until 1992, a 48-hour course of antibiotics was given preoperatively to patients thought to be at risk).
- During the past 40 years, certain antibiotics, namely penicillin and tetracycline, have been added to animal feed.
- Antibiotics are regularly used by the food industry to protect fruit and vegetables, and are also used in the fish industry.
- Over-prescribing has been widespread. In 1991, 240 million prescriptions for antibiotics were written in the USA, one for every person in the country.[4] This dropped to 110 million prescriptions for antibiotics in 1995, but 50 per cent of these were thought to be inappropriate for the disease that was being treated.[13]

Antibiotics are given to animals to increase growth. In some cases chickens fed with a broth of antibiotics have grown to be three times larger.[14] Although only minute amounts of antibiotics produce this growth, the consequence is that animals destined for human consumption regularly contain antibiotics, leading to a potential immunity or resistance of humans to those antibiotics. This immunity first manifested itself with an outbreak of salmonella in England in 1965. Normally, salmonella would have been swiftly brought under control with antibiotics. However, on this occasion, investigations showed that the bacterium was resistant, and six people died.[15]

Following this outbreak, the Swann Committee, which was composed of microbiologists and doctors, led an intensive enquiry. Their recommendation was the banning of antibiotics (used in human medicine) for promoting animal growth. Although the ban was agreed upon by England, Scandinavia, The Netherlands and most European countries, the USA government never approved the ban, and still uses the same antibiotics that are employed in human medicine as growth stimulants for animals.[4]

Shortly after penicillin was discovered, researchers found that some strains of *Staphylococcus* could manufacture an enzyme called *penicillinase*, which rendered penicillin inactive.[16] This resistant strain spread through hospitals and by 1955, 80 per cent of patients who were infected with *Staphylococcus* died if penicillin was the only antibiotic used to combat the infection.

Methicillin and cephalosporin were introduced in the 1960s in an effort to control penicillin-resistant *Staphylococcus*. They appeared to be effective, but then Gram-negative bacteria such as *Serratia* and *Klebsiella* began to show resistance to these new drugs. Another antibiotic, gentamycin, appeared on the market and seemed to have the situation under control until *Staphylococcus* reappeared – this time more resistant than before – the first methicillin-resistant *Staphylococcus aureus* (MRSA). The pharmaceutical business regrouped and produced a new antibiotic, ciprofloxacin, but MRSA quickly became immune to it. By 1980, MRSA was resistant to everything except vancomycin. This antibiotic had been held back, not only because it was toxic, but because it was feared that if MRSA became resistant to it there would be nothing else to throw at them. These fears became reality in the late 1980s, when hospitals began to report vancomycin-resistant infections.

Resistant bacteria are still often treated with cephalosporin, a fairly new antibiotic derived from a fungus. It was discovered by Giuseppe Brotzu, a bacteriologist from Cagliari in Sardinia.[4] The disadvantages of the cephalosporin group of antibiotics are the hypersensitivity that they cause in over 10 per cent of patients and their adverse effects on blood-clotting mechanisms.[9]

Many sexually transmitted diseases, including gonorrhoea and chlamydia, are now multiple resistant. *Shigella*, the cause of many faecal-contaminated gastric upsets, is multiple resistant, as are many respiratory infections.

Essential oils as potential antibacterial agents

Essential oils are not just pleasant aromas. They have antibiotic, antiviral and antifungal properties, which are mentioned in most aromatherapy courses and books. The responsibility for prescribing a proprietary antibiotic usually lies with a physician or nurse practitioner, and it would be inappropriate for an aromatherapist or another kind of nurse to take on this responsiblity. However, the use of an essential oil to enhance a prescribed synthetic antibiotic is acceptable and is already happening. However, what is perhaps needed in addition is a more detailed look at those antibacterial properties. Could they be used as prescription medicine? In a world where pathogens are mutating faster than we can create synthetic medicines to kill them, essential oils might have a very beneficial role to play. Perhaps they may turn out to be the antibiotics of the future.

There is a long history of essential oils being used against pestilence. Hypothetical examples that are often quoted include the large number of perfumers and glovemakers who appeared to have survived the Black Death. Indeed, it is documented that glove makers were licensed to impregnate their wares with essential oils, and often chose neroli and rose. Schweistheimer's research revealed that the town of Bucklesbury was spared from the plague – popular opinion was that this was because it was the centre of the lavender trade.[17] However, it is speculation to assume that essential oils were the sole reason for the survival of the inhabitants of Bucklesbury.

Nostradamus was supposed to have successfully treated the plague with pills of crushed roses placed under the tongues of plague victims. Rose contains *l*-citronellol, geraniol, nerol, *l*-linalol and phenylethyl alcohol.[18] Alcohols are thought to be strong anti-infection agents with antiviral properties.[19] Rose also contains eugenol (phenol), citral (aldehyde) and farnesol (asesquiterpenoid), all of which are thought to have strong antiseptic/antibacterial properties. However, the actions of Nostradamus seem to be logical, but the information is speculative.

About 58 per cent of all isolated antibiotics are produced from *Streptomyces* (a bacterium). Another 9 per cent are derived from other bacteria, 19 per cent from fungi, lichens and mosses, and 14 per cent from higher plants. Lewis writes that 'the total 909 antibiotics known in 1967 represent only a fraction of those found in nature. Not a single one, used therapeutically, is from the higher plants, even though these possess the largest single group of antibiotics for which there is no known use'.[20] Tamm reports on ansamycins – a group of antibiotics characterized by an aliphatic bridge linking two non-adjacent positions found in an aromatic nucleus.[10] An aromatic nucleus is found in essential oils.

Some of the plant groups and species known to have antibiotic properties include the following: yellow cypress; wild ginger; golden seal; poplar tree; turnip; wallflower; hops; cabbage; sweet clover; common bean; cashew; black walnut; potato; corn; garlic. All of these plants have been tested against bacteria, fungi, viruses or protozoa and found to be effective.[11]

Valnet suggests that if essential oils were used to treat pathogens then the surrounding tissue would not be adversely affected. Conventional medicines can sometimes destroy the surrounding tissue along with the infection, as antibiotics typically kill bacteria by puncturing their cell walls, which allows toxins to spill out.[21] In the case of burns, where the breakdown of tissue causes the body to reabsorb pathogenic toxins, Valnet suggests that the use of essential oils could be a more suitable method of treatment. The added bonus is the tissue-protecting properties of many essential oils, which prevent putrefaction.[22] Of course, essential oils with a high phenol content can cause dermal irritation, and would need to be avoided.

Research on the antibacterial properties of essential oils

In 1945, the Second National Symposium on Recent Advances in Antibiotic Research was held in Washington, under the auspices of the National Institutes of Health. During the proceedings, the effects of lupulon, a lipid-soluble antibiotic-like substance prepared from hops (*Humulus lupulus*) were discussed. The findings of Yin-Ch'ang Chin, Nai-Ch'u Chang and Hamilton H. Anderson were that lupulon inhibited the growth of *Staphylococcus aureus, Mycobacterium phlei* and *Mycobacterium tuberculosis in vitro* at concentrations of 1.56, 5.0 and 25 µg/ml, respectively. The research team further discovered that a 2 per cent solution of sodium chloride increased the antibiotic activity.[23] Hops produce an essential oil.[24] What is even more interesting is that 50 years ago antibiotic researchers were investigating possible plant alternatives.

In 1960, Maruzella presented an extensive report on the antibacterial activity of 133 essential oils *in vitro*. These were tested against six pathogens, namely *Escherichia coli, Staphylococcus aureus, Bacillus subtilis, Streptococcus faecalis, Salmonella typhosa* and *Mycobacterium avium*. In total, 71 per cent of the essential oils tested were shown to be effective against *Mycobacterium avium*, 19 per cent against *Bacillus subtilis*, 14 per cent against *Staphylococcus aureus*, 12 per cent against *Streptococcus faecalis* and 6 per cent against *Escherichia coli*.[25] Among the most effective essential oils were lemongrass, oregano, savory, red thyme and cinnamon. The research was conducted just 2 years after Maruzzella had published another paper with Henry Percival examining the antimicrobial activity of perfume oils.[26]

In a paper written in 1987, Deans and Svoboda reported that marjoram (*Oregano majorana*) was effective against *Pseudomonas aeruginosa, Salmonella pullorum* and *Yersinia enterocolitica, in vitro*, at a concentration of 1:10 in absolute ethanol. All three organisms are of significance in public health.[27]

The antimicrobial activity of 21 essential oils of eucalyptus was examined in a paper published in 1993.[28] The effects of the volatile constituents of *Eucalyptus citriodora* were found to be the most effective against *E. coli*, (Gram-negative), *Bacillus megaterium* and *Staphylococcus aureus* (both Gram-positive), although when the whole essential oil was used, *Eucalyptus cladocalyx* was most effective. This brings up the point, which has been paralleled in many other studies, that isolating the active common constituents of essential oils will not produce the same effects as using the whole essential oil. It was interesting that *E. globulus, E. smithi* and *E. radiata* were not among the eucalyptus types selected for testing, although they are regularly used in aromatherapy to treat infections.[29]

In a study conducted in 1992 by Ferdous *et al.* on the treatment of dysentery, *Nigella sativa* essential oil was shown to be effective against several multiple-drug-resistant organisms, such as *Shigella, Vibrio cholera* and *E. coli*.[30] The activity of the oil was compared with that of ampicillin, tetracycline, cotrimoxazole, gentamycin and nalidixic acid, and showed promising antibacterial activity against all of the bacterial strains tested, except for one strain of *Shigella dysenteriae* (strain 1548). *Nigella sativa* is commonly known as Roman coriander, nutmeg flower or fennel flower, although it is not in any way related to fennel. It actually belongs to the buttercup family. The French formerly used the seeds as a substitute for pepper, and in India the seeds are commonly used in curries.[31]

Helichrysum picardii, a member of the everlasting flower family, was shown to be effective against Gram-positive bacteria such as *Staphylococcus aureus, Bacillus subtilis, Bacillus cereus, Bacillus maegaterium* and Gram-negative *E. coli*, although the antibacterial activity was thought to be less potent than the classic antibacterial action of clove and thyme.[32] *Helichrysum* is used as a tobacco flavouring.

Much research on the antibacterial properties of essential oils has been carried out by Professor Stanley Deans of the Department of Biochemical Sciences, the Scottish Agricultural College, Auchincruive, Scotland. In one paper he presents the results of testing 50 essential oils against 25 genera of bacteria *in vitro*. His research revealed that the most effective essential oils were bay, cinnamon, clove, thyme, almond, marjoram, pimento, geranium and lovage.[33]

Artemesia dracunculus (French tarragon) was shown to be effective against *Pseudomonas aeruginosa, Staphylococcus aureus, Staphylococcus faecalis* and *Yersinia enterocolitica*.[34] In this study, the whole oil was tested against several of the main chemical constituents, such as eugenol, limonene, linalol, menthol, *cis*-omene, anisaldehyde and alpha-pinene. This same study produced firm evidence that the constituents of essential oils change, depending on the time of harvesting. In this instance tarragon plants harvested mid-season were the least potent.

The finding that the constituents of essential oils alter according to the time of harvesting is not new to aromatherapists, but this is one of the few studies which actually demonstrates the fact. Also of interest was the way in which the physical configuration of the molecule affected the essential oil (the difference between *cis* and *trans* isomers). In tarragon, the *cis* configuration produced a more antimicrobial plant. Tarragon is used as a flavour ingredient in many foods, as well as in alcoholic and soft drinks. It is also an important ingredient of Bearnaise sauce.

In another study in conjunction with the Instituto di Agronomia Gernerale e Coltivazioni Erbacee at the University of Bologna, Italy, Deans and his team tested hybrids (man-made cultivars) of four plants, namely lavender, sage, savory and thyme, against 25 bacteria *in vitro*. All four genera showed substantial antibiotic activity, but each was most potent against specific bacteria. These were:

- *Thymus* (thyme) against *Moraxella* spp. and *Clostridium sporogenes;*
- *Salvia* (sage) against *Acinetobacter calcoacetica, Brevibacterium linens, Clostridium sporogenes* and *Moraxella* spp.;
- *Satureja* (savory) against *Brevibacterium linens, Enterobacter aerogenes, Klebsiella pneumonia* and *Moraxella* spp.;
- *Lavandula* (lavender) against *Brevibacterium linens, Clostridium sporogenes, Moraxella* spp. and *Staphylococcus aureus.*

In yet another paper Deans tested the antibacterial properties of essential oils from Zimbabwe, demonstrating the highly potent oils of *Oregano officinalis* (a specially bred strain from Israel) and *Cymbopogon citratus* (West Indian lemongrass). Other essential oils which had antibacterial activity were tarragon, basil, sage, thyme and celery. Among the bacteria tested were *Salmonella pullorum, E. coli, Klebsiella pneumonia, Pseudomonas aeruginosa, Staphylococcus aureus, Streptococcus faecalis* and *Proteus vulgaris.*[35]

The antibacterial properties of lemongrass were the subject of a detailed investigation published in 1986.[36] This particular lemongrass was grown in Nigeria, where it was traditionally used for the treatment of rheumatism. Another study, this time of *Satureja hortensis* (summer savory), showed that the plant was also an effective antibacterial agent against the above organisms.[37] Cumin seed essential oil was found to be effective against *E. coli, Staphylococcus aureus* and *Streptococcus faecalis.*[38]

The plant family *Lamiacae* includes many plants which display antibacterial properties. Among these are *Rosmarinus officinalis* (rosemary), *Calamintha nepeta* (wild basil), *Thymus vulgaris* (thyme) and *Satureja montana* (savory). The effective chemical parts of these plants are thought to be carvacrol (in *Satureja montana*), alpha-pinene and cineole (in *Rosmarinus officinalis*) thymol (in *Thymus vulgaris*) and pulegone and *para*-cymene (in *Calamintha nepeta*).[39]

Balacs reports the results of some Polish research on *Matricaria recutitia* (German chamomile), renowned for its deep blue colour and anti-inflammatory properties. The research showed that the essential oil also had substantial antimicrobial activity, especially against Gram-positive bacteria such as *Staphylococcus aureus* and *Streptococcus faecalis.* Investigations into which component was producing this antibiotic effect pointed to alpha-bisabolol, which was more active than chamazulene.[40]

Essential oils were also tested against hospital pathogenic bacteria in a study by Benouda.[41] This study examined *Staphylococcus aureus, Streptococcus* C and D, *Proteus* (various species), *Klebsiella* spp., *Salmonella typhi, Haemophilus influenza* and *Pseudomonas aeruginosa.* Essential oils of *Artemesia herba alba*, *Thymus capitatus* and *Eucalyptus globulus* were found to have comparable action to standard antibiotics. Thyme was the most effective essential oil, although none of the oils had any impact on *Pseudomonas*.

A review paper by Carson showed that *Melaleuca alternifolia* (tea tree) was an effective antibiotic against *Staphylococcus*, *Streptococcus* or Gram-negative infections, and concludes that the full therapeutic potential of tea tree has not yet been realized.[42]

Manuka (*Leptospermum scoparium*) and kanuka, New Zealand's answer to tea tree, produced impressive results when investigated by Cawthron in 1994. This research, which was supported by Maori funds, covered the effects of these two essential oils against various bacteria and fungi. Manuka appeared to be very effective against *Staphylococcus aureus* and ringworm. It was felt that manuka could be a useful essential oil in cases of MRSA infection, although the paper stated that no clinical trials have yet been carried out.[43]

Finally, a further paper by Carson and her team in Western Australia showed that *Melaleuca alternifolia* (tea tree) was effective against MRSA. It was tested against 64 methicillin-resistant and 33 mupirocin-resistant isolates of *Staphylococcus aureus*, and was found to be effective in all cases, using dilutions of 0.25 per cent and 0.50 per cent. These results were duplicated in a UK study using similar methods. It should be noted that the tea tree used was chemotype terpineol. This is a monoterpenic alcohol which is present in this tea tree at levels above 30 per cent, and the cineol content (an oxide, and harsher on the mucous membrane) was present at less than 15 per cent.[44]

These examples are just a sample from many research papers which indicate the antibacterial potential of essential oils. Therefore aromatherapy should be viewed as something more than a 'pretty smell added to a massage'. Just because these oils are 'natural' does not mean they are not powerful. As Norman Farnsworth, Director of Pharmacognosy at the University of Illinois College of Pharmacy, says: 'there is not a dime's bit of difference between chemicals in plants and synthetics'.[45] All of the above research was conducted *in vitro*. However, if essential oils have pharmacologically active effects *in vitro*, as they evidently do, there is every reason to suppose that they will have *similar* effects *in vivo*.

Further research is obviously required, and normally this would involve extensive testing on animals. This method has already been used for potential toxicity. However, essential oils affect us on many levels, so to assess their therapeutic efficacy in humans may well mean that animal testing is not only unnecessary but also misleading. How can an animal tell the investigator if it feels nauseated or happy? How does the investigator know what the animal is feeling?

The drug industry can be relied upon to ask and investigate what could be the best drug solution to a specific medical problem. The specific drug under investigation is tested on laboratory animals, but perhaps we should be looking at essential oils in a different way, as they appear to have multiple properties and uses. If toxicity trials on human tissue slices and cell cultures indicate a safe level at which essential oils can be used (as many of the above trials have indicated), surely what is needed next is a series of tightly controlled trials of the efficacy and safety of essential oils in humans.

As Dr Peter Mansfield writes, 'Science is really a method for answering questions. If we ask stupid questions, scientific methods will faithfully produce for us a stupid answer'.[46]

Many essential oils, at a dilution known to be safe, have been shown to be effective against pathogens, several of which are resistant to synthetic drugs. Yet most of the research (to date) on humans in clinical situations is *not* about infection, but about subjective analysis of how relaxed the subjects are feeling. Aromatherapy is good for promoting relaxation, but essential oils have many other therapeutic properties that are waiting to be assessed clinically. Until this happens, nurses will use essential oils for their behavioural effect, which is evaluated subjectively, even though the same essential oil may have an antibacterial effect which could be measured objectively.

Finally, in 1994, at a special presentation on aromatograms and the use of essential oils as antibacterial agents at the Royal Society of Medicine, Michael Smith, a London-based pathologist gave an analysis of the antibacterial properties of several essential oils. *Every one tested on MRSA had shown itself to be effective against MRSA.* The list included *Origanum vulgare, Thymus vulgaris* CT3 (thymol), *Ormenis mixta, Lavandula intermedia* CT Super, *Cupressus sempervirens, Mentha piperita, Ravensara aromatica, Juniperus communis, Citrus limonum, Cymbopogon martini, Eucalyptus globulus* and *Eucalyptus smithii.* These are essential oils which aromatherapists use regularly, and they are generally accepted as being safe to use (with the possible exception of *Thymus vulgaris* CT3). Many of them are also used by nurses in a hospital or clinical setting for their other properties. The time is ripe to consider their use for *all* of their properties.

On the clinical aromatherapy course I teach to nurses in the USA, we have had some impressive case-study results using compresses on wound infections and infected bedsores. Swabs have been taken and a specific essential oil selected.

One particularly impressive case study was conducted by a nurse practitioner. One of her female patients had a chronically infected bedsore. This patient had been on systemic antibiotics, without effect. A wound swab showed that the infection had been caused by *Clostridium.* Searching through her monographs (which are given out in the course) the nurse practitioner found a reference to a paper by Ross.[47] After she had discussed the safety and potential efficacy of sweet marjoram with her consultant, and had shown him the monograph, he gave his consent for her to use this essential oil. The nurse also discussed this treatment with her patient, and obtained the patient's consent.

She applied a compress directly to the infected site, using a 5 per cent solution of *Origanum majorana* (sweet marjoram) in sterile water. The compress was re-applied three times a day. Within 24 hours there was a dramatic improvement, and within 5 days the wound was almost healed.

In other case studies, essential oils with antibacterial properties have been selected without a swab being taken. No case has shown any negative side-effects to date. In most instances, the infection has appeared to have healed more rapidly. It is hoped that the data from hundreds of similar case studies will be collated and published next year. This information will form part of the knowledge base which is so necessary for clinical aromatherapy to gain greater acceptance and to move forward.

The aromatogram

Just as with synthetic antibiotics, many essential oils are effective against particular pathogens. The skill lies in knowing which essential oil to use for which infection. Conventional medicine regularly takes wound or throat swabs, or urine or blood samples in order to cultivate a pathogen.

Gattefosse used exactly the same principle of this process, which is called an *antibiogram*, and named it an *aromatogram*. The whole procedure is similar to that which orthodoxy has used for many years, the only difference being that with an aromatogram an essential oil is added to the Petri dish instead of an antibiotic. A hypothetical example of an aromatogram is shown in Figure 7.5.

The Petri dish is lined with a culture medium such as agar-agar. Several small circles impregnated with an essential oil are interspersed in the dish. The pathogen is then added and the Petri dish is incubated for 24 hours.

If the essential oil is the correct antidote, an area of inhibition will occur in a circle around the drop. Sometimes an essential oil, not effective on its own, will be when it is close to a second essential oil. Sometimes two essential oils together will give the greatest area of inhibition. Much research has been done in France on the use of aromatograms, and Belaiche's book contains many tables illustrating the specific use of essential oils against specific bacteria, and their effects.[48]

In England, this technique has been used by Deans and Ritchie in a comprehensive and impressive study which examined 25 genera of bacteria and 50 essential oils.[33]

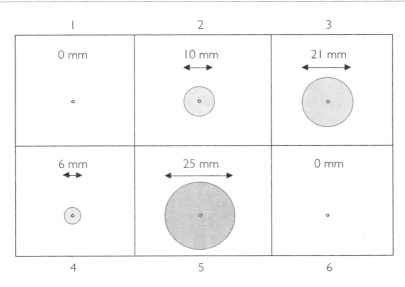

FIGURE 7.5 Hypothetical example of an aromatogram. Six different essential oils, here identified only by number, are being tested against one bacterial culture from the body of a patient. The shaded area is known as the 'area of inhibition' and shows how effective each oil is against the bacteria. In this case essential oils 3 and 5 would be used to treat the patient. Reproduced from Tisserand, R. (1988) *Aromatherapy for Everyone*, with the kind permission of Penguin Books, Harmondsworth.

This kind of sensitivity testing for essential oils in the treatment of bacterial infections is being carried out by several London hospitals. Although this facility is currently limited to London, there is active campaigning to increase the understanding of how aromatograms work.[49] It is hoped that this scientific method of selecting essential oils in sensitivity testing will become more widespread as it becomes better understood. (See Appendix 3 for contact addresses.)

Smith and Valnet both emphasize that standard organisms do not respond in exactly the same way as a host organism. Even though the pathogen is known and named, it may not respond in an identical way – the host must be taken into consideration. To illustrate this, Valnet points out that a colibacillus in one patient may respond to the essential oil of pine, whereas in another patient it may respond to the essential oil of lavender or thyme.[22] This is quite different to the Western approach to treating pathogens where everybody has the same antibiotic, usually a broad-spectrum one.

However, the selection of essential oils for testing in an aromatogram is based on the antibacterial properties reported in the literature.

Viruses, synthetic viricides and essential oils

A virus is different to any other pathogen. Sir Peter Medewar, a famous virologist, described it as 'simply a piece of bad news wrapped up in protein'. In fact, a virus is a coiled strand of nucleic acid protected by a protein coat, which can only survive and reproduce inside a host cell.[50] Because viruses are so small, their biology was not understood for many years. Only now, with electron microscopy, can viruses be seen. Many biologists would still not classify them as 'living' organisms in their own right – only when they are inside the infected host cell.

There are basically two different types of virus: those that attack bacteria and those that attack the cells of other living organisms, such as animals and humans. The basic structure of a virus is illustrated in Figure 7.6.

Viruses are classified as either DNA viruses or RNA viruses. The DNA viruses are subdivided into single-strand and double-strand viruses. RNA viruses also occur as single or double strands, with retroviruses (which include AIDS and HIV) in the single-strand group. A retrovirus contains an

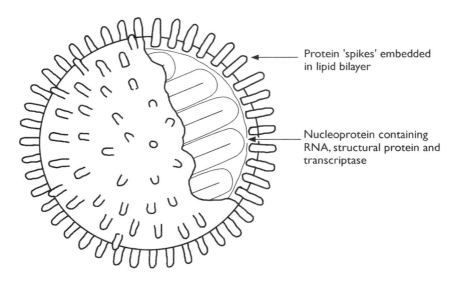

Protein 'spikes' embedded in lipid bilayer

Nucleoprotein containing RNA, structural protein and transcriptase

FIGURE 7.6 The structure of a virus. Diagram of enveloped virion showing arrangement of external proteins and internal nucleoprotein. The measles virus and influenza virus have this type of virion structure. Both viruses have a nucleoprotein which contains a single RNA molecule (measles virus) or 8 different RNA segments (influenza virus). Reproduced with permission from MacSween, R. and Whaley, K. (1992) *Muir's Textbook of Pathology*, 13th edn, published by Edward Arnold, London.

enzyme called reverse transcriptase which allows the RNA in the virus to be reverse-transcribed into DNA. Drugs such as zidovudine (AZT) and Retrovir (which contains zidovudine) are designed to inhibit production of reverse transcriptase. Resistance acquired by viruses during antiviral therapy has been well documented. It usually occurs by the virus mutating.[1]

Viruses such as those which cause glandular fever, influenza, warts, the common cold, mumps and measles are well known. Less common is the rabies virus. More recent additions are herpes and lassa fever. Of these viruses, only smallpox has been eradicated through immunization. A compulsory immunization programme in the West has controlled mumps and measles, although they remain potential killers in third world countries.

Patients with defective antibody production appear to be unable to cope with bacterial infections, although they seem to handle some viral infections normally. However, reduced T-cell functioning usually results in increased viral infections.[1]

Viral infections can be divided into:

- the highly virulent viruses which cause death in humans, e.g. rabies;
- host-deficiency-producing viruses (e.g. AIDS), where the death of the host is caused by a reduced immunological profile resulting in opportunistic infections.

Man-made viricides

Geoffrey Carr reports in the science pages of *The Economist* magazine that 'no viral epidemic has ever been stopped by drugs'.[51] Synthetic viricides are difficult to manufacture, and none of them appear to be totally effective to date. Most have moderate to severe side-effects. They work in one of three ways: through immunological control; through stimulation of the natural resistance mechanism of the host; or through chemotherapy. One of the most successful, AZT, stops the phosphate linkage being formed. This means that the virus cannot manufacture DNA.[52]

The controversy over AZT, and whether it is desirable to fight a disease which depletes white cells by using a drug that also reduces the number of white cells, remains unresolved. However, following AZT, protease inhibitors and stavudine (d4T) appear to be powerful weapons against an AIDS epidemic which may well turn out to be more devastating than the plague itself, and to have killed three times more Americans than the Vietnam war.[53]

After AIDS, however, more and more 'new' viruses are appearing for which there appears to be no antidote. Have these viruses always been around, unseen and undetected? Have they been waiting until our levels of immunity have fallen so low that they have gained entry? Or are they really new and, if so, where have they come from?

Essential oils as potential viricides

An investigation supported by the National Institutes of Health showed that *Melissa officinalis* (lemon balm) has antiviral properties.[54] These were tested on embryonic eggs and in tissue culture. The diseases tested were Semliki forest (mouse brain disease), Newcastle disease, vaccinia and herpes simplex. The results showed that *Melissa officinalis* protected the embryonic eggs against the lethal action of all of the viruses tested. It is thought that the antiviral action was produced by the tannin-like polyphenol. This activity was thought to be unrelated to that of tea tannins or tannic acid which are themselves known viricides and act on influenza A.[55]

A paper published by Kucera and Herrmann explored the antiviral effects further, this time including influenza A and B, mumps and three different strains of parainfluenza (1, 2 and 3). The results showed that melissa had an antiviral effect on mumps and the three parainfluenza strains, but had no effect on influenza A and B. Melissa is sold in commercial antiviral preparations in Germany.[56]

Peneol states in his paper on *Eucalyptus smithii* that many essential oils have a strong viricidal action. He suggests that the antiviral properties are possibly due to 1,8-cineol, (sometimes also called eucalyptol).[29] This compound is found in *Laurus nobilis* (bay laurel), *Ravensara aromatica*, *Lavandula latifolia* (spike lavender), *Rosmarinus officinalis* CT cineol (rosemary), *Salvia lavendulaefolia* (Spanish sage) and *Elettaria cardamomum* (cardamom). He writes further that limonene and alpha-pinene *reinforce* the antiviral action, whilst alcohols *strengthen* the antiviral action.

Cypress (*Cupressus sempervirens*) was the subject of a study of its viricidal properties. Obviously the investigators thought sufficiently highly of these properties, as they applied for a patent for some of its viricidal effects.[57]

Eucalyptus citriodora was found to be an effective viricide by Mendes in 1990.[58] This eucalyptus was also studied for its anti-HIV activities, together with eight other medicinal plants from Zaire.[59] In 1978, May and Willuhn found that *Eucalyptus globulus* had antiviral properties.[60] This is of particular interest to AIDS patients, as *Eucalyptus globulus* is also known to enhance the activity of streptomycin, isoniazid and sulfetrone in *Mycobacterium* TB, a common opportunistic infection in AIDS.[61] *Eucalyptus globulus* is also an effective treatment against herpes.[62]

May and Willuhn tested 178 species of medicinal plant belonging to 69 families for their virustatic properties. In total, 75 aqueous extracts appeared to have antiviral properties.[60] These were tested against polio, influenza and herpes viruses. *Laurus nobilis* (bay laurel), *Origanum vulgare* (oregano), *Rosmarinus officinalis* (rosemary) and *Salvia officinalis* (sage) were the most effective of the Lamiaceae family against all three viruses. *Juniperus communis* (juniper) also showed substantial antiviral action against herpes and influenza.

A less well known essential oil was used in a more recent Japanese study published in 1994. This showed the remarkable effects of *Houttynia cordata* against herpes simplex, influenza and HIV-1 (it was not effective against polio and coxsackievirus). These findings are very encouraging and appear to show that essential oils have the potential to interfere with the virus envelope. This results in the loss of infectivity of the virus, since the attachment to the cell surface must necessarily involve viral surface glycoproteins present in the envelope.[63]

Origanum majorana (sweet marjoram) was found to be antiviral in a study by Kucera and Herrmann.[64]

Garlic has been used against infections for centuries, and is the subject of almost a thousand research papers. Recent research has shown garlic to be effective against herpes virus types 1 and 2, parainfluenza virus type 3, vaccinia virus (cowpox) and human rhinovirus type 2 (which is a common cold virus). The active ingredients allicin and ajoene are thought to attack the virus inside the cell, possibly in the cell membrane.[65] Although garlic essential oil is available, it is unlikely to be used in a clinical setting because of its pervasive odour.

Franchomme lists three chemotypes of *Thymus vulgaris* (CT thymol, geraniol and linalol) as viricides in his textbook, *L'aromatherapie*.[66] Duke lists *Cinnamomum verum* (Ceylon cinnamon) as having antiviral properties,[67] and also *Syzygium aromaticum* (clove bud). The actual antiviral substance from the bud is called *eugeniin*.[68]

The above cases appear to suggest that essential oils could have a future role to play in the treatment of viral illness. Some of the essential oils are contraindicated (or carry cautions) for topical applications. Clove bud oil (used in baking, perfumes, lipsticks, soaps and dentistry) has caused hand dermatitis,[69] although clove bud essential oil is thought to be safe to use up to 5 per cent dilution.[70]

Cinnamon produces two essential oils – one from the leaf and one from the bark. The leaf essential oil contains less than 7 per cent cinnamic aldehyde (a known skin irritant), but the essential oil obtained from the bark contains up to 90 per cent cinnamic aldehyde.[69] The latter is therefore contraindicated for topical applications, as even at such low dilutions as 0.01 per cent, positive reactions have been found in patch testing.[71]

However, *Origanum majorana* (sweet marjoram), *Melissa officinalis* (melissa), *Cupressus sempervirens* (cypress), *Eucalyptus globulus* (eucalyptus) and *Juniperus communis* are generally thought to be safe to use. All essential oils with a high 1,8-cineol content should be used with caution, as they may cause skin sensitivity. These include *Eucalyptus smithii*, *Laurus nobilis* (bay laurel), *Ravensara aromatica*, *Lavandula latifolia* (spike lavender), *Rosmarinus officinalis* CT cineol (rosemary), *Salvia lavendulaefolia* (Spanish sage) and *Elettaria cardamomum* (cardamom). In addition, spike lavender and rosemary have accepted stimulatory properties.

Origanum vulgare (oregano) is a known skin irritant, and should not be used in topical applications above 2 per cent.[70]

Provided that safety guidelines are adhered to and patch tests are given, these essential oils could be used by nurses. In fact, several of these essential oils *are* already being used in the UK for their other therapeutic properties. Melissa and rosemary are listed by the Swiss Nursing Association (SBK) as being safe to use to treat conditions ranging from stress and pain to burns and mycoses (so long as their use has been approved by a doctor).[72] German nurses currently use rosemary for the treatment of headaches.

If an essential oil is already being used by a nurse, for some of its therapeutic effects, does a different protocol need to be drawn up for the use of its other therapeutic effects? In other words, do nurses need separate protocols for different therapeutic effects of the same essential oil? To be really safe and to avoid liability, possibly the answer is yes.

Fungal infections, synthetic fungicides and essential oils

A fungus is a primitive organism which is classified neither as a plant nor as an animal. Only a few fungi are pathogenic to man, and most cause superficial mild lesions.[1] Fungi are divided into three categories: superficial, subcutaneous and systemic, and fungal infections may be environmental in origin. The three categories are caused by:

- airborne allergens;
- elaborating toxins; and
- direct infection.

A disease or infection caused by fungi is called a mycosis.[73] With airborne allergens such as tinea (ringworm), the spores or hyphae of the fungus infiltrate the outer layers of the skin, causing destruction of the epidermis. With mycetoma, a localized infection occurs which may slowly spread. In candidiasis and cryptococcosis the infection can become systemic.

Cryptococcosis
This is primarily a respiratory disease which later spreads via the bloodstream to the lymph nodes and the brain. This fungus is abundant in pigeon droppings, and is usually only life-threatening to humans who are seriously immune-compromised.

Aspergillosis

Spores of this fungus are present in the atmosphere, and many species are infectious to man. The commonest is *Aspergillus fumigatus*. Whilst the effect of this fungus is not as rapid as that of *Cryptococcus*, the possible resulting bronchial asthma can be debilitating. The fungus may colonize a bronchial cavity and can result in necrotizing pneumonia. This tends to occur only in immune-compromised patients.

Candida albicans

Although *Candida albicans* is normally present in the intestines and on moist skin surfaces, this situation does not usually pose a problem. However, in certain circumstances, the fungus changes form and begins a mucocutaneous and systemic invasion. The mucosal change is caused by an alteration in the pH of the body tissue, producing an alkaline medium which allows the yeast fungus to proliferate. This is a fairly frequent side-effect of antibiotic treatment or immune-suppressive drugs. It can also occur in pregnancy and in diabetes.

From the mucosa, candida can invade surrounding surfaces such as nail beds, producing chronic granulomatous inflammation of the underlying tissue. It can also spread throughout the body, invading the heart valves, lungs, liver and kidneys with multiple small abscesses containing the fungus.[1] In the intestine, candida can change into a mycelial form, putting down thread-like roots which grow through the villi of the intestine. This results in macromolecules of food being absorbed with resulting multiple food allergies. This condition is known as candidiasis.

The common name for candidiasis is thrush. The symptoms may include vaginal itchiness with a profuse white curd-like discharge. Oral thrush is fairly common in babies. Frequently, patients have no symptoms other than abdominal bloating, tiredness and food intolerances. The incidence of candida overgrowth has increased dramatically during the last few years, and is thought to be related to immune depression, the use of the contraceptive pill and / or the over-use of antibiotics.[74]

Synthetic fungicides

It is more difficult to treat fungal infections than bacterial infections. Many fungal infections occur in tissues with a poor blood supply (if any), such as the nails, hair and skin. However, fungal infections are thought to be less difficult to treat (by orthodox medicine) than viral diseases. The drug of choice is fluconozole (Nystatin). Although topical application may keep the fungal infection at bay, systemic treatment is often given to reduce the incidence of recurrence following multiple infections. Fluconozole can affect kidney function. Of the other drugs used to treat fungal infection, many cause nausea, some induce skin rashes and a few can cause liver damage.[73]

Antifungal properties of essential oils

One of the earliest papers to be published on the antifungal properties of essential oils was by Myers in 1927.[75] He was prompted to investigate the fungicidal properties of essential oils following successful treatment of a lesion with a diluted solution of cinnamon oil which caused immediate relief of symptoms and rapid healing. He observed that thymol, carvacrol and oil of lemon destroyed yeast in less than a minute. His research involved nine yeast-like organisms which were isolated from infections in man, including two lung infections, two tongue infections, one infection involving a nail lesion, and various other patients with cutaneous ulcerations. Each infection rapidly became yeast-negative and was resolved with no recurrence.

Cryptococcosis

Specific essential oils that have been found to be useful against this opportunistic infection *in vitro* include *Rosmarinus officinalis* (rosemary)[76] and *Artemisia parviflora* (a member of the Indian tarragon family).[77] Whilst the latter is not in common use among aromatherapists or nurses, rosemary certainly is, and it is used topically for conditions such as muscle tension, or through inhalation for its antispasmodic effect on coughs.[72] In another paper Viollon and Chaumont suggest that geranium, palmarosa, savory and thyme might also be good choices.[78] If rosemary contains a high level of camphor, this oil should be used with care.[79]

Aspergillosis

Specific essential oils that have been found to be effective against aspergillosis *in vitro* are *Cymbopogon citratus* (West Indian lemongrass)[80] and *Cuminum cyminum* (cumin).[81] Cumin has a strong photosensitizing action and should not be used topically on patients who will be exposed to ultraviolet light within 12 hours. Dilutions should be kept to 0.04 per cent.[79] Others include *Artemisia dracunculus* (tarragon)[77] and *Eucalyptus citriodora* (lemon gum).[82] Of these, perhaps lemongrass and lemon gum are most commonly used by nurses, and neither of these essential oils has any adverse reactions known at dilutions of 1 to 5 per cent.[83]

Candida albicans

Specific essential oils that are effective against candida include *Melaleuca alternifolia*,[84] *Melissa officinalis* (melissa)[85] and *Eucalyptus citriodora* (lemon gum).[82]

Much has been reported about the antifungal effects of *Melaleuca alternifolia* from Australia.[86,87] However, several other essential oils that are commonly used have antifungal properties. Caraway, clove, geranium, lavender, lemon, lemongrass, neroli, peppermint, petitgrain, spearmint, coriander and sweet orange leaf are effective to varying degrees.[88] This might prove of interest to imbibers of the liqueurs Chartreuse and Benedictine, which contain coriander as a flavouring.[89]

Cymbopogon citratus (West Indian lemongrass) has been found to be an effective antifungal agent against *Aspergillus fumigatus*, various isolates of *Candida*, and *Trichophyton mentagrophytes*.[80] The most active component of lemongrass is citral (70 to 80 per cent), which is thought to be responsible for the antifungal activity of this plant. In another study, lemongrass was found to be effective against 15 fungi, including *Aspergillus terreus*, *A. flavus*, *A. ochraceus*, *A. parasiticus*, *A. fumigatus*, *A. ustus* and *A. niger* and *Penicillin nigricans*, *P. melin*, *P. chrysogenum*, *P. brevicompactum* and *Fusarium moniliforme*, and *F. oxysporum*.[90] Other plants with a high citral content are melissa, citronella, lemon verbena and *Eucalyptus citriodora*.

Cinnamomum camphora (camphor) was found to be as effective as Ceresan, copper oxychloride and Thiovit (all of which are synthetic, commonly used antifungal agents) against *Aspergillus flavus* – a common spoiler of stored food. However, essential oils of both brown and yellow camphor are contraindicated in human use, as they contain safrole, which is thought to be carcinogenic. White camphor may be used with caution.

Research from India shows that a great many Indian essential oils have antifungal properties.[91] Although these essential oils are not readily available, they can often be specially ordered from some of the leading essential oils distributors.

- *Piper longum* is a climbing shrub with heart-shaped leaves, and berries that fuse together to form spike-like cylindrical cones. The essential oil is pale green with an odour somewhere between that of black pepper and ginger. It is effective against *Candida albicans*.[18]
- *Ocimum sanctum*, otherwise known as holy basil, has a strong odour of cloves and contains 71 per cent eugenol, which has antifungal properties.
- *Trachyspermum ammi* (ajowan), which resembles the parsley plant although it has a totally different smell, is used in India to treat intestinal problems. The essential oil has a high thymol content and is used in Indian medicine to treat cholera as well as fungal infections.[18]

Melaleuca cajeputi (cajuput) was found to be effective against *Candida albicans* in a collaborative study between the Czech Republic and Vietnam.[92] The cajuput tree grows to a height of 45 feet. Its resilience has caused it to be something of an unwanted visitor in some parts of of the Far East, where it appears to resist burning and cutting. The principal constituent of the oil is cineole. Traditionally it has been used in Vietnamese medicine to treat skin diseases and lice and fleas.[18]

Origanum majorana (sweet marjoram) was shown to be effective against *Aspergillus niger* in research carried out in England in 1990.[93] It was also found to be effective, although to a lesser extent, against *Aspergillus flavus*, *A. ochraceus*, *A. parasiticus* and *Trichoderma viride*. *Candida albicans* was also inhibited by 21 different *Eucalyptus* species in a study by Faouzi, published in 1993.[94]

Lippia alba, which grows widely in Central and South America, has been shown to have strong antifungal activity against *Trichophyton mentagrophyes* var. *interdigitale* and *Candida albicans*. As several chemotypes of the plant exist, the essential oil from *Aruba* was thought to be most suitable as it contains 64 per cent citral.[95] *Lippia citriodoral* (lemon verbena) contains 30 to 35 per cent citral.

Melaleuca alternifolia (tea tree) has been shown to be very effective in the treatment of *Candida albicans*. In a study conducted by Belaiche, it was shown that deep nail infections (which are usually notoriously difficult to treat) responded well to tea tree. In all eight patients treated, mycosic degeneration stopped. In two of the cases the infective nail fell off but the regrowth was healthy. In the other six cases the nail changed colour. This effect disappeared as the regrowth progressed. Professor Belaiche noted that this has not been observed with any other antifungal agents. Another important facet of the study was that the treatment was pain-free and the skin appeared to be very tolerant of this method of treatment.[87]

Eugenia aromatica (clove) was shown to have fungicidal action at 0.4 per cent dilution against *Candida albicans* according to a study published in 1989.[96] In a study by Dube *et al.*, 22 species of fungi, including *Aspergillus*, were inhibited by the essential oil of *Ocimum basilicum* (basil).[97]

Melissa officinalis (lemon balm) was 100 per cent effective against *Candida albicans* in a study in 1991.[85] Melissa contains 30 per cent citral and 39 per cent citronella.[98] Finally, *Apium graveolens* (celery) and *Cuminum cyminum* (cumin) used together were effective in inhibiting the growth of 29 fungi tested, including *Aspergillus flavus* and *A. parasiticus*.

These are just a few examples of the hundreds of research studies (most of them conducted *in vitro*) carried out over the last few years on the antifungal properties of essential oils. Could using essential oils for their antifungal properties be seen to be part of our nursing brief? This is a difficult question to answer, as many of the essential oils mentioned above are not used for their antifungal properties (although they may have this therapeutic effect).

What happens if a patient likes the smell of melissa, for example, and the nurse has chosen melissa for its soothing and sedative effects? Together the nurse and the patient decide on an acceptable method of application. A daily foot massage is chosen and added to the nursing care plan. The patient is suffering from a fungal infection which appears to subside following a number of foot massages with melissa. Although the nurse has not been using melissa for its antifungal properties, she cannot stop melissa from working in this way. One could argue that this is acceptable. But what if the nurse *had* known about the antifungal properties and had chosen melissa primarily because of them? Would the nurse have overstepped her role? The International Council of Nurses states that, as nurses, 'our fundamental responsibility is to conserve life, to alleviate suffering and to promote health'.[99] Could using aromatherapy in this way be seen to be alleviating suffering?

Parasites

Temperate countries such as England do not have such a problem with parasites as their southern equivalents, where bilharzia and malaria can be endemic. Nevertheless, there *are* some parasites in northern climates which cause parasitic infections such as *Trichomonas vaginalis* (which causes vaginitis) and other amoebas which cause dysentery-like symptoms. Perhaps more common are infestations by worms (both roundworms and tapeworms) and lice, ticks and fleas.

Although several aromatherapy books suggest that various essential oils have anthelmintic properties which would be suitable for the removal of intestinal worms, very little research data is available. Currently, clinical trials are being completed on *Artemisia annua*. *In-vitro* trials using isolated biologically active substances (artemisinin and quinghaosu) obtained from this species of *Artemisia*, have shown them to have pronounced antimalarial properties.[100–103]

Because essential oils are absorbed into the blood system through the skin, oral administration is not always necessary for the treatment of parasites. Indeed, several of my students have used essential oils topically to kill sea-lice and remove the itching and erythema which accompanies infestations of this kind. The essential oil that they used was *Lavandula angustifolia* (true lavender), either undiluted or in 5 per cent dilution. The effect was 'almost instant'.

Eucalyptus citriodora (lemon-scented gum) has been found to be antiparasitic both for amoeba and for worms *in vitro*.[104,105] *Eucalyptus globulus* has been found to be effective against amoeba.

American wormseed (*Chenopodium ambrosioides* L. var. *anthelminticum*) has a long history of use among North American Indians, who used it to dispel all worms and parasites from the intestine. Sometimes called Jerusalem oak, the seeds from this plant produce an effective essential oil which has been used for hundreds of years and appears to be safe enough for children.[106] Grieve writes that this variety of *Chenopodium* is an effective remedy for hookworm and roundworm and was listed in the official *American Pharmacopoeia*.[107] However, there is often confusion between *Chenopodium ambrosioides* L. var. *anthelminticum* and *Chenopodium botrys* L., which contains a much higher percentage of ascaridole and can cause fatalities.

Wormseed lavant (*Artemisia cina*) also has a long history of use dating back to Dioscorides. Its anthelmintic action is thought to be caused by santonin, which accumulates in the flower-heads. It is an effective agent against roundworms and, to a lesser extent, against threadworms, but has no effect on tapeworms. Side-effects include vision disturbances which produce a yellow tinge to the world. There are three wormwoods, (common, sea and Roman) which belong to the genus *Artemisia*, which also includes tarragon, itself thought to be an anthelmintic.[108] All three (*Artemisia absinthium*, *Artemisia maritima* and *Artemisia pontica*) possess anthelmintic properties.

Spigelia marylandica (wormseed) is another North American plant used as a vermifuge. It was adopted by orthodox medicine in the nineteenth century.[20] However, this plant should not be confused with *Spigelia toxifera*, which contains a high percentage of the alkaloids strychnine and brucine, and was formerly used to make poison arrows by warring tribes.[20]

Thymus vulgaris (common thyme) and *Matricaria recutitia* (German chamomile) are traditionally thought to be effective against hookworms. In Mexico coconut milk is a common treatment for intestinal parasites.

Tea tree and lavender (either *Lavandula latifolia* or *L. angustifolia*) are common essential oils used to treat lice, ticks and fleas. They can also be safely used on children and animals (it is best to use tea tree diluted, as undiluted tea tree in cuts or scratches stings badly). Nelly Grosjean suggests geranium, sage or lavender for lice.[109] *Tagetes minuta* (marigold) was reported to have anthelmintic properties by Lawless.[108] Tisserand suggests the use of bergamot, chamomile, camphor, eucalyptus, fennel, hyssop, lavender, melissa or peppermint.[110] Valnet suggests all of the above, plus cajuput, caraway, cinnamon, clove, lemon, niaouli, savory, tarragon and thyme.[22] For the treatment of ticks, Lawless suggests sweet marjoram. For lice, she suggests cinnamon, eucalyptus (blue gum), geranium, spike lavender, Scotch pine, rosemary or thyme.

Whilst some of the above essential oils are difficult to obtain, or their use may be controversial, perhaps medicine should look closely at essential oils and their potential use as antiparasitic agents. Specifically, in the tropics or Third World countries where orthodox drugs are perhaps expensive and difficult to obtain, essential oils might bring some relief. I agree that, although the information provided here suggests that the essential oils mentioned could have antiparasitic effects, there is no guarantee of this. We need proper clinical trials.

Cross-infection

No discussion of infection would be complete without mentioning cross-infection. Although this might come under the heading of 'hospital-acquired infections', cross-infection can occur anywhere outside a hospital. It can become rampant in institutions or buildings, especially those which have a closed air-conditioning unit. Cross-infection includes bacterial, viral, fungal or protozoan infections.

In a study designed to investigate which essential oils would purify and deodorize the air, vaporized essential oils were observed for their capacity to destroy bacteria such as *Proteus*, *Staphylococcus aureus*, and *Streptococcus pyogenes*. It was found that 90 per cent of microbes were destroyed within 3 hours. The oils found to be most effective were clove, lavender, lemon, marjoram, mint, niaouli, pine, rosemary and thyme.[111]

In another study, six essential oils of *Artemisia*, *Coridothymus capitatus* and *Eucalyptus globulus* were tested against 16 resistant bacteria, with excellent results.[41] Perhaps essential oils could be studied for their potential role in antisepsis in operating theatres.

Finally, 'new' plants and thus 'new' essential oils are being discovered every week. The latest in the haul of nature's cornucopia are manuka and kanuka – the Maori answer to the Aboriginal tea tree. So far, both species of the *Leptospermum* genus look extremely promising in terms of their action against bacteria and fungi. Indeed, the *Cawthron Report Number 263*, published in September 1994, has led to clinical trials being run as this book is being written.[112]

PAIN

There are many possible causes of pain. A simple headache can have dozens of predisposing factors, ranging from low blood sugar, to hormonal imbalance or eye strain, to a brain tumour. In orthodox medicine we tend to treat all headaches initially in the same way, by taking an analgesic.

Pain is an emotional issue because it is so intensely personal. Whereas inflammation seems an acceptable reason for pain because it can be seen, often pain is hidden in some deep dark place, only accessible to the sufferer. Pain sufferers frequently feel guilty that somehow they should be able to bear their pain better.

Pain is closely linked to feelings. Many chronic pain suffererers talk of helplessness or vulnerability. Goleman writes that 'humanity is most evident in our feelings'.[113] Feelings such as despair and anxiety are known to heighten pain, and pleasure and relaxation appear to decrease pain. It is difficult to relax and feel pleasure unaided when one is in pain. It is all too easy to feel despair and anxiety. Changing one's perception of pain can be difficult. Pain sufferers need help to alter their feelings. Aromatherapy enables patients to get 'in touch with' feelings of relaxation and pleasure through smell and touch. These can facilitate the parasympathetic response, allowing patients to relax and 'let go' of their pain as much as possible.

Topical applications of dilute essential oils in the form of a compress or gentle massage can draw attention either to the site of the pain or away from it, depending on what the nurse feels will most help the patient's psychological need.

Pain is one of the most commonly addressed symptoms in a clinical setting. A survey of 2000 relatives of recently deceased cancer patients, carried out in 1994, showed that 88 per cent of those patients had experienced chronic and often severe pain before they died.[114] The author of this UK study concluded that hospital patients frequently did not obtain adequate pain relief in hospital, and went on to quote Ilora Finlay, chairman of the Association of Palliative Medicine, who said that 'narcotics are often so tightly controlled in hospitals that staff cannot get them when their patients most need them'. Perhaps the answer lies with patient-controlled analgesia (PCA), but with each device costing £2000, it will be a long time before every patient in need will have access to such a system.

People who live with pain on a daily basis have (what is to them) a clear way of describing what they feel. If the pain changes, they know it. However, describing pain to someone who does not experience it is subjective, and can pose a problem. Descriptions of pain vary greatly. Apart from the site of the pain (e.g. abdominal), one of the most important aspects to consider is the onset of pain. This onset clarifies which pain system is conveying the message of pain to the brain.

It is thought that there are two different pain systems.[115] It is important to state this, as only one system is particularly affected by opiates (or aromatherapy). More recently, a third system of pain has been identified.[116] This 'third' system is where disease or injury triggers crossed wires within the nervous system which stimulate the production of chemicals that encourage nerve growth. The crossed wires end up linking new nerve fibres which carry everyday messages of touch and pressure, triggering bouts of unpredictable and inexplicable pain.

The *fast pain system*, i.e. pain of sudden onset, is characteristically described by the patient as stabbing, cutting and well localized. This type of pain is not usually significantly affected by opiates. Fast pain is conducted via the oligosynaptic ascending system (OAS), which is closely associated with the primary somatic sensory system that mediates pressure and touch.

The *slow pain system* is commonly described as burning, aching pain, and is perceived to be in a more generalized area. This system uses a pathway known as the multi-synaptic ascending system, which is more complicated and tortuous and involves substance P (a peptide). Slow pain is thought to belong to an older pain system than fast pain, and the pain experienced via this system *is* usually blocked by opiates.[115] In fact, the body itself produces enkephalin, a penta-peptide that occurs in two forms, namely met-enkephalin and leu-enkephalin. These, together with endorphins (or brain opioids) are produced by the body in response to pain. Because aromatherapy works on the sensory system and appears to enhance the parasympathetic response, which is closely linked with endorphins,[117] it is thought that the slow pain system is the one in which aromatherapy might be most beneficial to patients.

Acute pain is associated with a sudden event which will end, e.g. renal colic or labour. Chronic pain goes on and on, and may not be associated with only one system of the body. Chronic pain is further divided into malignant pain (the pain produced by cancer) and non-malignant pain. We could try to clarify the situation even further, talking about superficial, intermediate and deep levels of pain, but not many patients are able to be this precise about where exactly the pain is located.

The intensity and depth of pain is influenced by external factors such as previous experience, attitude and culture. Some cultures are trained to tolerate levels of pain which would be intolerable in the West, so to some degree pain can be affected by mind. According to the *gate theory*, both skin receptors and the neural gate work in tandem. If one is not operational, pain is not felt. In other words, pain is not felt if the 'gate' to the brain receptors is closed by mental attitude. This theory explains why rubbing a hurt area, which will stimulate the critical fibres and close the gate, stops the sensation of pain.[115]

Pain is a warning system. By deadening it we lose our warning system. A headache pill does not make the cause of the headache go away – it merely allows us to carry on functioning.

Orthodox pain relief

All nurses know that analgesics are divided into narcotics and non-narcotics; narcotics are those in Schedule IV and in the Dangerous Drugs Act (DDA). Originally they were all opiate derivatives and all came from the plant *Papaver somniferum*. Recent advances in pharmacology have resulted in the development of several synthetic painkillers which have opiate-like effects. These reduce the perception of pain by acting on the opioid receptors in the brain. As mentioned above, opioids are not successful in treating fast pain.

Narcotic/opiate drugs

Morphine is possibly the most common analgesic in this category. Derived from the opium poppy, morphine works by depressing the cerebral cortex, resulting in reduced powers of concentration as well as reduced pain. However, the respiratory and cough centres are also depressed by morphine, as is the neurotransmitter, acetylcholine. *Cananga odorata* var. *genuina* (ylang ylang) is purported to have opiate-like properties, and can be used to enhance the effect of opiate drugs.

Codeine is another popular but milder narcotic, also derived from the phenanthrene series of the opium poppy.[118] Codeine is frequently used to suppress dry coughs or for the relief of general pain. Morphine, codeine and opiate-like drugs are addictive, although they are less likely to be addictive for someone in severe or chronic pain. Such a patient's chances of addiction then fall to 1 in 3000.[114] One of the side-effects of opiates is constipation. However, despite their side-effects, narcotic drugs have an extremely important role to play in health care.

Common non-opiate/narcotic drugs

There are two important drugs in this category.

- Aspirin (acetylsalicylic acid), as well as having anti-inflammatory effects, is a recognized analgesic. Originally this analgesic was derived from herbs (from *salacin*, a glycoside found in willow tree bark). Aspirin blocks prostaglandin synthesis in the central nervous system (CNS) and peripheral nervous system.
- Paracetamol (acetaminophen) is a painkiller that has no anti-inflammatory effects because it blocks prostaglandin synthesis only in the CNS.[73]

Chronic pain syndrome

This has been described as one of the most complex emotional, financial, social and physical dysfunctions, and is extremely difficult to treat. Orthodox medicine treats it with a mixture of opiate and non-opiate drugs backed up with tricyclics or Valium-type drugs which are not antidepressants, although they are used for that purpose in this instance. However, it is commonly recognized that touch, relaxation and pleasure play an important part in determining how we perceive our circumstances, and that includes pain.[119] Aromatherapy massage is exceedingly gentle, and is in fact very different from classic massage.

The gentle application of diluted essential oils in sequenced movements is known to be extremely relaxing. The odour of the essential oils is pleasurable. So already, not even taking into account the possibility that any essential oil might have analgesic properties, aromatherapy could play an important role in the management of pain, including chronic pain syndrome.

Essential oils with analgesic effects

Two thousand years ago, man used the plants *Salix* (willow) or *Populus* (poplar) to cure his pain.[20] Although Gatefosse states in his book that 'almost all essential oils have analgesic properties',[120] some give more pain relief than others. So, too, does the manner of giving them, touch in this case being an excellent medium.

Analgesic essential oils include the following:

- lemongrass;
- rosemary;
- frankincense;
- juniper;
- rose;
- ginger;
- verbena;
- spike lavender;
- peppermint;
- myrrh;
- clove bud;
- ylang ylang;
- true lavender;
- sweet marjoram;
- black pepper.

Lemongrass has a direct analgesic effect similar to that of peripheral-acting opiates.[121] In one paper by Lorenzetti, lemongrass (*Cymbopogon citratus*) was found to have an analgesic effect on a peripheral area, not on the CNS, which was remarkable as the essential oil was administered orally. The analgesic effects did not lead to tolerance over a period of 5 days (which would have occurred with a narcotic). The isolated component was myrcene, a terpene which is found in a number of essential oils, e.g. rosemary, frankincense, juniper, rose, ginger and verbena,[122] all of which have traditional analgesic qualities. The paper concludes by suggesting that terpenes should be investigated with a view to the 'possibility of developing a new class of analgesic' with myrcene as the prototype.

The idea that terpenes may have analgesic properties is repeated in Price's latest book and in Franchomme's textbook,[19] paracymene being quoted by Price.[72] Cymene is found in lemon, angelica, frankincense, eucalyptus and sweet marjoram. Paracymene is found in thyme and cumin, and the methyl ether, p-cymene-8-ol, is found in black pepper. However, terpenes occur in almost all essential oils, so it is difficult to separate their actions.

Ginger (*Zingiber officinale*) is a classic peripheral analgesic essential oil possibly because of its topical rubefacient effect. Gingerol, one of the components of ginger, is traditionally thought to provide the analgesic effects, although gingerol does not occur in the essential oil.[123]

Jeanne Rose lists benzoin, camphor, clove, coriander, ginger, hops, lemongrass, marjoram, black pepper, pine, savory and ylang ylang as being analgesics.[124] Price mentions white birch, chamomile, frankincense, wintergreen, clove, lavender and mint in the text. However, wintergreen and white birch are contraindicated due to their toxicity – they both contain a large amount of methyl salicylate.[79] Franchomme lists Roman chamomile, ylang ylang and mandarin as being useful in the treatment of pain.[19]

A review of clinical research into the mixture *Oleum spica* showed it to be an effective analgesic. *Oleum spica* contains 1 part spike lavender to 4 parts of turpentine. It is thought that the analgesic effect of turpentine is enhanced by the presence of spike lavender.[125]

Peppermint was the subject of a study on headaches in 1994. Pain was induced in healthy humans using pressure, thermal and ischaemic stimuli. The intensity of the pain, neurophysiology, performance-related activity and mood states were monitored. Peppermint diluted in ethanol and applied topically produced a significant analgesic effect.[126] In another paper, the analgesic properties of *Mentha rotundifolia* and *Mentha longifolia* are cited by Perez Raya *et al.*[127]

During the pre-Christian era myrrh was given to provide pain relief to those about to be crucified.[128] Myrrh contains terpenes, esters and a phenol called eugenol, reputed to be an analgesic.[19] Eugenol is found in West Indian Bay (*Pimenta racemosa*) with myrcene, and in clove (*Syzygium aromaticum*). It is important that it is clove bud oil (which also contains esters) and not the leaf or stem which is used. Clove oil can cause skin and mucous membrane irritation, and should be used with care.

Borneol (an alcohol) and myrcene (a terpene) were found to be effective antagonists of acetylcholine in a study by Cabo *et al*. This study was conducted on isolated duodenum to counter contractile tissue.[129] Acetylcholine is a central and peripheral nervous system transmitter.[130]

Artemisia caerulescens was found to have an analgesic effect on rats in a study published in 1989.[131]

Some pain is caused by muscle spasm. Several essential oils have antispasmodic effects. Esters belong to the group of components thought to produce this therapeutic effect. Franchomme writes that the greater the number of different esters, the greater the antispasmodic effect.[132] Roman chamomile has more esters than any other essential oil (up to 310), including esters from angelic and tiglic acid (Roman chamomile is also a recognized analgesic).[123]

Antispasmodic essential oils include the following:

- *Chamaemelum nobile* (Roman chamomile);[19]
- *Citrus aurantium* var. *amara* (petitgrain);[133]
- *Eucalyptus citriodora* (lemon-scented eucalyptus);
- *Salvia officinalis* (sage).[134,135]

Sometimes, in cases of arthritic pain, heat can help. If this is the case, there are essential oils which have rubefacient effects. The following essential oils have this property:

- *Piper nigrum* (black pepper);
- *Zingiber officinale* (ginger).

It is important to allow your patients to smell the mixture before you apply it – they will have to live with it, after all! Be very gentle and slow. Allowing someone actually to touch a painful area takes courage, and that courage needs to be rewarded with respect. All of the essential oils mentioned (with the possible exception of sage) are safe to use for relief of pain. Make a 1 to 5 per cent solution with a carrier oil, and gently apply to the area, or add 1 to 5 drops to a bowl of warm water, wring the compress out and apply it to the painful area.

Finally, the pain experienced by patients with sickle cell anaemia (SCA), an inherited disease, may be relieved with an essential oil. *Pelargonium graveolens* (geranium) has been used successfully to revert sickled cells *in vitro*.[136] It is thought that the active parts of *Pelargonium* are quercetin and kaemferol (flavonoids). Fennel has also been shown to reverse sickling.[137]

There is no suggestion that essential oils should be used instead of conventional analgesia. However, topical applications of dilute essential oils might enhance orthodox analgesia either through the placebo response, through the effect of touch and smell on the parasympathetic nervous system, or because of pharmacologically active ingredients within the essential oils which may have an analgesic effect.

Despite the fact that there have been few clinical trials, perhaps there is still sufficient evidence to suggest that essential oils might have a role in augmenting conventional analgesia. As nurses, part of our job is to alleviate pain and suffering. Perhaps using aromatherapy and selecting one of the essential oils covered in this section might be helpful in the treatment of pain.

NAUSEA AND VOMITING

Nausea and vomiting are symptoms which should be addressed separately, as nausea does not always lead to actual vomiting. However, the causes of nausea are similar to those of vomiting.

Vomiting is activated by the vomiting centre in the brain which triggers nerves supplying the stomach and chest muscles. Vomiting can have numerous causes.

Gastrointestinal causes

These include the following:

- stomach or intestinal irritation, gastro-enteritis;
- appendicitis;
- obstruction;
- hypertrophic pyloric stenosis.

Central nervous system (CNS) causes

These include the following:

- loss of sense of balance due to middle/inner ear trauma, labyrinthitis;
- sensory responses in the brain activated by smell, sight or emotion;
- raised pressure in the brain (due to tumours, haemorrhage, meningitis);
- head injury;
- migraine;
- psychiatric disorder;
- chemoreceptor trigger areas, which respond to either chemicals produced by the body (e.g. kidney, pancreas) or motion sickness.

Metabolic causes

These include the following:

- pregnancy;
- uraemia;
- alcohol;
- chemoreceptor trigger areas responding to drugs absorbed by the body.[9]

Orthodox approaches

As the vomiting centre of the brain is stimulated by the neurotransmitter acetylcholine, one of the most direct ways of inhibiting vomiting is to use anticholinergic drugs such as atropine, hyoscyamine or scopolamine. Transdermal scopolamine provides up to 72 hours of anti-emetic treatment. However, long-term use of these drugs can cause side-effects such as poor digestion, dry mouth, blurred vision and constipation.

Antihistamines such as dramamine affect the organ of balance as well as the vomiting centre of the brain. These drugs also have an impact on the chemoreceptor trigger zone (CTZ), as well as blocking the histamine and dopamine receptors. In addition, they inhibit acetylcholine. Antihistamines work by reducing the sensitivity of the vomiting centre to input from the inner ear, although they do not directly affect the inner ear.

The neurochemical that stimulates the chemoreceptor trigger zone (CTZ) is dopamine. Dopamine blockers work by stopping dopamine-mediated transmission, so relieving nausea. This group includes phenothiazines, of which one of the most commonly used is chlorpromazine. (Chlorpromazine is used extensively in psychiatric medicine as a sedative.) Phenothiazines prevent the CTZ from stimulating vomiting. Corticosteroids can help to reduce nausea associated with chemotherapy. Haloperidol and droperidol block stimulation of the CTZ.

Essential oils with anti-emetic properties

Cardamom

Cardamom is listed in the *Indian Materia Medica* as checking vomiting and nausea,[138] and it is one of the oldest essential oils known.[139] It has been reported by Tisserand to relieve nausea.[140] Cardamom contains 50 per cent alpha-terpinyl acetate and 1,8-cineole, with small amounts of borneol, alpha-terpineol and limonene. Borneol was shown to be an effective antagonist of acetylcholine in a study by Cabo,[129] and perhaps it is this compound that imbues cardamom with its anti-emetic property.

Peppermint

Peppermint has been a classic choice for the treatment of nausea for hundreds of years. However, too much peppermint can cause nausea (too much of any essential oil can exacerbate symptoms – only a few drops are needed). Used primarily to treat nausea, rather than actual vomiting, *Mentha piperita* has carminative effects both *in vitro* and *in vivo*. Peppermint also has recognized antispasmodic effects, and in a study of endoscopy spasm, peppermint was found to relieve colonic spasm within 30 seconds.[141]

In another study, patients were given peppermint following colostomies. Among these patients, 18 out of 20 individuals displayed reduced postoperative colic.[142] Valnet states that peppermint is useful for the treatment of nervous vomiting, quoting Trousseau.[22] Franchomme also states that peppermint is an anti-emetic. Peppermint is an active ingredient of babies' gripe-water.

Ginger

Ginger (*Zingiber officinale*) was introduced into Europe in the Middle Ages. The essential oil, which does not smell anything like the dried root or candied ginger, contains zingiberene. In China, ginger is classically given to new mothers following the birth of their children. Although it is often used in the treatment of pain, ginger is a very effective remedy for nausea, either through inhalation or diluted in a foot or hand massage. Ginger is particularly suitable for pregnancy nausea and nausea associated with CNS disturbances.

Clove (*Eugenia caryophyllata*) is listed in Potter's *New Cyclopaedia of Botanical Drugs and Preparations* as an anti-emetic.[123] Trease and Evans suggest that cardamom (which has an antispasmodic action on the gastro-intestinal tract) and peppermint are both suitable as carminatives.[132] Fennel (*Foeniculum vulgare*) and aniseed (*Anethum graveolens*) are also mentioned (more as carminatives than as anti-nausea essential oils).

Acetylcholine-affecting essential oils

In a study investigating the activity of major components of various essential oils of aromatic plants from Granada, borneol and myrcene were found to be active against acetylcholine. In this instance, borneol and myrcene were found in essential oils of *Thymus granatensis* and *Salvia lavendulaefolia* (Spanish sage). The experiment was carried out with isolated duodenum.

However, if these components of essential oils display anti-acetylcholine activity, it would be logical to try other essential oils which contain these compounds in order to provide relief from nausea and to inhibit vomiting. Myrcene and borneol are found in many essential oils.

Borneol (an alcohol) is found in the following:

- *Lavandula angustifolia*   True lavender
- *Lavandula x intermedia*   Lavandin
- *Lavandula latifolia*   Spike lavender
- *Rosmarinus officinalis*   Rosemary
- *Boswellia carterii*   Frankincense
- *Pinus sylvestris*   Scots pine
- *Origanum majorana*   Sweet marjoram
- *Cananga odorata*   Ylang ylang
- *Juniperus communis*   Juniper

Myrcene (a terpene) is found in the following:

- *Boswellia carterii*   Frankincense
- *Piper nigrum*   Black pepper
- *Juniperus communis*   Juniper
- *Rosa damascena*   Rose
- *Melaleuca alternifolia* Tea tree
- *Origanum majorana*   Sweet marjoram
- *Pinus sylvestris*   Scots pine

All of the above essential oils would be safe to use in clinical aromatherapy, with a precaution on the use of rosemary and spike lavender, which are both stimulants and therefore contraindicated in hypertension. My students have recently completed an informal study of nausea using ginger and peppermint, and found that patients tended to prefer one or the other of these. The essential oil that the patient preferred was more effective against their nausea and vomiting than the one that they did not like. This highlights the importance of learned memory and involving the patient in choosing their oils. The method of choice would usually be inhalation. However, a gentle tummy rub can be very beneficial to a child or anxious patient who is more sick with worry than nauseous for physical reasons.

INFLAMMATION

Inflammation is the body's defensive response to infection, trauma or occasionally, allergic reaction. This response produces changes in the tissue if the injury or infection does not cause death of the affected part. As such, inflammation is a fundamentally protective mechanism,[143] and has been called 'the most important of the body's defence mechanisms'.[1] Derived from the Latin, '*inflammare*', meaning 'to burn', the function of inflammation is to restore the body to normal functioning as quickly as possible.

Inflammation can be either acute (of sudden onset, e.g. as with a contusion or around a fracture) or chronic (when the tissue granulates).

There are specific and well-recognized symptoms of acute inflammation. These are redness, swelling, heat and pain. These symptoms are further listed by Mills in *Out of the Earth* as 'rubor', 'tumor', 'calor' and 'dolor'.[144] A further state of *functio laeso* (loss of function) is added in *Modern Pharmacology*.[145] The redness and heat are caused by increased vascular flow and permeability, as the blood flow increases by up to tenfold during the first 15 minutes. The swelling and pain result from the escape of leucocytes from blood vessels into the tissue, taking with them oedema fluid and fibrin. This protective fluid mixture has a high content of plasma proteins (35–50 g/l).

The leucocytes that are predominant during the first 24 hours are neutrophils. Their role is to remove insoluble tissue debris, either by enzyme action or by phagocytosis.

Whilst it is dependent on the site of inflammation, the acute response by the body is essentially beneficial. The damaged cells are readily supplied with nutrients, any toxins present are diluted, antibodies arrive quickly at the scene and protective fibrin is produced together with plasma to maintain the response. In the case of inflammation caused by infection, the immune response occurs within a few days and can be maintained for several years.

However, if it occurs in a site such as the trachea, acute inflammation can be serious. A child's stridor is indicative of inflamed mucous membrane. This is acute inflammation and requires rapid hydration with steam. A wasp-sting in the neck could produce an acute inflammation due to allergic reaction which would need much more than steam.

Chronic inflammation occurs when the response continues for months, becoming counter-productive to health at the tissue level. Inflammation and repair occur at the same time. Viewed histologically, difference lies in greater tissue destruction and fewer neutrophils. There is also greater production of fibrous tissue. Chronic inflammation occurs:

- when there is a foreign body at the site, such as a splinter;
- in certain diseases, such as TB, leprosy, and brucellosis;
- in autoimmune diseases.

Inflamed systems of the body are referred to by specific names, e.g. bronchitis, salpingitis, neuritis, dermatitis (all names end in '-itis').

Orthodox treatment

Conventional medicine has proved to be life-saving in many acute inflammatory conditions, especially those connected with acute allergic response. However, chronic inflammation does not respond well (in the long term) to the synthetic medicines available.

Anti-inflammatory drugs are usually aspirin- or steroid-based, both of which cause problems with long-term use. However, on a short-term basis they ease the pain and discomfort which is basically all they can do (they treat the symptoms, not the cause of those symptoms). However, they are without doubt extremely helpful in alleviating suffering and are widely used. A further group of drugs blocks the production of prostaglandins, so reducing the level of inflammation, but again not addressing the cause. Non-steroidal anti-inflammatory drugs (NSAIDs) can be purchased over the counter, and are to be found in most homes. Many, but not all, are aspirin-based. Aspirin is an NSAID, but it also blocks prostaglandin synthesis. The others work like aspirin but are not based on that drug structurally.

Corticosteroid drugs are particularly effective in conditions in which eosinophils and lymphocytes predominate as the inflammatory cells.[145] Sometimes antihistamine or immunosuppressant drugs are given.

Adverse effects of some anti-inflammatory drugs

Goodman-Gilma listed the undesirable side-effects of anti-inflammatory drugs in 1985 in his standard textbook.[146] It may be helpful to divide these further into the two main categories, namely non-steroidal and steroidal.

NSAIDs

At present the action of non-steroidal anti-inflammatory drugs is not fully understood. The most likely hypothesis is that they somehow inhibit the production of prostaglandins, as it has been shown that prostaglandins of the E and F series are capable of evoking local and systemic inflammation. However, the actual inhibition of prostaglandin synthesis can give rise to specific side-effects.

All NSAIDs, including aspirin-based (salicylic acid) anti-inflammatories, can increase gastric bleeding in patients with gastric ulcers, due to the inhibition of prostaglandin PGE2, which suppresses gastric acid secretion. They can also prolong bleeding, due to the inhibition of thromboxane 2. They can upset the fluid balance, decreasing excretion due to inhibition of renal blood flow. They can cause bronchospasm and nasal polyposis in susceptible individuals, and they can delay the onset of labour due to loss of contractile effects of prostaglandins on the uterine muscles.[147] Indomethacin is often used when salicylates are not tolerated. However, in arthritic patients, they can lead to a high incidence of CNS effects if the dose is extremely high.

Phenylbutazone-like drugs can cause gastro-intestinal irritation, hepatitis, vertigo and headaches. With prolonged usage, they can also depress the bone marrow, leading to leukaemia and aplastic anaemia.[145]

Steroid-based anti-inflammatory drugs

Despite being superior in effect to NSAIDs (and affecting the inflammatory process at each level), steroid-based anti-inflammatory drugs can also have many side-effects, and as a long-term treatment they are not to be recommended. Most doctors will agree that they should be avoided if possible.

The side-effects of long-term treatment can include hyperglycaemia leading to diabetes, myopathy, increased intra-ocular pressure with the potential for glaucoma, electrolyte imbalance leading to hypertension, thinning of the skin with an increased tendency for poor healing and skin breakdown, hirsutism, insomnia, depression and psychosis.[145] Despite this, these drugs have provided both relief and release for many sufferers of chronic inflammatory conditions, and will continue to be used until other drugs with fewer side-effects are found.

Other orthodox treatments

Gold should be mentioned here. Now infrequently used, it was a common treatment for rheumatoid arthritis in the 1970s. The majority of gold applications were given intramuscularly as, except in the case of auranofin, gold is poorly absorbed through the digestive tract. There was evidence that inflamed joints accumulated twice as much gold as non-inflamed joints, and that gold in some way inhibited certain lysosomal enzymes which were involved in the inflammation process. Fatalities due to gold treatment have been reported.[145]

Anti-inflammatory essential oils

In an Italian paper published in 1987, 75 species of plant were selected, based on medicinal folklore, and their extracts were investigated for possible therapeutic effects on inflammation.[148] The experiments were performed on rats with carrageenan-induced foot oedema. The control drug was indomethacin, a commonly used NSAID. Herbal extracts (not essential oils) from the plants were administered orally. However, many of the plants selected also produce essential oils which are used for anti-inflammatory purposes in aromatherapy.

This is an interesting study, not only because some of the herbs were more effective than the control, *but also because the route of choice was oral*. In aromatherapy, if an inflamed joint is being treated, a dermal application would be the route of choice. Why lose vital effects due to first-pass metabolism in the liver if this is not entirely necessary? Although it is recognized that much less essential oil is absorbed through the skin, the effects of the essential oils are being directly applied to the inflamed area.

Many of the plants tested produce essential oils which are regularly used in aromatherapy. *Coriandrum sativum* (coriander), *Foeniculum vulgare* (fennel) and *Juniperus communis* (juniper) all produced 45 per cent inhibition, comparable with the control. These essential oils are all used to treat anti-inflammatory conditions.[89] However, aromatherapists would apply the essential oils directly to the inflamed area. In the case of internal inflammation, inhalation or application to the skin would still allow the essential oil to reach the internal inflamed part. Only in the case of intestinal inflammation is oral application considered. Several clinical trials have shown that essential oils are absorbed through the skin, with 70 per cent of the oil being absorbed within 24 hours.[149] Blood levels may remain low because the essential oils will be continually eliminated.

Roman chamomile (*Anthemis nobilis*) was the focus of a comparative study in 1988. Again the study was performed on rats with carrageenan-induced oedema, and again the control was indomethacin, only this time three essential oils of chamomile were used. White-headed double-flowered chamomile flowers showed a greater anti-inflammatory action than the yellow-flowered variety. Nevertheless, all three essential oils of Roman chamomile produced significant anti-inflammatory effects. In this study the chamomile was given subcutaneously into the peritoneal cavity.[150]

Jakovlev demonstrated the anti-inflammatory effect of German chamomile, and suggested that the antiphlogistic effects were due to bisabolol and bisabolol oxides.[151] In another study, when German chamomile (*Matricaria recutita*) was applied topically to mouse ears, with hydrocortisone as the control, the chamomile showed an anti-inflammatory action, although the effect was only half as strong as that of the steroid.[152]

Turmeric (*Curcuma longa*) is a less well-known essential oil, but none the less used in cases of arthritic inflammation. Due to the fact that it contains a high level of tumerone, a ketone, Lawless suggests that it should be used only for limited periods,[89] although in their latest *Safety Data Manual* Tisserand and Balacs note that there is no oral or dermal toxicity.[79]

Nutmeg (*Myristica fragrans*) may have been the inspiration for Nostradamus and his prophesies, but it also has proven anti-inflammatory activities which are attributed to the activity of eugenol, one of the main constituents of nutmeg. In a study published in 1988, the greatest effect was observed after 4 hours, and was comparable to the effects of phenylbutazone and indomethacin.[153]

In a German study, various essential oils were screened which had traditionally been used in the treatment of inflammation. It was concluded that eugenol, eugenyl acetate, thymol, capsaicin, curcumin and carvacrol were present in most of the essential oils, and that antiphlogistic effects were closely linked to the vascular reaction of early inflammation. In herbal medicine this is called the counter-irritant effect. In this study, clove and cinnamon had the strongest effect. Dwarf pine (*Pinus mugo* var. *pumilo*) and eucalyptus (*Eucalyptus aetherolum*) oil also had a mild effect.[154] *Matricaria aetherolum* had a weak anti-inflammatory effect.

Traditionally, aromatherapists have used many essential oils to treat inflammatory conditions. In Shirley Price's *Aromatherapy for Health Professionals*, she lists 28 essential oils, ranging from the common ones such as *Lavandula angustifolia* (true lavender) to *Boswellia carterii* (frankincense) and *Pogostemon patchouli* (patchouli).[72] Sylla Sheppard-Hanger lists 66 essential oils.[122] Jeanne Rose lists just nine oils[124] and Patricia Davis suggests only three oils, namely chamomile, myrrh and lavender.

Whatever the preference of the aromatherapist (who will not be addressing merely the inflammation, but also the whole package that the patient represents), essential oils can and do play an important role as anti-inflammatories. After thousands of years of use, perhaps we should give them a try.

Contraindications

Of the essential oils suggested above, cumin, lavender, chamomile (both German and Roman), juniper, turmeric, patchouli and myrrh are non-toxic in topical application. Frankincense is very mildly irritant to the skin, and fennel is moderately irritant to the skin. All of the essential oils were tested at concentrations of 1 to 30 per cent. When fennel was used at 4 per cent dilution, no skin sensitization was observed.

INSOMNIA

Today's society is a fast-moving, achievement-oriented one in which thousands of people travel daily, many across time zones. Regularity and sleep patterns are constantly disturbed as new sounds and unfamiliar surroundings compound the sense of timelessness caused by continuous movement. Sleep has become a commodity to be bought and sold.

Patients in hospitals are separated from everything that makes them relaxed and sleepy, in a strange bed, with a strange routine, and a sense of fear. It is hardly surprising that sleeping pills are almost *de rigueur*. However, perhaps there could be another way, especially in the case of long-stay patients who take sleeping tablets regularly.

Sleepless nights can affect us all at some time in our lives. Trauma, worries and jet lag can all cause insomnia. However, repeated sleepless nights result in a poor attention span and, ultimately, in poor health, both physical and mental.

Sleep is defined as an 'altered state of consciousness from which a person can be aroused by stimuli of sufficient magnitude'.[155] Why we sleep is unclear, but this period of 'opting out' is essential for healthy living. Going without sleep produces varying degrees of symptoms, ranging from feeling irritable to psychosis. For a patient in hospital sleep deprivation is just one more stressor.

It is known that sleep occurs in two modes:

- rapid-eye movement sleep (REM), when dreaming occurs;
- orthodox sleep.

Both types of sleep are important. It is believed that sleep may be controlled by a natural chemical called melatonin, which is secreted by the pineal gland. It is possible to buy this compound over the counter as a supplement, although it has recently been banned in the UK.

Insomnia affects almost everyone at some stage in their life, but it is usually transitory, and after the trauma causing the insomnia has passed, normal sleep rhythms return. However, chronic insomnia threatens to destroy normal functioning. This kind of sleep problem can occur in two forms – failure to drift off to sleep, or waking up after a short period of time. Both can be caused by being in a hospital, where strange noises and smells permeate through dreams, or prevent sleep from occurring. A bedtime routine is also very difficult to maintain in hospital.

Sleeping tablets

Orthodox treatment of insomnia involves two types of drugs, namely sedatives (anxiolytics) and sedative-hypnotics. The commonest sleeping tablet is a benzodiazapine (which is both sedative-hypnotic and anxiolytic) such Valium, Ativan or Mogadon. It is known that dependency can occur within weeks.

Benzodiazepines

Benzodiazepines have a basic structure consisting of a benzene ring coupled to a seven-membered heterocyclic structure containing two nitrogen atoms (diazepine) at positions 1 and 4.[156] This molecule binds to specific macromolecules within the central nervous system at receptors closely associated with γ–aminobutyric acid (GABA) transmission. GABA is the main inhibitory neurotransmitter in the brain. Research has indicated that benzodiazepines potentiate GABA transmission.

Benzodiazepines depress the central nervous system, and in low dosages produce a feeling of calmness. As the dose is increased, a feeling of drowsiness is followed by hypnosis and muscle relaxation. The interval between feeling drowsy and potential death through overdose is a large one. Because these drugs have a large therapeutic index they are extremely useful for many patients, although their long-term use can be problematic. Benzodiazepines have almost replaced the previously favourite sleeping pill, which was the barbiturate.

Barbiturates

Barbiturates are used to treat intractable insomnia, and are increasingly rarely prescribed. They, too, bind to receptors associated with GABA transmission. However, this class of drug prolongs rather than intensifies the GABA effect. Pink tablets of soneryl and striped capsules of tuinal, once a regular part of the night drug round, are less common. Public awareness of the dangers of barbiturate dependence was heightened in the 1970s by books such as *Valley of the Dolls*.

Barbiturates have significant drug interactions. Several of the drugs that they react with are in common use, e.g. the contraceptive pill, digoxin, beta-blockers, and anticoagulants. Barbiturates accelerate the metabolism of these drugs, necessitating an increased dosage. In addition, if the patient is on anti-coagulant therapy, when barbiturates are discontinued a dangerous reaction resulting in severe haemorrhage can occur.[156] This type of reaction can also occur with other drugs because the induction of GABA metabolism has stopped.

Essential oils with sedative effects

'Lavender beats Benzodiazepines' was the headline in an aromatherapy journal published in 1988.[157] In this article, the use of essential oils as sedatives, in a hospital setting, was outlined. Of particular note were lavender, marjoram, geranium, mandarin and cardamom. Helen Passant, possibly *the* most holistic nurse after Florence Nightingale, introduced aromatherapy into the Churchill Hospital, Oxford, where she was in charge of a ward for the elderly. Remarkably, Helen reduced her original drug bill by one-third by gradually replacing analgesia and night sedation with essential oils. She found that her patients seemed to 'get off to sleep just as easily, if not better, with oils of lavender or marjoram, either vaporised or applied by massage'.

In the same article another hospital was mentioned. The Radcliffe Infirmary introduced aromatherapy into Beeson Ward at about the same time. Patients were given the option of aromatherapy instead of night sedation or analgesics. Nearly all of the patients chose aromatherapy.

Traditionally, *Lavandula angustifolia* (true lavender) has been used in aromatherapy to promote sleep and relaxation and to relieve anxiety. In 1973, in a paper published in Bulgaria, linalol and terpineol were suggested to be the active components that cause lavender to have a depressing effect on the central nervous system.[158]

That lavender has sedative effects was also the conclusion of a French paper published in 1989. This paper also pointed out that lavender potentized barbiturate sleep time.[159] Although this is a standard test for sedative activity, it could be argued that for a patient on barbiturate medication who also inhaled lavender the effect of the barbiturate would probably be potentized.

A paper published in 1991 substantiated the beliefs of aromatherapists and provided evidence for the sedative effect of true lavender (*Lavandula angustifolia*) when *inhaled* by mice. Interestingly, the more agitated the animal was initially (as a result of the injection of caffeine), the more effective was the calming effect of *Lavandula angustifolia*.[160]

This inhaled sedative effect was replicated with human subjects in a study conducted in Newholme Hospital, Bakewell and published in 1994. In this study, the effects of night-time diffusion of lavender were monitored in a ward of dementia patients. The trial ran for 7 weeks and showed that lavender had a statistically significant sedative effect when inhaled.[161]

Neroli was reported to have sedative properties in a paper published in 1992. In this study, the sedative effects were observed during the first 30 minutes of exposure to the aroma. This study also investigated the sedative effects of citronella and phenylethyl acetate, both of which were found to have sedative properties.[162] Citronella is found in *Citronella*, *Eucalyptus citriodora* and *Eucalyptus radiata*, lemon, rose, melissa, lemongrass, basil and geranium. Phenylethyl acetate is found only in neroli, but phenylethyl alcohol is also found in geranium (bourbon) and rose.[122]

Passiflora incarnata (passionflower) and *Tilia cordata* (lime-blossom) essential oils were reported to have sedative properties in a paper published in 1992. Lime-blossom and its major component, benzyl alcohol, decreased the motility of animals in both normal and induced-agitation states. *Passiflora incarnata* and its main components, maltol and 2-phenylethanol, only reduced motility when the animals were in an agitated state.[163]

Nigella sativa was shown to have a demonstrable sedative effect in a study cited by Balacs. This study demonstrated that the essential oil was more sedating than chlorpromazine (Largactil), and as it was also found to be analgesic, it was proposed that *Nigella sativa* contains an opioid-like component.[164]

Finally, whilst conducting routine toxicity investigations of Tastromine, it was observed that the animals used in the study became sedated.[165] Further investigation revealed that significant central nervous system depressant activity appeared when the basic ethers involved were derived from thymol. Isomers of thymol, namely cavacrol and isothymol, were relatively inactive. It was noted that the structural requirements of morphine-like analgesics were similar to the structure of thymol ether. Thymol is found in thyme, winter savory, sweet marjoram and several essential oils from the Labiatae family.[122]

Most people enjoy the smell of roses. Indeed, rose is perhaps the most popular aroma in the world. Despite the fact that essential oils of rose are very expensive, perhaps the cost is justified where chronic insomnia is concerned. There have been no studies, as yet, which have demonstrated that rose is effective in promoting sleep in humans. However, some studies have shown that *Rosa damascena* (rose) has a sedative effect.[166,167] Certainly my personal experience, as well as that of my students and patients, would suggest that rose is a strong contender and certainly an essential oil to try for the treatment of insomnia.

STRESS MANAGEMENT

It could be argued that, as this is a book about aromatherapy, there is no need to write a section on stress. However, aromatherapy is one of the most effective ways of relieving, avoiding and removing stress, not just for patients, but also for staff and relatives.

There are many definitions and types of stress, but it is generally agreed that the *idea* of stress was conceived by Hans Selye of McGill University in 1935. He was carrying out research on rats and discovered that those which had been injected with various hormonal extracts developed enlarged adrenal glands, shrunken lymphatic glands and bleeding gastro-intestinal ulcers. He called this 'the stress syndrome'.[168]

Further research performed in the 1950s and 1960s by Thomas Holmes and Richard Rahe, both psychiatrists at the University of Washington School of Medicine, showed that the more stress a person experienced, the more likely it was that he or she would fall ill.[169] Holmes and Rahe interviewed over 5000 people and devised what was to become a classic systematized method for correlating the events in people's lives with their illnesses.[170] Until that time it had been assumed that only adverse stress would have a significant effect. However, in the tests carried out by Rahe and Holmes, *any* change in the normal pattern of life was found to produce symptoms of stress.

Today, 'stress' is a modern buzz-word – the cause of all ills which cannot be explained in any other way, even though the meaning of the word is unclear. An article in the *British Medical Journal* called stress a 'chimera' – an unreliable word to be used sparingly.[171]

In the early 1980s a major conference was funded to bring together leading psychologists, immunologists and physicians in Arizona, to discuss stress and to try to define it. After heated debate, it was agreed there was no *absolute* definition of stress. What was agreed was that stress was caused by 'things' outside people. These 'things' were labelled as stressors. It was suggested that people reacted and adapted to stressors differently. Some individuals seemed to be able to cope, while others did not, and there was no way of telling who would cope and who would not.

The conference delegates agreed that stressors had measurable psychological and physiological effects. This was borne out by Cohen's later research on stress and human susceptibility to the common cold,[172] which showed that individuals under stress were more likely to 'catch' a cold than those who were not under stress.

There is a history of knowledge of the anticipated physiological effects of stress in China, where individuals suspected of lying would be forced to chew rice powder and then spit it out. The Chinese believed that the stress of lying would render a person incapable of salivation.[168] Indeed, perhaps this is the origin of the saying 'the dry mouth of fear'.

Selye listed several common stressors as follows.

- *Extreme stimuli – too much or too little of almost anything.* Consider a patient in a hospital, perhaps in a high dependency unit. It is obvious that the patient *is* frequently receiving extreme stimuli in the form of bright lights (no darkness in which to recover) and too much noise (not enough peace).
- *Extreme deficiency, including social deficiency incurred during solitary confinement, blindness, deafness, etc.* We call this sensory deprivation, but some patients are physically isolated when they are barrier-nursed for either their own protection, or that of others. However, it can be argued that there are some patients who are made to feel outsiders to society because of their illness – not just those with AIDS, HIV or hepatitis, but also those patients who are partially paralysed or in a wheelchair. Perhaps a semi-conscious patient would also fit into this category.
- *Stressors are often injurious, unpleasant or painful.* Hospital personnel do not set out to injure their patients in the accepted sense of the word. However, some medical (and nursing) procedures are unpleasant or painful.
- *Stressors are things which an individual perceives to be a threat, whether real or imaginary.* It is well known that many hospital and nursing procedures could be perceived to be threatening, e.g. injections, lumbar punctures.
- *Stress is an intangible phenomenon.* It cannot be tasted, heard, smelled or measured directly.
- *Stressors are individual.* What is stressful today may not be so tomorrow, and what is stressful to one patient may not be so to another.

Some indicators of stress can be easily measured, e.g. blood pressure rise, tachycardia, pupil dilation etc. But how often are they measured for stress? And what do hospital staff do about removing their causes?

Perhaps we should divide stress into that which is necessary for us to survive and that which will eventually make us break down emotionally and physically. Selye divides the physiological response to stressors into three stages: alarm, resistance and exhaustion. We know that our alarm response to certain stressors can be life-saving – the fight or flight phenomenon. Alarm, or acute stress, is vital to our survival, because it gives us the physical ability for flight or fight. Those physiological changes (produced by receptors in the brain) increase our heart-beat and respiration rate.

Unnecessary metabolism, such as digestion, is curbed, while blood and oxygen are swiftly redirected to the more vital centres of the body. This is all to our benefit. Who needs to digest curry when the sabre-toothed tiger is chasing him? However, when the danger is over, the body very quickly returns to its original state. Sweaty, clammy hands and cold feet become warm and dry again. Our respiration and pulse slow down to a more comfortable level, and digestion recommences.

However, as has been pointed out by Dr Peter Nixon, a respected cardiologist, when the stressor continues, it reaches a point of no return. This is called *chronic stress*. Nixon's famous curve (Figure 7.7) indicates when a person under chronic stress would break down.[173] Nixon considers that if you isolate that person and encourage him or her to sleep, you will be removing the stressors and the body will have a chance to mend itself. I was fortunate to see many individuals treated successfully in this way when I worked with his patients in the 1970s.

In chronic stress, the arousal state of a person is never completely ameliorated, and the measurable levels of stress in the body do *not* return to

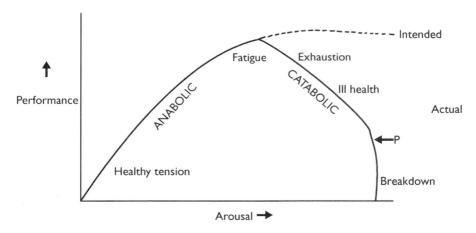

FIGURE 7.7 The human function curve: a performance arousal curve used as a model for a systems or biopsychosocial approach to a clinical problem. Reproduced from Nixon, P.G.F. (1976) The Human Function Curve, *Practitioner* 217: 76: 769, 935–44, with the kind permission of the author.

normal, cortisol levels remaining above average. Over a period of time, discreet but damaging physiological changes occur – blood sugar is raised, blood pressure is raised, hormonal functions change, and digestion and elimination are affected. The effects of chronic stress are frequently produced by psychological stressors, although many of those effects are measurable physiological reactions. Lactate concentrations in the blood have been found to increase in patients with increased levels of psychological stress, producing anxiety neurosis.[174] Barasch has written of prolonged stress causing excessive clotting which can create 'fibrin cocoons' that prevent T-cells from attacking cancerous metastases.[175]

Stress is now recognized as being one of the most serious health issues of the twentieth century, although the work-force still continues to push itself to the limit, often unnecessarily. It is almost as though being stressed is the acceptable face of modern life. No one wants to consider changing their lifestyle. However, stress will win in the end, often forcing us, through breakdown, to alter that which we would not otherwise change.

If a person is unable to 'switch off, either physically or mentally,' they may eventually break down. It may be slow in coming, but break down they will because the body cannot maintain that level of stress. It was never intended to. As the psychologist Elizabeth McCormick writes in her book on breakdown, 'if we start to break down in our bodies with symptoms that don't seem to have an organic cause, it is a message to us from the unconscious that we need to be taken into areas we have not yet explored or made conscious'.[173] In today's world it is much easier to attribute the responsibility for our own stress to someone else. In the end, however, we shall be forced to face the real cause.

Occasionally, some individuals who have undergone stringent training in the handling of potentially stressful situations (e.g. army personnel, firefighters or paramedics) will only show signs of stress when the situation is over, almost as if their body is allowing them to 'let go' when it is safe. Only then do they experience the palpitations and interrupted sleep patterns that their colleagues experienced whilst in the stress situation.

Sir William Osler stated that 'the care of tuberculosis depends more on what the patient has in his head than what he has in his chest'.[170] TB may not be the threat that it used to be, but the principle of 'how a patient feels affects how he recovers' is very relevant to how we look after a patient in hospital. Perhaps we should re-evaluate the word *treatment* when we use it in connection with patients. Are they receiving a treatment which helps them to *feel* better as well as to *get* better?

We can further subdivide stressors into several categories as follows:

- physical;
- emotional;

- behavioural;
- environmental;
- cultural;
- political.

A patient in hospital could be experiencing physical, emotional, behavioural and environmental stress. We know that physiological stress is usually accompanied by some psychological stress. We also know that psychological stress leads to physiologically measurable changes. Even though psychophysiology has researched a wide range of physiological responses to psychological stress, very little is done in hospitals to address anything other than the physical stress of patients.[168]

Physiological responses to stress are governed by the hypothalamus, which is conveniently positioned next to the pituitary for easy hormone control.[176] As the hypothalamus controls the autonomic nervous system and forms part of the limbic system, it is immediately apparent that stress will have a direct effect on almost all bodily functions, from temperature to hormone imbalance. It also becomes obvious that anything which affects the sensory systems, e.g. an odour, has a direct pathway to the limbic system (in particular to the amygdala). Recent research suggests that this pathway 'does not allow for cortical processing and may be responsible for emotional responses a person does not understand'.[177]

The secretion of almost every hormone is altered in response to stress, and the altered chemical signals immediately affect the immune system. The immune system governs our ability to repair and heal.[178] Therefore the suggestion that aromas, such as essential oils, might affect our response to stress is a very important one.

Common measurable physical responses to stress include the following:

- increased concentrations of adrenaline/noradrenaline (in the blood and urine);
- an increase in the rate and force of the heart-beat;
- a rise in systolic blood pressure;
- dilation of the pupils;
- a decrease in the number of white blood cells (eosinophils and lymphocytes), leading to immunosuppression and decreased resistance to infection;
- an increase in the level of blood adrenocorticoids – aldosterone, thyroxine and glucagon – which increases the level of blood glucocorticoids; an increase in cortisol levels, affecting carbohydrate, lipid and protein metabolism – this leads to muscle wasting, thinning of the skin and depression of immune responses; raised blood cholesterol levels and a reduction in vitamin D levels and calcium absorption, leading to osteoporosis;

■ an increase in the level of lactate in the blood;

■ an increase in the level of urinary adrenocorticoids.

Much of the way in which stressors affect us is determined by whether we become angry or frightened. It is thought that the proportions of adrenaline and noradrenaline are directly related to the emotion which we display.[176] Predatory animals produce more noradrenaline, whereas domestic animals produce more adrenaline. Patients in hospital tend to become frightened rather than angry, but whether this is a cultural trait or one indicative of the parent–child role so often assumed by patient and doctor or patient and nurse, is difficult to assess. It might be interesting to measure the levels of adrenaline and noradrenaline in patients in order to determine which is higher and therefore what the stress response might be.

Symptoms of stress

Physical symptoms of stress include the following:

■ clenched jaw, leading to bruxism and referred neck pain;

■ hostility, depression, introspection, over-emotionalism, nervous twitches, nail-biting;

■ sweating for no obvious reason;

■ inability to sit still;

■ frequent crying or wish to cry;

■ lack of appetite or unnatural craving for food;

■ dyspepsia, indigestion/heartburn, constipation, diarrhoea;

■ constant tiredness;

■ insomnia, vivid dreams, sleep disturbances;

■ headaches, migraines;

■ breathlessness without exertion, palpitations, tachycardia;

■ dry mouth, dysphagia;

■ hypertension;

■ infertility, impotence.

Mental symptoms of stress include the following:

■ constant irritability;

■ loss of sense of humour;

■ difficulty in concentrating;

■ lack of interest in life.

■ feeling unable to cope;

■ depression, being unable to show one's feelings;

■ dreading the future;

■ being afraid of being alone.

Recognized stress-related illnesses include the following:

- eczema, psoriasis, acne, skin disorders;
- asthma;
- dysmenorrhoea, premenstrual syndrome, hormonal imbalance, alopecia;
- pruritus;
- diabetes mellitus;
- overactive thyroid;
- colitis, irritable bowel syndrome.[179]

In Pitts's paper entitled 'The Biochemistry of Anxiety' he lists the following 26 symptoms of anxiety which are affected by prolonged stress: palpitation; tires easily; breathlessness; nervousness; chest pain; sighing; dizziness; faintness; apprehensiveness; headache; paresis; weakness; trembling; breath unsatisfactory; insomnia; unhappiness; shakiness; fatigued all the time; sweating; fear of death; smothering; syncope; nervous chill; urinary frequency; vomiting and diarrhoea; anorexia.[174]

Stress and immunology

The immunological effects of stress are not always clear because each person deals with them in his or her own way, and because the effects are cumulative. However, there is a growing body of published evidence (both scientific and anecdotal) to show that specific stressors are linked to depressed immune function.

A decrease in immunoglobulin A (S-IgA) was measured in a study of dental students during their first year. A similar study of medical students prior to and during the first day of their final examinations repeated those findings, the students' ability to produce interferon being drastically reduced. Bartrop's study on bereavement also showed a lower lymphocyte function during the first 8 weeks following bereavement.[180] Quinn used this knowledge for her research on bereavement, looking at lowered immunological function and the effects of therapeutic touch.[181]

The research results of molecular biologist Candace Pert suggest that all neuropeptides may be composed of one molecule, and that changes in the configuration of this molecule would result in new information that could differentiate one neuropeptide from another.[180] She describes immunology as a network of information, with the mind flowing along it. Karl Pribram, who carried out neurophysiological research at Stanford University for many years, describes the brain as a hologram storing information which is available to all of its different parts. In this case, could it be that when a person becomes stressed, this hologram is affected, and communication between the neuropeptides becomes blocked?

It would appear that certain types of people could be protected from feelings of chronic stress. Achterberg noted that, at two institutions for the criminally insane, those inmates who had carried out horrendous crimes had been 'unusually' protected from life-threatening diseases such as cancer, despite poor health habits such as heavy smoking. Further studies showed that mentally handicapped people were less likely to die from cancer. On the basis of these studies it was suggested that a higher level of intelligence could be linked to a higher incidence of chronic diseases such as cancer.[175] Do intelligent people tend to suppress their feelings, which then suppress their immunological systems?

Stress and patients

One of the most stressful situations in anyone's life is to be institutionalized. To many people a hospital can seem like a prison. For them, the most stressful thing that could happen to them would be to be hospitalized. This attitude is well documented.[182] Patients lose their identity and become a number, exchange a business suit for a nightgown, and become a condition in a bed. Without personality, family or job, the patient can feel anonymous. This feeling of anonymity is not helped by Western medicine, which appears to treat the medical condition rather than the patient. An appendix is removed, a cancer is irradiated, with little regard for the gender, age or weight of the person in which it occurs. Yet if we are all different and indeed unique individuals, how can such a 'blanket' treatment be right?

Patients in hospital are encouraged to conform – to agree to the process of institutionalization. Questioning of procedures often labels them as 'difficult'. The medical profession has been trained to diagnose, not to discuss. Responsibility and choice of treatment is taken over from the patient by the medical model, insistent that its way is right. Cases are frequently discussed in front of the patient almost as though he or she was either deaf or stupid. Some patients are never asked how they feel about their situation.

It is generally accepted that one of the most stressful things about being a hospital patient, or indeed any patient, is the loss of control. This is not just the loss of control produced by an alien environment (unable to determine when they can sleep and when they can eat), but also the loss of control of intimate bodily functions. The more seriously ill the patient, the more severe will be the loss of control, and the ensuing stress. Compounding this is the sense of invasion felt by many patients, whether they are in a surgical or a medical ward.

Privacy is invaded, personal space is invaded and, in surgery, flesh is invaded. Of all surgery, perhaps heart surgery is the most feared. Research shows that a high percentage of patients experience psychological disturbances following open-heart surgery.[183] This may be due to the heart-lung machinery used during theatre time, but it may have a closer correlation with the relentless stressors which intensive-therapy units imbue – loss of privacy, loss of sleep, bright lights and continuous noise.[184] Perhaps it is the innate recognition that what is required by orthodox medicine in a high-dependency unit actually compounds the stress of patients, which has allowed complementary therapies, such as aromatherapy, into critical-care units long before they were accepted on the wards.

Aromatherapy and stress

At a basic level, smells that we recognize and associate with a happy memory will make us feel happy when we encounter them. This is usually the case with essential oils from plants and flowers, so essential oils have the power to de-stress us instantly if we select an aroma that is both pleasing and a reminder of a less stressful time. Certain essential oils, such as lavender, rose, neroli and petitgrain, are known for their ability to reduce anxiety.

Each hospital department, whether oncology, organ transplant or out-patients, carries its own particular brand of stress and fear. One of the most common, but least life-threatening, stressors in oncology is the patient's fear of hair loss. For women, especially, this does produce understandable anxiety and, with it, considerable stress. These patients need a great deal of reassurance that their hair will regrow, often thicker than before, after therapy. The simple act of a gentle head massage with a calming and very diluted essential oil such as lavender (*Lavandula vera*) can do a tremendous amount to literally 'touch the spot' and assuage the angst.

Organ transplant brings with it intense relief, but also feelings of guilt and anger. Sometimes these two emotions are not fully addressed, although many hospitals have counselling facilities. For the patient receiving the transplant, it is not the fact that another human being has had to suffer, or indeed die, for them, but that a part of their own self has been 'thrown away'. In the case of heart transplants, when a patient has literally 'lost their heart', aromatherapy can introduce smell (and, where appropriate, touch) to help to release these feelings of grief and 'soul pain'. Essential oils such as frankincense, ylang ylang, angelica and neroli can be gentle tools in the healing process.

Out-patient departments are associated with long waits, dark corridors, fraught staff, and doctors who rarely have time to look up from their notes. If patients have travelled long distances and fear that they will fail to catch public transport home, the wait is very stressful. A vaporizer containing rose (*Rosa damascena*) or eucalyptus (*Eucalyptus globulus*) would gently uplift patients and staff[185,186] and reduce cross-infection.[187] More specific problems which nurses often encounter in different hospital departments will be covered in Chapter 8.

Stress and hospital staff

Stress in hospitals is not confined to patients. The nursing staff are under tremendous stress – their numbers have dwindled in recent years, even though their workload has remained as heavy. Hospital managers also show symptoms of stress, as they are trying to save an out-of-balance monolith which appears to be careering down a steep precipice. Doctors are depressed and stressed. They have been forced into the role of God by the public, and are then frequently accused of getting it wrong. If stress leads to dis-ease and this leads to illness, then it would appear that a very large number of health workers are not healthy.

From the junior doctors, many of whom still work an 80-hour work, to the consultant surgeons who dash between operating theatres, the comment could be made that 'there is no way these people could *not* be stressed'. Show me a doctor who lingers over his or her food, or who does not answer the telephone by the second ring. Stress is something accepted along with medicine, but frequently a doctor's manner of dealing with his or her stress is hardly what he or she would prescribe for someone else, or one hopes so. Alcoholism, drug abuse and suicide are on the increase in the medical profession,[188] and perhaps the situation is similar among nurses.

Despite the huge body of knowledge held by health professionals, they do not look after themselves or each other. Whilst I am sure that Western culture would not take too kindly to a sudden display of touching or massage between nurses and doctors on the wards, there *are* solutions which might lessen the load. Take the junior houseman's on-call room, which is often musty and full of stale air. Simply inhaling a soothing oil such as mandarin (*Citrus reticulata*), lavender (*Lavandula angustifolia*) or chamomile (*Chamaemelum nobile*) for 5 minutes in order to relax, or breathing in a few drops of peppermint (*Mentha piperita*), black pepper (*Piper nigrum*) or rosemary (*Rosmarinus officinalis*) oil on a tissue, to revive and stimulate, might make those long nights more tolerable.

Nurses have to lay out patients who have died. This is always deeply distressing, regardless of how experienced the nurse may be. However, usually there is no way of ameliorating the emotional distress that the nurse feels other than a cigarette at her next break. A 5-minute hand massage with some neroli (*Citrus aurantium* var. *amara*) by a colleague would be a practical, effective and therapeutic alternative.[189] Angelica, petitgrain or rose would be possible substitutes. Touch and smell may be as old as the hills, but they can be deeply comforting.

Stress and visitors

Visiting a sick relative is stressful. What is one to say? What is one to do? Where should one sit? Frequently, the patient has insufficient energy to carry on much conversation, and the silences become longer and longer. The sicker the patient the more stressed the visitor and yet they come, sometimes long distances, if only for a few moments, to show that they care. Learning a simple hand or face massage, and using very dilute gentle oils will empower the visitor and make the patient feel wanted and cared for. No words are necessary – touch can say it all.

It does not matter how ill the patient is – they still need this kind of compassion, especially from their loved ones. We know that the sicker the patient, the less likely they are to be touched by their relatives who are frequently afraid to upset the complicated equipment around the patient. Research has shown that patients with the poorest prognosis, or who are the most acutely ill, are often touched least,[190] although one of the most basic human emotional needs is to feel physical contact.[191]

As nurses, we represent a reservoir of professional people who touch other people throughout life, from birth and paediatrics through to hospice work. Surely we should demonstrate to others what comes naturally to ourselves in our profession. There can be no simpler, more acceptable way of showing how much we care than by gentle aromatic touch, especially as we know that in times of stress everyone's need for physical contact is increased.

Children, in particular, can benefit from learning how to give a very gentle aromatherapy massage to elderly relatives, such as grandparents, who have been hospitalized. Frequently, child visitors are restless and awkward, feeling desperately ill at ease in the hospital environment, and longing to be back home where everything is normal. This kind of massage is easy both to teach and to learn. It is a loving and simple thing to do, it costs very little in terms of money, time or energy, but it communicates a great deal. It can also be empowering to both giver and receiver. It is often the little things in life which are important, and in hospital the little things become even more significant – fresh air, natural light, plants, peace, kindly touch and pleasant smells. Perhaps this is what Florence Nightingale was alluding to when she said that the least fortunate were those who found themselves nearest to a hospital, as many of these things were not to be found there.[192]

Relaxation

Relaxation is not just the opposite of stress. It is the *answer* to stress, and however we manage to achieve it, through meditation, stress management, visualization, exercise, chanting, or whatever, relaxation is relevant to our quality of life and to our survival. However, it can sometimes be extremely difficult to 'switch off'. The more 'uptight' a person is, the more impossible it becomes to achieve a state of peace. The harder a person tries, the more elusive relaxation seems to be. Modern life is geared to *doing*, not *being*. What do you *do*? What do you want to *do*? These are the questions we use, not who are you, or who do you want to *be*? As a patient, the ability to *do* is to an increasing degree replaced with enforced '*being*'. This in itself is stressful to someone who has spent most of their life in a *doing* mode. However, as Larry Dossey states in his book, 'the most effective way to reverse illness is sometimes to focus primarily on *being*'.[193]

As nurses, we frequently ask the impossible. 'Just relax', we murmur, before plunging a hypodermic needle deep into the upper outer quadrant. 'Just relax', we encourage, before inserting one finger high into the rectum with a suppository. 'Just relax', we whisper, as the gowned, masked and gloved surgeon inserts a cardiac catheter into the femoral artery, aimed at the heart. 'Just relax'. The question is, what do we do to help patients to relax?

Relaxation brings with it manifold benefits both for our patients and for ourselves. Indeed, in Benson's book, *The Relaxation Response*, he suggests that a relaxation break should replace a coffee break.[194] However, relaxation or stress management for patients, or for staff, is not currently part of a nurse's or doctor's training.

In a discussion of massage and aromatherapy as supportive therapies in health care, Sheena Hildebrand quotes from Wang Wei, writing in the eighth century 'Look in the perfumes of flowers and of nature for peace of mind and joy of life'.[195] Certainly on looking at the photographs of the young child being massaged by Sheena, one is immediately drawn to the conclusion that here is a therapy that allows the recipient to *be*, and through *being* comes relaxation, but there is more. Perhaps it would be appropriate to quote from a poem by Drury in *Visions of Nursing*:

> Caring, loving, touching,
> Absence of connection to stress factors,
> Being a part of reality but
> Being centred in caring
> for the whole person, Functioning with a positive
> confident, loving presence.[196]

Pleasure, relaxation and endorphins

Many people find it pleasant and soothing to be stroked gently (for that is all we are really doing) with a pleasantly smelling aromatic. For those who have disturbing memories of either sexual abuse or other forms of physical cruelty, touch can be threatening. In some cases such memories are deeply hidden, only emerging later in life, sometimes during an aromatherapy session. This is not the place to discuss these cases, although many have found great comfort and peace through a systematic, carefully controlled aromatherapy programme. On the whole, though, most people find touch pleasant.

In *Caring Touch*, reference is made to Sidney Simon, who speaks of 'skin hunger', and writes that 'every human being comes into the world needing to be touched, and the need for skin contact persists until death, despite society's efforts to make us believe otherwise.'[197] He continues 'touch is quite distinct from sexual contact', and he calls for 'touch nourishment strategies'.

Massage presents a large body of reference suggesting a relaxation response. In *Palliative Care for Patients with Cancer*, Victor Brewer, a patient with advanced cancer, is quoted as describing the effects of massage as follows: 'You unwind with the gentleness of the human touch. It would be marvellous if nurses could do it in hospital. . . . With massage, *as soon as the hands go on*, you know she's there, she's calm, she has time for you'.[198] The type of massage carried out by nurses is different to that performed by beauty therapists. It is much lighter and slower, and is not intended to address muscle tone, but to address soul tone.

Stress and pain

It is known that massage aids the release of endorphins, neurochemicals which are triggered in response to touch and smell. Some endorphins, called enkephalins, are known to be more powerful than morphine, and they work by blocking the release of the pain transmission 'substance P'. These opiate receptors are distributed throughout the pleasure (and pain) systems of the body.

According to the gate theory of pain control, pain is alleviated by the effect of rubbing (massaging) the skin, which stimulates large diameter afferent (LDA) sensory fibres which in turn excite the interneurones, causing enkephalin release. Enkephalin release inhibits the release of substance P from activated unmyelinated C-fibres. This prevents T-cell activation and closes the pain gate. The pain most affected by massage is that which is classified as slow pain – burning, aching pain which is poorly localized.[115] This type of pain can be associated with many chronic conditions and with post-operative recovery, although not with immediate post-operative care. Although deep massage is contraindicated following recent surgery, the gentleness of aromatherapy massage around the affected area is highly appropriate, and very useful as an adjunct to pain control.

Some fragrances have deeply relaxing effects. Japanese research has shown that contingent negative variation (CNV), namely the upward shift in the brain waves recorded by electrodes attached to the scalp, occurs in situations where subjects are expecting something to happen. CNV alters in response to odour. Following experiments with diazepam and caffeine to cause CNS depression and stimulation, research showed that lavender had a depressing effect and jasmine had a stimulating effect. Further investigation revealed that, although odour had an effect on the brain, it did not appear to affect physiological functions.[199] It is interesting to note that even in individuals who have no sense of smell (asmosis), a chemical reaction to odours can be shown to occur in the brain.

In conclusion, the effects of touch and smell add up to two of the most powerful relaxation tools available to us. It would be a waste not to use them.

Stress, relaxation and psychoneuroimmunology (PNI)

The American doctors Siegal and Dossy have done much to raise awareness of the importance of psychoneuroimmunology (PNI). Perhaps the term first started to become popularized in 1978, with the publication of Siegal's book, *Love, Medicine and Miracles*, in which he writes of patients who had survived cancer. He calls them 'exceptional cancer patients' (ExCaps).[200] In one famous address to eminent, staunchly orthodox doctors (many of whom were openly hostile to his views), he read aloud from *Lady Chatterley's Lover*. He read for some time, until the darkly suited men in front of him were wriggling and red-faced. Then he paused, closed the book, and said quietly 'now then, gentlemen, don't tell me that your mind has not affected your body!'

PNI is a medical subspeciality that involves the study of the connection between the mind ('psycho'), the brain ('neuro') and the body's ability to defend itself against disease ('immune'), in other words, a person's ability to get in touch with his or her immune system. It is becoming increasingly obvious that humans *do* have the capacity to affect their 'wellness', or disease, through the power of thought. This finding has not been accepted readily within orthodox medicine. Indeed, Siegal quotes from Dostoevsky, right at the beginning of his book 'A new philosophy, a way of life, is not given for nothing. It has to be paid for dearly and only acquired with much patience and great effort'. Perhaps this quote is as relevant to aromatherapy in nursing as it is to PNI.

Norman Cousins decided to apply the principle of PNI to himself. Diagnosed as having a sudden onset of ankylosing spondylitis, he was told that his spinal connective tissue was dissolving.[201] Medication consisting of 26 aspirin and 12 phenylbutazone tablets *daily* resulted in hives all over his body, but no pain relief. Appalled by his hospital treatment, where on one day he had to give four separate samples of blood for the same test because the pathology laboratory was so unco-ordinated, he checked out of the hospital and into a hotel. Cousins knew that pain could be affected by attitude, and he instinctively chose to try laughter instead of medication.

It was a brave and desperate move, but one which showed him that 10 minutes of genuine belly-laughter had an anaesthetic effect and gave him 2 hours of pain-free sleep. Wanting 'real' proof, Cousins then undertook blood tests which confirmed that his ESR fell by at least five points following laughter 'therapy'. Better still, the effect was cumulative. It seemed that laughter *was* stimulating the production of endorphins, which resulted in a profound reduction in his joint inflammation. Bolstered by this discovery, he refused to let his friends see him unless they could bring a new joke, cartoon or film to make him laugh. Norman Cousins understood that how he felt would affect how he was, and that meant his illness.

It would be interesting to see if laughter could become a commodity provided by hospitals. True, some get-well cards can be slightly amusing, but *laughter therapy*, although indisputably shown to be effective, is not an approach conducive either to a Western medical model or to the Western temperament. Illness is serious business and, in the private sector, serious illness means serious money and long faces. No wonder no one wants to be seen to belittle it. Although perhaps they would all agree with Wilde-McCormick, who writes in her book on changing one's life through self-help psychotherapy, 'Make sure you laugh every day'.[202]

The relationship between an emotional reaction brought on by an illness and the survival rate of a patient is highlighted in Fiore's article on fighting cancer.[203] Nurses are in a unique position to encourage the use of PNI amongst their patients, because 'as care givers they have the power to be dispiriting or inspiring to their patients'.[204] How many nurses use this power to enhance their patients' ability to draw on their own self-healing mechanisms?

Aromatherapy is a perfect way of utilizing PNI. Many patients find themselves lulled by repeated stroking movements, which encourage a series of endorphins into play. The pleasant smell of an essential oil may enhance this effect. Together, smell and touch can produce a synergy of social, physical, psychological and neurological interactions in the patient. The most common comment made by patients is how relaxing they find the treatment, and how the feeling of relaxation *remains for several days*. This may be highly relevant. Although it is recognized that smell is instant, the effect of smell wears off very quickly as our olfactory neurones become inured to the odour. Perhaps by administering the 'smell' transdermally, we are giving *slow-release smell*, which produces a longer-lasting effect.

Research on PNI and HIV has shown that relaxation 'may influence the immune function of those patients with HIV, and retard disease progression among early HIV-1 seropositive individuals'.[205] Psychologist Sandra Levy at the University of Pittsburgh found that *supportive* personal relationships improved the immune function of women with breast cancer.[206] A similar finding was reported in Dean Ornish's study on reversing heart disease through diet, exercise and *stress management*. He wrote that he was 'increasingly convinced that the root of chronic stress is a sense of isolation – from oneself, from others and from something spiritual'.[207]

In Jacqui Farrow's 6-week trial of massage on an acute medical ward, her conclusions were that massage reduced anxiety in patients who were receiving morphine pump therapy for pain, during the period when the pump was being changed, that it enabled a woman who had undergone lumpectomy to relax whilst awaiting the results of the biopsy, and that it enabled a teenager to cope better with her disfiguring post-operative ileostomy tubes and drains.[208] Three patients with three very different needs and conditions were thus all helped by massage, but in different ways.

Robert Tisserand writes about the emotionally uplifting and comforting oils that can be used with cancer patients.[209] King writes about the ability of odour impressions to 'produce effects partly through mood changes', and concludes that 'fragrance provides a useful adjunct for relaxation and has considerable potential for future development'.[210]

Birchall, writing for the *New Scientist*, asks whether aromatherapy matches the potency of valium and librium, stating that many of aromatherapy's claims are now being validated by research.[211] In fact, as early as May 1988, the *Journal of Aromatherapy* bore the headline 'Lavender beats benzodiazepines'.[157]

In Reed and Norfolk's study, they found that 36 out of 38 patients experienced a feeling of relaxation following aromatherapy.[212] This study was carried out at an Ipswich hospital by two midwives who were investigating the possibility that lavender might reduce pain during childbirth. Patients were asked to take baths with 5 drops of lavender during labour. There was no control to this study. However, the results suggested that aromatherapy did alter pain perception in 30 women, and 36 women felt that their ability to relax during labour was enhanced. Relaxation was also enhanced in a further trial involving 586 women in labour (see next page).

Stevenson's study on patients concludes that 100 per cent of the patients in her aromatherapy trial found the effects of a foot massage with essential oil to be beneficial.[189] She was investigating the effects of neroli (*Citrus aurantium* subsp. *aurantium flos*) on 100 patients in The Middlesex Hospital cardiac intensive-care unit following open-heart surgery. This was a controlled, randomized study using a modified Spielberger State Trait Anxiety Inventory for Adults (STAI) State Evaluation Questionnaire to measure pain, anxiety, tension, calmness, rest and relaxation. Physiological measurement showed a decrease in respiration, suggesting an increased parasympathetic response, a conclusion which was supported by the psychological measurements. Stevenson showed that patients who received a neroli foot massage felt that their anxiety decreased more than the patients who received a foot massage without the neroli essential oil.

In total, 91 per cent of the patients in Woolfson's study experienced a reduction in their heart rate of between 11 and 15 beats per minute, showing a relaxation response.[213] This study was also conducted in an intensive-care unit, this time at the Royal Sussex County Hospital. A total of 36 patients were allocated to one of three groups: those who received massage with essential oils, those who received massage without essential oils, and a control group who just rested. The results of this study appear to agree with Stevenson's findings that massage with an essential oil, in this case lavender, was more effective in reducing stress than massage without an essential oil.

Dunn's study of 122 patients showed anxiety reduction following aromatherapy massage.[214] Dunn led one of the first formal trials to be conducted in a hospital, and which paved the way for further trials. Her study was carried out in an intensive-care unit and investigated the effects of lavender.

Burns and Blamey studied over 585 women in labour in order to determine whether aromatherapy with any of 10 essential oils could reduce anxiety, increase contractions and reduce pain.[215] The oils used were lavender, clary sage, peppermint, eucalyptus, mandarin, chamomile, jasmine, rose, frankincense and lemon. The study was set up when the two investigators discovered that aromatherapy was part of the curriculum and examination syllabus for all student midwives in Germany. Their results showed much satisfaction expressed by the mothers and the delivery team concerning the reduction of stress with all of the essential oils used. The study was not randomized or controlled, but was an important investigation nevertheless as it looked at many essential oils, and has led the way for other maternity units which have been looking at aromatherapy as a possible effective method of stress management in labour.

There have been, and currently are, many other trials looking at the use of aromatherapy in the treatment of stress and anxiety. Perhaps one could summarize by quoting from Wise's article published in the *Nursing Times* in 1989: 'aromatherapy helps to take the anxiety out of being in hospital and quickens the patient's return to self-care'.[216]

Whether we choose the inhalation of drops of essential oil on a pillow, or floating on a bowl of warm water, or whether we opt for aromatic massage for our patients, colleagues or visitors, there is no doubt that *aromatherapy as a method of stress therapy is a very valid and important part of our work to promote healing*.

Spontaneous remission

Finally, no chapter that refers to PNI would be complete without a mention of spontaneous remission. The Institute of Noetic Sciences, USA, was founded in 1973 by astronaut Edgar D. Mitchell following his experience of walking on the moon. It is a research foundation and an educational institution, and has 30 000 members world-wide. The word *'noetic'* comes from the Greek, *'nous'*, meaning 'mind', intelligence and transcendental knowing.

In 1993, the Institute of Noetic Sciences and the Fetzer Institute published a book documenting the results of a 10-year research programme on the healing response. Their programme was 'based on the belief that the ability of the physician to promote health, and to heal the sick in the future, may be as dependent on the deeper understanding of the mind–body relationship as on the development of new technologies'.

Their study revealed that there is a large body of evidence which suggests that extraordinary healing, including regression of normally fatal tumours, takes place, with no currently available scientific explanation.[217] This discovery was not new to medicine. In 1909, Handley wrote in the *British Medical Journal* that 'the recorded cases of natural repair of cancer, far from being anomalous and exceptional, merely illustrate more strikingly than usual the natural laws which govern every case of the disease'.[218]

However, the Institute of Noetic Sciences study was the largest investigation ever carried out on spontaneous remission, and it concluded that 'the evidence suggests this kind of healing can be triggered by a variety of stimuli, diverse in nature, including signals, suggestions and guidance from the physical, mental and/or spiritual realm of every individual'.

Sadly, Brendan O'Regan, the visionary responsible for the programme, died in 1992 before the programme was completed, but his efforts helped to establish what is now one of the most exciting and rapidly growing areas of mind–body healing – PNI. Without doubt, his is one of the most far-reaching achievements in medicine. Although a great part of the book was completed in 1990, over 300 additional references to spontaneous remission from cancer and other diseases, which were published in medical journals between 1990 and 1992, have been collated subsequently.

Whilst it would be impossible, and also immoral, to suggest that aromatherapy could result in spontaneous remission, nevertheless there is sufficient anecdotal evidence to suggest that aromatherapy *does* enhance the mind–body link. It would be interesting indeed to measure immune levels before and after an aromatherapy treatment. A recent survey conducted among patients who had used 'a complex of traditional medical and alternative treatments suggests that as many as 10 per cent of them undergo spontaneous remission'. One wonders if any of them had been receiving aromatherapy. To quote the Institute of Noetic Sciences, 'We are at the threshold of a new field of inquiry'. Ralph Waldo Emerson wrote that 'thought is the blossom, language the bud, action the fruit behind it'.[219] I hope that this book will serve as the bud to encourage a little fruit!

REFERENCES

1. **MacSween, R.N.M. and Whaley, K.** 1992: *Muir's textbook of pathology*, 13th edn. London: Edward Arnold.

2. **Ward K.** 1993: Care of the person with an infection. In Hinchcliff, S., Norman, S. *Nursing practice and health care*. London: Edward Arnold, 402–34.

3. **Gasgoigne, S.** 1993: *Manual of conventional medicine for alternative practitioners. Volume 1.* Richmond: Jigme Press.

4. **Fisher, J.** 1994: *The plague makers.* New York: Simon & Schuster.

5. **Meers, P.O.** *et al.* 1981: Report on the National Survey of Infection in Hospitals. *Journal of Hospital Infection* **2 (Suppl.),** 1–51.

6. **Department of Health and Social Services/Public Health Laboratory Service Hospital Infection Working Group.** 1988: *Hospital infection control: guidance on the control of infection in hospitals.* London: HMSO.

7. **Rubinstein, E., Green, M. and Molan, M.** 1982: The effects of nosocomial infections on the length and costs of hospital stay. *Journal of Antimicrobial Chemotherapy* **9 (Suppl.),** 93.

8. **Sleigh, J.D., Pennington, T.H. and Lucas, S.B.** 1992: Microbial infection. In MacSween, R.N.M. and Whales, K. (eds), *Muir's textbook of pathology.* 13th edn. London: Edward Arnold, 301–2.

9. **Hope, R.A., Longmore J.M., Hodgetts, T.J. and Ramrakha, P.S.** 1993: *Oxford handbook of clinical medicine,* 3rd edn. Oxford: Oxford University Press.

10. **Tamm, C.H.** 1971: Recent advances in the field of antibiotics. In Wagner, H. and Wolffe, P. (eds), *New natural products and plant drugs with pharmacological, biological or therapeutic activity.* Berlin: Springer-Verlag, 82–136.

11. **Lewis, W.H. and Elvin-Lewis, M.P.** 1977: Antibiotics, antiseptics and pesticides. In *Medical Botany.* New York: Wiley Interscience, 360–4.

12. **Blaschke, T. and Bjornsson, T.** 1995: Pharmacokinetics and pharmacoepidemiology. *Scientific American* **8,** 1–14.

13. **Schmidt, M.A.** 1995: Antibiotics: the promise and the peril. In *Conference Proceedings. Holistic Aromatherapy.* San Francisco: Pacific Institute of Aromatherapy, 81–8.

14. **Jukes, T.H.** 1973: Public health significance of feeding low levels of antibiotics to animals. *Advances in Applied Microbiology* **16,** 1–29.

15. **Corpet, D.E.** 1987: Antibiotic residues and drug resistance in human intestinal flora. *Antimicrobial Agents and Chemotherapy* **31**, 587–93.

16. **Abraham, E.P. and Chaine, E.** 1940: An enzyme from bacteria able to destroy penicillin. *Nature* **3713**, 837–8.

17. **Deinenger, E.** 1995: The spectrum of activity of plant drugs containing essential oils. In *Conference Proceedings. Holistic Aromatherapy*. San Francisco: Pacific Institute of Aromatherapy, 15–43.

18. **Guenther, E.** 1952: *The essential oils*. Malabar, FL: Krieger.

19. **Franchomme, P. and Peneol, D.** 1991: *L'aromatherapie exactement*. Limoges: Roger Jollois.

20. **Lewis, W.H. and Elvin-Lewis, M.P.F.** 1977: *Medical Botany*. New York: Wiley Interscience.

21. **Service, R.F.** 1994: *E. coli* scare spawns therapy search. *Science* **265**, 475–6.

22. **Valnet, J.** 1980: *The practice of aromatherapy*. Saffron Walden: C.W. Daniel.

23. **Chin, Y.C., Chang, N.C. and Anderson, H.** 1949: Factors influencing the antibiotic activity of lupulon. Paper presented at the Second National Symposium on Recent Advances in Antibiotic Research, 11–12 April, 1949, Washington, DC: National Institutes of Health.

24. **Budavari, S. (ed.)** 1996: *Merck Index*, 12th edn. Whitehouse Station, NJ: Merck Co. Inc.

25. **Maruzella, J.C. and Sicurella, N.A.** 1960: Antibacterial activity of essential oil vapors. *Journal of the American Pharmaceutical Association (Scientific Edition)* **49**, 693–5.

26. **Maruzella, J.C. and Percival, H.** 1958: Antimicrobial activity of perfume oils. *Journal of the American Pharmaceutical Association* **XLVII**, 471–6.

27. **Deans, S.G. and Svoboda, K.P.** 1990: The antimicrobial properties of marjoram (*Origanum majorana*). *Flavour and Fragrance Journal* **5**, 187–90.

28. **Zakarya, D., Fkih-Tetouani, S. and Hajji, F.** 1993: Antimicrobial activity of twenty-one *Eucalyptus* essential oils. *Fitoterapia* **LXIV**, 319–31.

29. **Peneol, D.** 1991/92: *Eucalyptus smithii* essential oil and its use in aromatic medicine. *British Journal of Phytotherapy* **2**, 154–9.

30. **Ferdous, A.J., Islam, S.N. et al.** 1992: *In vitro* antibacterial activity of the volatile oil of *Nigella sativa* seeds against multiple drug-resistant isolates of *Shigella* spp. and isolates of *Vibrio cholerae* and *E. coli*. *Phytotherapy Research* **6**, 137–140.

31. **Grieve, M.** 1931: *A modern herbal*. Harmondsworth: Penguin.

32. **de la Puerta, R., Saenz, M. and Garcia, M.D.** 1993: Cytostatic activity against HEp-2 cells and antibacterial activity of essential oils from *Helichrysum picardii*. *Phytotherapy Research* **1**, 378–80.

33. **Deans, S.G. and Ritchie, G.A.** 1987: Antibacterial properties of plant essential oils. *International Journal of Food Microbiology* **5**, 165–80.

34. **Deans, S.G. and Svoboda, K.P.** 1988: Antibacterial activity of French tarragon (*Artemisia dracunculus*) essential oil and its constituents during ontogeny. *Journal of Horticultural Science* **63**, 503–8.

35. **Deans, S.G., Svoboda, K.P.** *et al.* 1992: Essential oil profiles of several temperate and tropical aromatic plants: their antimicrobial and antioxidant activities. *Acta Horticulturae 306: Medicinal and Aromatic Plants*, 229–33.

36. **Onawunmi, G.O. and Ogunlana, E.O.** 1986: A study of the antibacterial activity of essential oil of lemon grass. *International Journal of Crude Drug Research* **24**, 64–8.

37. **Deans, S.G. and Svoboda, K.P.** 1989: Antibacterial activity of summer savory (*Satureja hortensis*) essential oil and its constituents. *Journal of the Horticultural Society* **64**, 205–10.

38. **Jain, S.H. and Purohit, M.** 1992: Pharmacological evaluation of *Cuminum cyminum*. *Fitoterapie* **6314**, 291–4.

39. Balacs, T. 1993: Antimicrobial Lamiaceae. *International Journal of Aromatherapy* **5**, 34.

40. **Kedzia, B.** *et al.* 1991: Antimicrobial activity of oils of *Chamomilla* and its components. *Herba Polonica* **37**, 29–38.

41. **Benouda, A., Hassar, M.** *et al.* 1988: *In vitro* antibacterial properties of essential oils tested against hospital pathogenic bacteria. *Fitoterapia* **59**, 115–19.

42. **Carson, C.F. & Riley, T.V.** 1993: Antimicrobial activity of essential oil of *Melaleuca alternifolia*. *Letters in Applied Microbiology* **16**, 49–55.

43. **Cooke, A. and Cooke, M.D.** 1994: *Cawthron Report Number 263: An investigation into the antimicrobial properties of manuka and kanuka oil*. Nelson, New Zealand: Cawthron.

44. **Carson, C.F., Cookson, B.D., Farrelly, H.D. and Riley, T.V.** 1995: Susceptibility of methicillin-resistant *Staphylococcus aureus* to the essential oil of *Melaleuca alternifolia*. *Journal of Antimicrobial Chemotherapy* **35**, 421–4.

45. **Sears, C.** 1995: How to sell drugs. *New Scientist* **Nov 4**, 37–40.

46. **Mansfield, P.** 1996: Animal experiments are an obstacle to health. *Holistic Health* **No. 50**, 4–7.

47. **Ross, S.A., El-Keltawi, N.E. and Megella, S.E.** 1980: Antimicrobial activity of some Egyptian aromatic plants. *Fitoterapia* **51**, 201–5.

48. **Belaiche, P.** 1979: *Traite de phytotherapie et d'aromatherapie. Tome 1. l'aromatogramme*. Paris: Maloine.

49. **Blackwell, R. and Smith, M.** 1995: Aromatograms. *International Journal of Aromatherapy* **7**, 22–7.

50. **Roberts, M.B.V.** 1986: *Biology: a functional approach*, 4th edn. Walton on Thames: Nelson.

51. **Carr, G.** 1996: The profit and loss of AIDS. *The Economist* **340**, 85–6.

52. **Craig, C. and Stitzel, R.** 1994: *Modern pharmacology*, 4th edn. Boston, MA: Little, Brown & Co.

53. **Sullivan, A.** 1995: When plagues end. *The New York Times Magazine* **Nov 10**, 52–84.

54. **Kucera, L.S. and Herrmann, E.C.** 1967: *Proceedings of the Society for Experimental Biology and Medicine* **124**, 865–969.

55. **Cohen, R.A., Kucera, L.S. and Herrmann, E.C. Jr.** 1964: Antiviral activity of *Melissa officinalis. Proceedings of the Society for Experimental Biology and Medicine* **117**, 431–4.

56. **Foster, S. and Duke, J.A.** 1960: *A field guide to medicinal plants (Eastern/Central).* New York: Houghton Mifflin Co.

57. **Cariel, L. and Jean, D.** 1990: *Antiviral compositions containing proanthocyanidols.* Patent – PCT. In appl. 90. 13 304. In *Chemical Abstracts* **114**, 53.

58. **Mendes, N.M. Araujo, N., De Souza, C.P. and Katz, J.** 1990: Molluscicidal and carcaricidal activity of different species of *Eucalyptus. Revista Societe Brasilia Medicinale Tropicale* **23**, 197–9.

59. **Muanza, D.N., Euler, K.L., Williams, L. and Newman, D.J.** 1995: Screening for antitumor and anti-HIV activities of nine medicinal plants from Zaire. *International Journal of Pharmacology* **33**, 98–105.

60. **May, G. and Willuhn, G.** 1979: Antiviral activity of aqueous extracts from medicinal plants in tissue cultures. *Arzneimittel-Forschung* **28**, 1–7.

61. **Kufferath, F., Mundualgo, G.M.** 1954: The activity of some preparations containing essential oils in TB. *Fitoterapia* **25**, 483–5.

62. **Takechie, M. and Tanaka, Y.** 1985: Structure and antiherpetic activity among the tannins. *Phytochemistry* **24**, 2245–50.

63. **Kyoko, H., Kamiya, M. and Hayashi, T.** 1994: Viricidal effects of the steam distillate from *Houttynia cordata* and its components on HSV-1, influenza virus and HIV. *Planta Medica* **61**, 237–41.

64. **Kucera, L.S. and Herrmann, E.C.** 1967: Antiviral substances in plants of the mint family (Labiatae). 1. Tannin of *Melissa officinalis. Proceedings of the Society for Experimental Biology and Medicine* **124**, 865, 874.

65. **Weber, N.D. et al.** 1992: *In vitro* viricidal effects of *Allium sativum. Planta Medica* **58**, 417–23.

66. **Franchomme, P. and Peneol, D.** 1990: *L'aromatherapie.* Limoges: Jollois.

67. **Duke, J.A.** 1985: *Handbook of medicinal herbs.* Boca Raton, FL: CRC Press.

68. **Takechi, M. and Tanaka, Y.** 1981: Purification and characterisation of antiviral substance eugenin from the bud of *Syzygium aromatica aromaticum. Planta Medica* **42**, 69–71.

69. **Lovell, C.** 1993: *Plants and the skin.* Oxford: Blackwell Scientific Publications.

70. **Opdyke, D.L. (ed.)** 1979: *Monographs on fragrance raw materials.* Oxford: Pergamon Press.

71. **Mathias, C.G.T.** *et al.* 1980: Contact urticaria from cinnamic aldehyde. *Archives of Dermatology* **116**, 74–6.

72. **Price, S.** 1995: *Aromatherapy for health professionals.* London: Churchill Livingstone.

73. **Parish, P.** 1991: *Medical treatments: the benefits and the risks.* Harmondsworth: Penguin.

74. **Zarno, V.** 1994: Candidiasis. *International Journal of Aromatherapy* **6**, 20–23.

75. **Myers, H.** 1927: An unappreciated fungicidal action of certain volatile oils. *Journal of American Medical Association* **Nov 26**, 1834–6.

76. **Soliman, F.N., El-Kashoury, E.A., Fathy, M.M. and Gonald, M.H.** 1994: Analysis and biological activity of essential oil of *Rosmarinus officinalis.* *Egyptian Flavour and Fragrance Journal* **9**, 29–33.

77. **Mehrotra, S., Rawat, A.K.S.** *et al.* 1993: Antimicrobial activity of the essential oils of some Indian *Artemisia* species. *Fitoterapia* **14**, 65–8.

78. **Viollon, C. and Chaumont, J.P.** 1994: Autifungal properties of essential oils and their main components upon *Cryptococcus neoformans.* *Mycopathologia* **128**, 151–3.

79. **Tisserand, R. and Balacs, T.** 1995: *Essential oil safety.* London: Churchill Livingstone.

80. **Onawunmi, G.O.** 1989: Evaluation of the antifungal activity of lemongrass oil. *International Journal of Crude Drug Research* **27**, 121–6.

81. **Garg, S.C. and Dengre, S.I.** 1988: Antifungal activity of some essential oils. *Pharmacie* **43**, 141–2.

82. **Hmamouchi, M., Tantaoui-Elaraki, A., Es-Safi, N. and Agoumi, A.** 1990: Illustrations of antibacterial and antifungal properties of *Eucalyptus* essential oils. *Plantes Medicinales et Phytotherapie* **24**, 278–9.

83. **Opdyke, D.L.J.** 1976: Inhibition of sensitization reactions induced by certain aldehydes. *Food and Cosmetics Toxicology* **14**, 197–8.

84. **Belaiche, P.** 1985: Treatment of vaginal infections of *Candida albicans* with essential oils of *Melaleuca alternifolia.* *Phytotherapy* **15**, 13–14.

85. **Larrondo, J.V. and Calvo, M.A.** 1991: Effects of essential oils on *Candida albicans*: a scanning electron microscope study. *Biomedical Letters* **46**, 269–72.

86. **Shemesh, A.** 1991: Australian tea-tree: a natural antiseptic and fungicidal agent. *Australian Journal of Pharmacy* **12**, 802–3.

87. **Belaiche, P.** 1985: Treatment of skin infections with essential oils of *Melaleuca alternifolia.* *Phytotherapy* **15**, 15–17.

88. **Galal, E.E., Adel, M.S. and El-Sherif, S.** 1973: Evaluation of certain volatile oils for their antifungal properties. *Journal of Drug Research* **5**, 235–45.

89. **Lawless, J.** 1992: *Encyclopedia of essential oils.* Shaftesbury: Element.

90. **Agarwal, I., Kharwal, H.B. and Methela, C.S.** 1980: Chemical study

and antimicrobial properties of essential oil of *Cymbopogon citratus*. *Bulletin of Ethnobotanical Research* **1**, 401–7.

91. **Satinder, K. and Sinha, G.K.** 1991: *In vitro* antifungal activity of some essential oils. *Journal of Research into Ayerveda and Siddha* **12**, 200–205.

92. **Cuong, N.D.** *et al.* 1994: Antibacterial properties of Vietnamese cajuput oil. *Journal of Essential Oil Research* **6**, 63–7.

93. **Deans, S.G. and Svoboda, K.P.** 1990: The antimicrobial properties of marjoram (*Origanum majorana*) volatile oil. *Flavour and Fragrance Journal* **5**, 187–90.

94. **Faouzia, H., Fkih-Tetouani, S. and Tantaoui-Elaraki, A.** 1993: Antimicrobial activity of twenty-one *Eucalyptus* essential oils. *Fitoterapia* **LXIV**, 1.

95. **Fun, C.E. and Svendsen, A.B.** 1990: The essential oils of *Lippia alba*. *Journal of Essential Oil Research* **2**, 265–7.

96. **Briozzo, J., Nunez, L.** *et al.* 1989: Antimicrobial activity of clove oil. *Journal of Applied Bacteriology* **66**, 69–75.

97. **Dube, S., Upadihay, P.D. and Tripathi, S.C.** 1989: Antifungal, physiochemical and insect-repelling activity of the essential oil of *Ocimum basilicum*. *Canadian Journal of Botany* **67**, 2085–7.

98. **Wagner, H.** 1984: *Plant drug analysis*. Berlin: Springer-Verlag.

99. **Hector, W.** 1982: *Modern nursing: theory and practice*, 7th edn. London: Heinemann.

100. **Klayman, D.L.** 1985: Qunghaosu (artemisin): an antimalarial drug from China. *Science*. **228**, 1049–55.

101. **Cubukcu, B., Bray, D.H. and Warhurst, D.C.** 1990: *In vitro* antimalarial activity of crude extracts and compounds from *Artemisia abrotanum*. *Phytotherapy Research* **4**, 203–4.

102. **Liu, K.C., Yang, S.L. and Roberts, M.F.** 1992: Antimalarial activity of *Artemisia annua* flavonoids from whole plants and cell cultures. *Plant Cell Reports* **11**, 637–40.

103. **Chalchat, J.C., Garry, R.P. and Lamy, J.** 1994: *Influence of harvest time and composition of Artemisia annua. Journal of Essential Oil Research* **6**, 261–8.

104. **De Blasi, Debrot, S.** *et al.* 1990: Amoebicidal effect of essential oils *in vitro*. *Journal of Clinical Toxicology and Experimental Therapeutics* **10**, 351–73.

105. **Gilbert, B. and Mors, W.B.** 1972: Anthelmintic activity of essential oils and their constituents. *Anais da Academia Brasileira de Ciencias* **44**, 423–8.

106. **Erichsen-Brown, C.** 1979: *Medicinal and other uses of North American plants*. New York: Dover.

107. **Grieve, M.** 1931: *A modern herbal*. Harmondsworth: Penguin.

108. **Lawless, J.** 1992: *Encyclopedia of essential oils*. Shaftesbury: Element.

109. **Grosjean N.** 1992: *Aromatherapy from Provence*. Saffron Walden: C.W. Daniel.

110. **Tisserand R.** 1989: *The art of aromatherapy*. Saffron Walden: Daniel.

111. **Bardeau, F.** 1976: The use of essential oils to purify and deodorise the air. *Chirugien-Dentiste de France (Paris)* **46**, 53.

112. **Cooke, A. and Cooke, M.D.** 1994: *Cawthorn Report Number 263. An investigation into the antimicrobial properties of manuka and kanuka oil.* Nelson, New Zealand: Cawthron.

113. **Goleman, D.** 1996: *Emotional intelligence.* New York: Bantam.

114. **Carter, R.** 1996: Give a drug a bad name. *New Scientist* **6 April**, 27–9.

115. **Sofaer, B. and Foord, J.** 1993: Care of the person in pain. In Hinchcliff, S. *et al.* (eds), *Nursing practice and health care.* London: Edward Arnold, 374–401.

116. **Pennisi, E. and Nowark, R.** 1996: Racked with pain. *New Scientist* **9 March**, 27–9.

117. **Weil, A.** 1996: *Spontaneous healing.* New York: Fawcett.

118. **Martin, B.** 1994: Opioid and nonopioid analgesics. In Craig, C. and Stitzel, R. (eds), *Modern pharmacology*, 4th edn. Boston, MA: Little, Brown & Co., 431–50.

119. **Beck, D. and Beck, J.** 1987: *The pleasure connection – how endorphins affect our health and happiness.* Anaheim, CA: Synthesis Press.

120. **Gattefosse, R.M.** 1937: *Gattefosse's aromatherapy* (translated in 1993 by R. Tisserand. Saffron Walden: C.W. Daniel).

121. **Lorenzetti, B., Souza, G. and Sarti, S.** 1991: Myrcene mimics the peripheral analgesic activity of lemongrass tea. *Journal of Ethnopharmacology* **34:** 43–8.

122. **Sheppard-Hangar, S.** 1995: *Aromatherapy practitioner reference manual. Volume II.* Tampa, FL: Atlantic School of Aromatherapy.

123. **Wren, R.C.** 1988: *Potter's new cyclopaedia of botanical drugs and preparations.* London: Churchill Livingstone.

124. **Rose, J.** 1992: *The aromatherapy book.* San Francisco: North Atlantic Books.

125. **Von Frohilche, A.** 1968: A review of clinical, pharmacological and bacteriological research into *Oleum spicae. Wiener Medizinische Wochenschrift* **15,** 345–50.

126. **Gobel, H., Schmidt, G. and Soyka, D.** 1991: Effect of peppermint and eucalyptus oil preparations on neurophysiological and experimental algesimetric headache parameters. *Cephalalgia* **14,** 228–34.

127. **Perez–Raya, M.D., Utrilla, M.P., Navarro, M.C. and Jimenez, J.** 1990: CNS activity of *Mentha rotundifolia* and *Mentha longifolia* essential oil in mice and rats. *Phytotherapy Research* **4,** 232–4.

128. **Lawless, J.** 1994: *Aromatherapy and the mind.* London: Thorsons.

129. **Cabo, J., Crespo, M.E., Jimenez, J. and Zarzuelo, A.** 1986: The spasmolytic activity of various aromatic plants from the province of

Granada. The activity of the major components of their essential oils. *Plantes Medicinales et Phytotherapie* **20,** 213–18.

130. **Craig, C.** 1994: Introduction to CNS pharmacology. In Craig, C. and Stitzel, R. (eds), *Modern pharmacology*, 4th edn. Boston, MA: Little, Brown & Co., 329–36.

131. **Moran, A., Martin, N.K.** *et al.* 1989: Analgesic, antipyretic and anti-inflammatory activity of essential oil of *Artemisia caerulescens* subsp. *gallica. Journal of Ethnopharmacology* **3,** 307–17.

132. **Evans, W.C.** 1994: *Trease & Evan's pharmacognoscy*, 13th edn. London: Baillière Tindall.

133. **Reiter, M. and Brandt, W.** 1985: Relaxant effect on the trachea and ilea of smooth muscle of the guinea pig. *Arzneimittel-forschung (Aulendorf)* **35,** 408–14.

134. **Taddei, I., Giachetti, D., Taddel, E. and Mantovani, P.** 1988: Spasmolytic activity of peppermint, sage and rosemary essences and their major constituents. *Fitoterapia* **LIX,** 463–8.

135. **Giachetti, D., Taddei, E. and Taddei, I.** 1988: Pharmacological activity of essential oils on Oddi's sphincter. *Planta Medica* **54,** 38–40.

136. **Fakim, G. and Sewaj, M.D.** 1992: Studies on the antisickling properties of extracts of *Sideroxylon puberulum, Faujariopsis flexuosa, Cardispermum halicacabum* and *Pelargonium graveoleus. Planta Medica* **58 (Suppl.),** A648–9.

137. **Fakim, G.A., Sofowora, E.A., and Sewaj, M.D.** 1990: Reversal of sickling and crenation in erythrocytes by aqueous extracts of *Pelargonium × asperum, Foeniculum vulgare* and *Sideroxylon puberulum. Revue Agricole et Societe de I'll Maurice* **69,** 91–3.

138. **Nadkarni, K.M.** 1992: *Indian Materia Medica. Volume 1.* Prakashan: Bombay Popular.

139. **Arctander, S.** 1994: *Perfume and flavor materials of natural origin.* Carol Stream, IL: Allured Publishing.

140. **Tisserand, R.** 1989: *The art of aromatherapy.* Saffron Walden: C.W. Daniel.

141. **Leicester, R.J. and Hunt, R.H.** 1982: Peppermint oil to reduce colonic spasm during endoscopy. *Lancet* **2,** 989–90.

142. **McKenzie, J. and Gallacher, M.** 1989: A sweet-smelling success: use of peppermint oil in helping patients accept their colostomies. *Nursing Times* **85,** 48–9.

143. **Betts, A.** 1993: An overview of pathology. In Hinchcliff, S., Norman, S. and Schober, J. (eds), *Nursing practice and health care.* London: Edward Arnold, 148–9.

144. **Mills, S.** 1991: *Out of the earth.* London: Viking Arkana.

145. **Craig, C.R. and Stitzel, R.** 1994: Lipid mediators of homeostasis and inflammation. In *Modern pharmacology*, 4th edn. Boston, MA: Little, Brown & Co.

146. **Goodman-Gilma A., Goodman, L.S. and Murad, F.** (eds) 1985: *The pharmacological basis of therapeutics*. New York: Macmillan.

147. **Kvam, D.C.** 1994: Anti-inflammatory and anti-rheumatic drugs. In *Modern pharmacology*, 4th edn. Boston, MA: Little, Brown & Co., 485–500.

148. **Mascolo, N., Autore, G. and Capasso, F.** 1987: Biological screening of Italian medicinal plants for anti-inflammatory activity. *Phytotherapy Research* **1**, 28–31.

149. **Bronaugh, R.L., Wester, R.C.** *et al.* 1990: *In vivo* percutaneous absorption of fragrance ingredients in Rhesus monkeys and humans. *Food and Chemical Toxicology* **28**, 369–73.

150. **Rossi, T., Melegari, M.** *et al.* 1988: Sedative, anti-inflammatory and anti-diuretic effects induced in rats by essential oils of varieties of *Anthemis nobilis:* a comparative study. *Pharmacological Research Communications* **20 (Suppl.)**, 71–4.

151. **Jakovlev, V., Isaac, O., Thiemer, K. and Kunde, R.** 1979: Pharmacological investigations with compounds of chamomile. II. New investigations on the antiphlogistic effects of a bisabolol and bisabolol oxide. *Planta Medica* **35**, 125–40.

152. **Tubaro, A., Zillia, C., Redaeli, C. and Loggia, R.** 1984: Evaluation of anti-inflammatory activity of chamomile extract topical application. *Planta Medica* **50**, 359–60.

153. **Benet, A., Stamford, F. and Tavares, I.A.** The biological activity of eugenol, a major constituent of nutmeg: studies on prostaglandins, the intestine and other tissues. *Phytotherapy Research* **2**, 125–9.

154. **Wagner, H., Wierer, M. and Bauer, R.** 1986: *In vitro*-Hemmung der Prostaglandin-Biosynthe durch etherische Ole und phenolische Verbindungen. *Planta Medica* **4**, 185–6.

155. **Manley, K.** 1993: Care of the acutely ill. In Hinchcliff, S., Norman, S. and Schober, J. (eds), *Nursing practice and health care*, 2nd edn. London: Edward Arnold, 1067–72.

156. **Dailey, J.W.** 1994: Sedative-hypnotic and anxiolytic drugs. In Craig, C.R. and Sitzel, R.E. (eds), *Modern pharmacology*, 4th edn. Boston, MA: Little Brown & Co., 369–77.

157. **Tisserand, R.** 1988: Lavender beats benzodiazepines. *International Journal of Aromatherapy* **1**, 1–2.

158. **Atanassova-Shopova, S., Roussinov, K.S. and Boycheva, I.** 1973: On certain central neurotropic effects of lavender essential oils. II. Communications: studies on the effects of linalol and of terpineol. *Bulletin of the Institute of Physiology* **XV**, 149–56.

159. **Guillemain, J., Rouseeau, A. and Delaveau, P.** 1989: Effects neurodepresseurs de l'huile essentielle de *Lavandula angustifolia. Annales pharmaceutiques francaises* **47**, 337–43.

160. **Buchbauer, G., Jirovetz, L. and Jager, W.** 1991: Aromatherapy: evidence for sedative effects of the essential oil of lavender after inhalation. *Archiv der Pharmazie (Weinheim)* **46C,** 1067–72.

161. **Henry, J., Rusius, C.W., Davies, M. and Veazey-French, Y.** 1994: Lavender for night sedation of people with dementia. *International Journal of Aromatherapy* **6,** 28–30.

162. **Jager, W., Buckbauer, G. and Jirovetz, L.** 1992: Evidence of the sedative effect of neroli oil, citronella and phenylethyl acetate on mice. *Journal of Essential Oil Research* **4,** 387–94.

163. **Buchbauer, G., Jirovetz, L. and Jager, W.** 1992: Kurzmitteilungen: *Passiflora* and lime-blossoms – motility effects after inhalation of the essential oils and of some of the main constituents in animal experiments. *Archiv der Pharmazie (Weinheim)* **325,** 247–8.

164. **Khanna, T. et al.** 1993: CNS and analgesic studies on *Nigella sativa. Fitoterapia* **64,** 407–10.

165. **Ashford, A.A., Sharpe, C.J. and Stephens, F.F.** 1993: Thymol basic ethers and related compounds: central nervous system depressant action. *Nature* **No. 4871,** 969–71.

166. **Nacht, D.I. et al.** 1921: Sedative properties of some aromatic drugs and fumes. *Journal of Pharmacology and Experimental Therapeutics* **18,** 361–72.

167. **Rovesti, P. and Columbo, E.** 1973: Aromatherapy and aerosols. *Soap, Perfumery and Cosmetics* **46,** 475–7.

168. **Anthony, G. and Thibodeau, G.** 1983: *Textbook of Anatomy and Physiology.* London: CV Mosby.

169. **Rahe, R.H.** 1975: Epidemiological studies of life change and illness. *International Journal of Psychiatry in Medicine* **6,** 133–46.

170. **Pelletier, K.R.** 1992: Mind-body health: research, clinical and policy implications. *American Journal of Health Promotion* **6,** 345–8.

171. **Wilkinson, G.** 1991: Stress: another chimera? *British Medical Journal* **302,** 191–2.

172. **Cohen, S., Tyrrell, D.A.J. and Smith, A.P.** 1991: Psychological stress and susceptibility to the common cold. *New England Journal of Medicine* **325,** 606–12.

173. **Wilde McCormick, E.** 1992: *Healing the heart.* London: Optima Books.

174. **Pitts, F.** 1969: The biochemistry of anxiety. *Scientific American* **Feb.** 69–75.

175. **Barasch, M.** 1993: *The healing path.* New York: Putman.

176. **Clark, E. and Montague, S.** 1993: The nature of stress and its implications for nursing practice. In Hinchcliff, S., Norman, S. and Schober, J. (eds), *Nursing practice and health care.* London: Edward Arnold, 214–47.

177. **LeDouz, J.** 1996: *The emotional brain.* New York: Simon & Schuster.

178. **Linn, B.S., Linn, M.W. and Klimas, N.G.** 1988: Effects of

psychophysical stress on surgical outcomes. *Psychosomatic Medicine* **50**, 230–44.

179. **Wilson-Barnett, J. and Carrigy, A.** 1978: Factors influencing patients' emotional reactions to hospitalization. *Journal of Advanced Nursing* **3**, 221–9.

180. **Pelletier, K.** 1992: *Mind as healer, mind as slayer*. New York: Delta.

181. **Quinn, J.** 1993: Psychoimmunologic effects of therapeutic touch on practitioners and recently bereaved recipients. *Advanced Nursing Science* **15**, 13–26.

182. **Jamison, R.N., Parris, W.C.V. and Maxson, W.S.** 1987: Psychological factors influencing recovery from outpatient surgery. *Behavioural Research Therapies* **25**, 31–7.

183. **Layne, O.L. and Yudofsky, S.C.** 1971: Postoperative psychosis in cardiotomy patients. *New England Journal of Medicine* **11 March**, 518–20.

184. **Roberts, R.** 1991: Preventing PDD (post-pump delirium) after surgery. *Nursing* **4**, 28–31.

185. **Tasev, T., Toleva, P. and Balabanova, V.** 1969: The neuro-psychic effect of Bulgarian rose, lavender and geranium. *Folia Medica* **11**, 307–17.

186. **Sugano, H. and Sato, N.** 1991: Psychophysiological studies of fragrance. *Chemical Senses* **16**, 183–4.

187. **Muruzzella, J.C. and Sicurella, N.A.** 1960: Antibacterial activity of essential oil vapors. *Journal of the American Pharmaceutical Association (Scientific Edition)* **49(11)**, 692–5.

188. **Bennett, G.** 1987: *The wound and the doctor*. London: Secker & Warburg.

189. **Stevenson, C.** 1992: Orange blossom evaluation. *International Journal of Aromatherapy* **4**, 22–4.

190. **Ashworth, P.M.** 1984: Staff-patient communication in coronary care units. *Journal of Advanced Nursing* **9**, 35–41.

191. **Weiss, S.** 1979: The language of touch. *Nursing Research* **28**, 76–80.

192. **Landsdown, R.** 1994: Living longer? Qualitative survival. *Journal of the Royal Society of Medicine* **87**, 636.

193. **Dossy, L.** 1993: *Healing words*. San Francisco: HarperSanFrancisco.

194. **Benson, H.** 1975: *The relaxation response*. New York: Avon.

195. **Hildebrand, S.** 1994: Massage and aromatherapy. In Wells, R. (ed.), *Wells' supportive therapies in health care*. London: Baillière Tindall, 110–11.

196. **Drury, M.** 1989: Caring. In McGuire, C. (ed.), *Visions of nursing*. Sedona: Light Technology, 44.

197. **Pratt, J. and Mason, A.** 1981: *The caring touch*. London: Heyden.

198. **Penson, J.** 1991: Complementary therapies. In Penson, J. and Fisher, R. (eds), *Palliative care for people with cancer*. London: Edward Arnold, 233–46.

199. **Torii, S., Fukuda, H., Kanemoto, H., Miyanchi, R., Hamauzu and Kawasaki, M.** 1988: Contingent negative variation (CNV) and the

psychological effects of odour in perfumery. In Van Toller, S. and Dodd, G. (eds), *Psychology and biology of fragrance*. London: Chapman & Hall, 107–20.

200. **Siegal, B.** 1986: *Love, medicine and miracles.* New York: Arrow.

201. **Cousins, N.** 1979: *Anatomy of an illness as perceived by a patient.* New York: W.W. Norton.

202. **Wilde McCormick, E.** 1990: *Change for the better.* London: Unwin.

203. **Fiore, N.** 1979: Fighting cancer – one patient's perspective. *New England Journal of Medicine* **300,** 284–9.

204. **Young, S.** 1990: The exceptional cancer patient support group: coping with cancer. In Clements, S. and Martin, E.J. (eds), *Nursing and holistic wellness*. Dubuque, IA: Kendall/Hunt Publishing, 233–47.

205. **Antoni, M.H., Fletcher, M.A., Goldstein, D.A., Ironson, G. and Laperiere, A.** 1990: Psychoneuroimmunology and HIV-1. *Journal of Consulting and Clinical Psychology* **58,** 38–49.

206. **Kiecolt-Glaser, J.K. and Glaser, R.** 1993: Mind and immunity. In Goleman, D. and Curin, J. (eds), *Mind-body medicine*. New York: Consumer Reports Books, 39–65.

207. **Ornish, D.** 1991: Reversing heart disease through diet, exercise and stress management. *Journal of the American Dietetic Association* **91,** 162–5.

208. **Farrow, J.** 1990: Massage therapy and nursing-care. *Nursing Standard* **4,** 26–8.

209. **Tisserand, T. and Balacs, T.** 1988/1989: Essential oil therapy for cancer. *International Journal of Aromatherapy* **1,** 20–25.

210. **King, J.** 1993: Have the scent to relax. *World Medicine* **1 Oct,** 29–31.

211. **Birchall, A.** 1990: A whiff of happiness. *New Scientist.* **25 Aug,** 44–7.

212. **Reed, L. and Norfolk, L.** 1993: Aromatherapy in midwifery. *International Journal of Alternative and Complementary Medicine* **11,** 15–17.

213. **Woolfson, A. and Hewitt, D.** 1992: Intensive aromacare. *International Journal of Aromatherapy* **4,** 12–13.

214. **Dunn, C., Sleep, J. and Collett, D.** 1995: Sensing an improvement: an experimental study to evaluate the use of aromatherapy, massage and periods of rest in an intensive-care unit. *Journal of Advanced Nursing* **21,** 34–40.

215. **Burns, E. and Blamey, C.** 1994: Soothing scents in childbirth. *International Journal of Aromatherapy* **6,** 24–8.

216. **Wise, R.** 1989: Flower power. *Nursing Times* **85,** 45–7.

217. **O'Regan, B. and Hirshberg.** 1993: *Spontaneous remission.* Sausalito, CA: Institute of Neotic Sciences.

218. **Handley, W.S.** 1909: The natural cure of cancer. *British Medical Journal,* 582–9.

219. **Emerson, R.W.** 1996: Quotation. In *Noetic Sciences Review* **No. 37,** 1.

8

CLINICAL USE IN SPECIALIZED DEPARTMENTS

My aim in writing this clinical section is to make nurses aware of the potential of aromatherapy for treating recognized problems within specific departments. It is also hoped that nurses might draw the attention of doctors to the potential of medical applications of aromatherapy within the following specific departments:

- cardiology;
- care of the ageing;
- critical care;
- dermatology;
- endocrinology;
- gynaecology;
- immunology;
- oncology;
- paediatrics;
- palliative and terminal care;
- respiratory care.

'Ultimately it is the physician's respect for the human soul that determines the worth of his science' (Norman Cousins, 1993).[1]

CARDIOLOGY

Many advances have been made in cardiology since I trained as a nurse in the 1960s. Transplants are no longer newsworthy. Despite incredible life-saving achievements, there are still a great many patients with cardiac problems. I have decided to select one potential 'problem' from the medical side and one from the surgical side: myocardial infarction and post-pump depression (PPD).

Myocardial infarction

This life-threatening condition occurs when a blood clot obstructs one or more of the coronary arteries, preventing blood from reaching the heart muscle. The ischaemic heart causes severe pain, often accompanied by nausea and sometimes with loss of consciousness. Depending on the severity of muscle damage, the patient will live or die. The number of deaths from heart attacks each year is equal to the number of babies born[2] – a staggering thought.

Many patients arrive in a coronary-care unit full of fear. They have been swept away from the life they knew into a nightmare situation where every blip on the monitor is watched. Their privacy and dignity are left behind, along with unattended business meetings and unreturned telephone calls. Patients in such a unit find it extremely difficult to relax. It is accepted that anxiety can extend infarction areas or precipitate further arrhythmias.[3] These patients, it is suggested, are more likely to experience severe or chronic psychological distress. Rowe discovered that patients' anxieties tend to be focused on their own illness.[4] However, the severity of the infarction and also how close to death patients perceive themselves to be will influence the level of psychological distress that they experience. Vlay and Fricchione reported on the emotional disturbances of these patients, which are often expressed in the form of depression, anger, frustration and fear.[5]

Attempting to alleviate these feelings, to reduce anxiety and to enhance patient care is the key to using aromatherapy in a coronary-care unit. Because patients may be nursed together in an open environment, it is important to select essential oils which will be acceptable to all who have to smell them. Aromas of citrus and herbs are usually acceptable. Single rooms may be used by patients as they progress. However, although their anxiety level may be reduced, they will still be stressed from their experience.

Although Tisserand and Balacs state that 'it is extremely unlikely that an essential oil could exacerbate hypertension or hypotension',[6] it might be advisable to avoid any essential oil which is thought to have hypertensive or stimulating properties. This would rule out essential oils such as *Rosmarinus officinalis* (rosemary) and *Lavandula latifolia* (spike lavender). However, rosemary was shown to have slight anxiety-reducing effects in a study at the University of Wolverhampton. Unfortunately, the botanical name and chemotype were not stated.[7]

Peppermint is traditionally thought of as having stimulating properties, but one study showed that two particular mints, *Mentha rotundifolia* and

Mentha longifolia, which grow wild in Spain, had sedative properties in rats and that both potentiated sodium barbitone-induced sleep.[8] l-menthol is supposed to dilate systemic blood vessels when given intravenously.[9] Menthol-flavoured cigarettes and peppermint confectionery have led to atrial fibrillation in cardiac patients who were on cardiac stabilizers.[10] Peppermint also has a pervasive smell and is difficult to live with long term.

Essential oils which could have relaxing effects include the following:

- *Melissa officinalis* (melissa);[11, 12]
- *Lavandula angustifolia* (lavender);[13, 14]
- *Anthemis nobilis* (Roman chamomile);[15]
- *Citrus aurantium* subsp. *aurantium flos* (neroli);[16, 17]
- *Aniba rosaeodora* (rosewood);[18]
- *Origanum majorana* (marjoram);[18]
- *Rosa damascena* (Rose).[18, 19]

Although *Salvia sclarea* (clary sage) and *Matricaria recutitia* (German chamomile) also have relaxing qualities, it is best to avoid them on a cardiac ward. They both have very powerful aromas, and many people do not like them. Clary sage can occasionally cause headaches in a confined space. The colour of German chamomile makes it impractical to use, and its aroma can sometimes cause nausea, especially among patients who are mildly allergic to chamomile tea.

It is important to ask your patients which aromas remind them of pleasant memories, and use only those. Remember that gentle touch is one of the most soothing actions we can offer to another human being in distress. Nursing is about being there for our patients – completely and holistically. Aromatherapy can put the heart back into nursing.

Post-pump depression (PPD)

Many patients arriving in a critical-care unit have undergone *elective* surgery, so they have known (and to a certain extent have been prepared for) the ordeal that awaits them. This is unlike the situation for patients in a coronary-care unit, which mainly admits medical emergencies. Although emergency surgical operations obviously do occur, the majority of patients admitted to a cardiac critical-care unit are predetermined.

Consequently, critical-care units are more geared towards the orientation and preparation of patients. This preparation includes a tour of the unit, an explanation of the monitoring equipment, and a brief description of what will happen to the patient when he or she returns from theatre. In her book, *Healing the Heart*, Elizabeth McCormick suggests that 'preparation by the feeling heart for the worker heart's surgery is essential'.[2] I believe that she is right.

Indeed, it is understood that patients who are prepared in this way are better able to cope with their condition post-operatively.[20] Fear of surgery is a factor which can strongly influence a patient's emotional response to hospitalization.[21] Of all the operations that are performed, possibly open-heart surgery is the most feared.

Post-pump depression (PPD), sometimes called post-pump delirium, occurs in 30 to 40 per cent of cardiotomy patients.[22] PPD is characterized by hyperventilation, tachycardia, auditory hallucinations, disorientation and paranoid delusions. The symptoms are distressing for the patient, their relatives, and the nurses who care for them.

Although there are several theories concerning the pathogenesis of PPD, nothing is clear-cut. It is thought that older patients, those undergoing aortic valve replacement and male patients are more at risk. However, a reduction in post-operative psychosis was achieved in 50 per cent of patients by a pre-operative psychiatric interview. This interview allowed and encouraged patients to ask questions about their disease and surgery, and to discuss openly any worries they had.[22] Pre-operative psychological preparation is now recognized as being important not just for the patient, but also for the relatives who will be supporting the patient post-operatively.[20]

Discussing current or potential marital or relationship problems can help to indicate which patients are more likely to succumb to PPD.[23] It is recognized that any illness will force a relationship to change, and open-heart surgery will certainly test the strength of every relationship.

Utilizing the preparation time, aromatherapy can set a safe, gentle pattern which, when repeated post-operatively, could affect the patient positively through learned memory. If a patient feels relaxation and pleasure when he or she receives a foot, hand or face massage with a favourite smell pre-operatively, then the chances are that he or she will feel the same sensation of relaxation and pleasure when the aromatherapy is repeated post-operatively.

It is thought that this 'pleasure memory' could have an effect even when the patient is not fully conscious. What the patient is receiving is care in a manner he or she can recognize, even in this critical state. When I was conducting a pilot study on post-cardiotomy patients, one of the most striking remarks a patient in the study made to me was 'you were the first person who didn't hurt me'. That has stayed with me. As nurses, we do not want to hurt our patients, but sometimes we do all the same.

Talk with your patient about the smells they enjoyed in their childhood and about the smells they did not like. Were they brought up in the country, near a wood? Have they travelled to far-away places? What kind of perfumes do they enjoy? The answers to all of these questions will provide guidelines as to which essential oils to use. This is a situation where, apart from trying to reduce the patient's anxiety, we are also trying to give pleasure in circumstances in which pleasure is not often experienced.

Patients frequently experience a 'high' of survival immediately after open-heart surgery. This is often followed by a 'low' of exhaustion. Touch and smell allow a recognition of this rite of passage. Post-cardiotomy patients need to feel celebrated, whole and held. They have survived one of the greatest miracles orthodox medicine has to offer. Now it is time to help them to heal through the comforts of gentle touch and familiar smell.

Essential oils to choose for the possible reduction of PPD include the following:

- *Citrus aurantium* subsp. *aurantium flos* (neroli);[24]
- *Angelica archangelica* (root) (angelica);[25]
- *Lavandula angustifolia* (lavender);[26]
- *Aniba rosaeodora* (rosewood);[18]
- *Origanum majorana* (marjoram);[18]
- *Rosa damascena* (rose);[18, 27]
- *Melissa officinalis* (melissa);[11, 12]
- *Anthemis nobilis* (Roman chamomile);[15]
- *Pelargonium graveolens* (geranium).[7]

CARE OF THE ELDERLY

It perhaps appropriate to include a section on care of the elderly, as Helen Passant, recognized as one of the first nurses to use aromatherapy in a hospital, was the ward sister of a geriatric unit.[28]

Improved diet and medical breakthroughs have allowed the human race to survive longer and longer – the oldest surviving woman, Jeanne Calment, lived to the age of 121 years. Therefore it is hardly surprising that many of these older people will need care and, in some instances, supervision. It is a sad part of our Western culture that age is not revered, and those who could have imparted so much information and life experience to the younger members of society are frequently sent off to institutions. This is not to denigrate institutions for the elderly, as they are obviously much needed, but to question why we either cannot or do not want to look after our own.

Sheltered housing seems to be a good compromise. The world has become such a busy place that there appears to be no time to nurture or just 'be' with those whose sense of time has gone. It would appear that dementia and Alzheimer's disease are on the increase. Whether this increase is because we are all living longer or because factors which may contribute to dementia are becoming more widespread is difficult to say. At present, 20 per cent of those over 80 years old suffer from dementia. Alzheimer's disease is possibly the most difficult condition to accept. Recently, I was in New Mexico and met a physician investigating dementia among the Native American population. She said that there is no record of Alzheimer's disease among the Navaho – it just does not occur. This is not because the Nahavo have no name for Alzheimer's, but she felt that it was possibly because of genetic or environmental factors.

I have friends who run a beautiful home for the elderly in the New Forest. The average age of the inmates is 88.4 years. However, the 82-year-old mother of one of the owners regularly comes in to help out at weekends – a sprightly, immaculately dressed lady, she is older than some of the residents she cares for. This would seem to indicate that age often has little to do with ageing. That residential home uses aromatherapy regularly, and one is immediately struck by the wonderful atmosphere and lovely smells that prevail.

It is recognized that there are classic problems which can occur among elderly patients. These include the following:

- sleep pattern alteration;
- dementia;
- constipation;
- skin ulcers and poor healing;
- osteoarthritis.

Sleep pattern alteration and insomnia

There have been a few published studies which have shown that *Lavandula angustifolia* (true lavender) can be helpful in facilitating sleep.[29] The *Lancet* published a letter explaining one of the studies.[17] Despite the lack of hard data, lavender is being used to promote relaxation and sleep in many hospitals in the UK. However, it is important to use the right lavender.[30]

It is equally important to remember that too much (even of the right lavender) can have a negative effect, causing patients' insomnia to increase. There can be problems with 'overdosing' if electric nebulizers are kept constantly switched on.

For some elderly people, lavender is a much disliked smell, associated with death. This learned memory can be triggered, raising images of dying relatives and friends from times long ago, when the bed-linen smelled strongly of lavender. Linen chests were liberally stacked with lavender bags. In all cases, but especially with care of the elderly, it is really important to allow patients to choose their aromas. Memories are very individual and personal, and they are easily triggered by smells.[31]

Other possible essential oils which could be used to promote sleep would include the following:

- *Citrus aurantium* subsp. *aurantium flos* (neroli);[16]
- *Citrus reticulata* (mandarin);[25]
- *Cymbopogon citratus* (lemongrass);[32]
- *Angelica archangelica* (angelica).[25]

I personally have also found *Chamaemelum nobile* (Roman chamomile) and *Origanum majorana* (sweet marjoram) to be useful for gently promoting sleep in patients.

Dementia

Dementia is present in 20 per cent of individuals over 80 years of age.[33] Although there are over 50 different causes of dementia, some of which are reversible, the majority are progressive, leading to premature death. The most common cause of dementia in the developed world is Alzheimer's disease. Although Alzheimer's can affect patients as young as 35 years of age, the most recent view is that this disturbing disease is part of a pathological cascade process linked with ageing.[34] In total, 70 per cent of patients aged over 65 years with dementia will have Alzheimer's disease. Currently there is no cure.

Whilst it is recognized that aromatherapy is not a cure for dementia, smell and touch are powerful messengers, often penetrating the fog of amnesia in a way in which words do not. In cases where patients cannot or will not remain stationary, walking alongside them whilst simultaneously conducting a gentle hand massage can lead to some positive changes in the patient, such as renewed eye contact and speech coherence. Where patients are confined to bed and incapable of walking, or are violently resistant to any form of touch, vaporizers and nebulizers can be used. Even in instances such as these, when it seems that the patient will be unable to help with the selection of an aroma, offering a choice of two different smells can elicit a response.

Suitable essential oils would be ones that the patient might be familiar with either from his or her childhood or from life experiences. For example, Trumpers, possibly the oldest gentlemen's hairdressers in London, has traditionally used essential oil of geranium (Bourbon) in their pomades for over a 100 years (G. Freeman, personal communication).

Rosmarinus officinalis CT cineole or borneol (rosemary) is useful, as rosemary will be remembered by most elderly patients as a common ingredient in cooking and from gardening. 'There's rosemary – that's for remembrance' may have been quoted by Ophelia, but it is a valid comment. Rosemary is traditionally thought to be helpful as a memory aid. (As it is acknowledged to be a hypertensive, it should not be used on patients with diastolic blood pressure above 100 mmHg. The chemotypes champhor and verbenone, which contain ketones, should be avoided.)

Other aromas with which the elderly may be familiar could include the following:

- *Pelargonium graveolens* (geranium);
- *Lavandula angustifolia* (lavender).

If a patient has lived in the tropics, offer an essential oil such as lemongrass, ylang ylang or sandalwood.

Aromatherapy is used by the Dales Occupational Therapy Service in Derbyshire to improve the quality of life of patients with Alzheimer's disease. Essential oils that have been found to be useful include the following:

- pine, eucalyptus and peppermint to trigger conversation and memory;
- lavender and geranium to trigger thoughts of cooking and plants.[35]

Constipation

The slowed-down passage of food through the large intestine may be a result of reduced exercise or insufficient roughage in the diet. The latter could be due to poor appetite for various reasons ranging from ill-fitting dentures to boredom with institutional food. Another cause of constipation is regular use of sleeping pills.

One of the simplest and most gentle ways to ease constipation of early onset is through abdominal massage using essential oils, although it is emphasized that this is suitable for constipation of a few days' duration only. A slight improvement was documented in a study by Klauser, although in that instance no essential oils were used.[36] In the residential home I mentioned earlier, this form of massage has produced significant results!

Possible essential oils to choose would include the following:

- *Piper nigrum* (black pepper);
- *Zingiber officinale* (ginger);
- *Foeniculum vulgare* (fennel);
- *Origanum marjorana* (marjoram);
- *Citrus × paradisi* (grapefruit).[37]

Use only two drops of either essential oil, and let your patient choose which oil is used. Work slowly and rhythmically up the ascending colon, along the transverse colon and down the descending colon, paying attention to both hepatic and splenic flexures. This gentle massage only takes 5 minutes, but can be really useful, and is best repeated up to five times a day or until relief is obtained.

Skin ulcers and slow healing

As we age our ability to heal becomes slower. Our skin becomes thinner and more fragile, and the slightest knock can cause a deep bruise. Very gentle massage with linoleic-acid-rich carrier oils can aid the elasticity of ageing skin. Certain essential oils have the ability to help skin to mend. Possibly the most extensive clinical data (although it is not in the form of a randomized trial) comes from Alan Barker, an aromatherapist employed by the National Health Service. He uses the following floral waters to irrigate wounds:

■ *Melaleuca viridiflora* (niaouli);
■ *Citrus limon* (lemon);
■ *Melaleuca alternifolia* CT terpineol (tea tree);
■ *Matricaria recutitia* (German chamomile);
■ *Citrus paradisi* (grapefruit).[38]

Wounds can be irrigated with floral waters and compresses applied. Areas immediately around the sore can be gently wiped with macerated oils such as *Hypericum perforatum* (St John's wort), *Calendula officinalis* (calendula) or just plain carrier oil of evening primrose. *Matricaria recutitai* (German chamomile) was found to be effective in a controlled double-blind study of slow-healing wounds in 14 patients in 1987. A further article reported two case-studies in the *Journal of Tissue Viability* in 1993, using lavender and tea tree.[39]

Osteoarthritis

Degenerative joint pain is frequently part of the ageing process, especially if there is a family history of rheumatism. As secondary changes occur in the underlying bone, so pain and impaired function make life a misery for those who were once agile. This is particularly the case if one of the affected joints has been injured. Macdonald wrote about elderly patients and osteopathic pain,[40] and the following essential oils were used in her research:

■ eucalyptus;
■ juniper;
■ marjoram;
■ rosemary.

Unfortunately, no botanical names were given, so it is impossible to assess which essential oils were actually used (there are 400 different types of *Eucalyptus!*). Traditional essential oils for this osteoarthritis pain are warming, encourage blood circulation, or have an analgesic-like action. Franchomme and Penoel state that *p*-cymene has analgesic properties that are particularly suited to osteoarthritis.[25] Paramycene is found in the following essential oils: lemon, savory, coriander, angelica, frankincense, tea tree, *Eucalyptus globulus*, cypress and oregano.[41]

I personally have found *Cymbopogon citratus* (lemongrass) to be useful for treating this kind of pain, possibly because of its myrcene content,[42] and *Satureja hortensis* (summer savory), which contains myrcene and also 1 per cent damascenone – a ketone with papaverine-like properties.[43]

Perhaps I should end this section with a mention of the anti-ageing potential of essential oils. Professor Stanley Deans has conducted substantial research into the properties of polyunsaturated fatty acids (PUFAs) which form part of plant oils and are used by the human body to make cellular components and steroid hormones. It has been shown that ageing is associated with a decline in PUFAs. In research on ageing rats, essential oils were found to restore PUFA levels almost to the levels observed in young mice. Of the essential oils tested, thyme and clove appeared to give the most impressive results.[44] This research involved feeding the rats essential oils by mouth. There is no suggestion that we should do the same to our patients or ourselves, but the anti-ageing properties of essential oils may turn out to be an exciting area.

CRITICAL CARE

Critical care can encompass both medical and surgical emergencies and elective post-operative patients. Frequently, the medical and surgical departments are separate, but in a small hospital the unit may include a large cross-section of different types of patient. The one common factor may be the brevity of their condition. However, each patient is someone's child, no matter how old he or she may be. Each patient belongs, in some capacity, to another, and it is the others who are so often in need of nurturing. Critical-care units can be very frightening to those seeing them for the first time, with so many tubes and so much complicated machinery around motionless bodies – but the motionless body has the face of a loved one.

I remember seeing my father in a critical-care unit not so long ago, and experiencing some of the feelings of helplessness that many visitors feel. I felt this even though I had trained and worked in critical care for many years. Often relatives feel that there is nothing they can do except wait and pray. In one sense they are right, but aromatherapy does present a wonderful opportunity if a critical-care nurse is open to using it. The gentle stroking movements used in aromatherapy touch (especially in the hand massage) are extremely simple both to teach and to learn.

I have taught them to a 5-year-old granddaughter, who spent almost an hour lovingly stroking her grandfather's hands. Her sad cross little face softened as she sang gently under her breath, moving her hands in time to her lullaby. Her parents watched her as she worked, amazed at the transformation. This little girl knew that she had been given an important task which not only empowered her but was actually of therapeutic value.

Teaching relatives to touch in this way does not take very long – probably only 5 minutes. We can all find that amount of time. Talking with relatives about the aromas that patients enjoyed before they came into hospital allows dialogue on a safe subject, but one that is still linked to the patient. Finding an aroma which relatives feel could help their loved one gives them something to think about, and a way of becoming involved. It is best to offer just a few aromas that are known to have relaxing effects. The floral aromas are usually popular. Relatives can choose the aroma in the privacy of a day-room or at the bedside. Just because a patient is intubated does not mean that aromatherapy will have no effect – essential oils are absorbed through the skin. The aromas will also be inhaled by the patient's relatives.

The two conditions I have chosen to illustrate the use of aromatherapy in critical care are shock and pressure area sores.

Shock

When nurses talk about 'shock', they mean circulatory collapse, when the arterial blood pressure is too low to maintain an adequate supply of blood to the tissues.[45] Physical shock induces cold sweating skin, a weak rapid pulse and irregular breathing. However, if individuals other than nurses talk about shock, they are usually referring to the emotional impact of a bad experience (e.g. someone who has received bad news, or who has returned home to find it burgled). These events produce emotional shock which has similar, although not so extensive, effects to the physical shock that we know as nurses.

Patients who are in a critical-care unit have suffered immense shock, both physical and emotional. Modern medicine will ensure that the physical symptoms are addressed with adrenaline drips and fluid replacement, but what about the emotional shock? Where is the hug and the cup of hot sweet tea? These are offered to conscious people who have 'had a shock.' As nurses, we are responsible for the totality of our patients – to relieve the whole shock, emotional as well as physical. This means giving comfort. We may not be able to give a cup of hot sweet tea, but we can touch gently and soothingly with hands that smell of familiar and pleasant memories.

Essential oils to offer in shock include the following:

- *Citrus aurantium* var. *amara flos* (neroli);[24]
- *Lavandula angustifolia* (lavender);[26]
- *Chamaemelum nobile* (chamomile);[46]
- *Rosa damascena* (rose);
- *Angelica archangelica* (root) (angelica);
- *Melissa officinalis* (melissa).

Although I have found no references in the literature on the use of rose and angelica to treat shock in humans, I have used both essential oils on many patients, to tremendous effect. I have yet to find someone who does not like the smell of either of them. Angelica is a useful aroma for patients who dislike floral smells – it is woody and slightly earthy. The root is more pungent than the seed, but has a wonderful 'after-smell' that most people find very comforting. I have suggested that the root be used even though it contains furanocoumarins, which require caution when patients are likely to be exposed to ultraviolet light. Critical-care patients are unlikely to be exposed to ultraviolet light in the unit, but nurses and relatives might be, and they will also be inhaling the aroma of the essential oil. However, photosensitivity to the essential oil is only manifested when it is applied to the skin, not when it is inhaled.

Rose was the subject of some research carried out on the motor activity of white mice.[47] Rose appeared to sedate the animals without causing ataxia, whilst the control substance (reserpine) produced ataxia. Gentle sedation is another term for calming. Perhaps this study demonstrates that animals can be calmed by smelling roses, just as humans can. The rose aroma *is* very soothing and, I feel, under-utilized in critical-care units. It gives a special kind of comfort, even if this is only from learned memory.

Pressure area wounds

Critically ill patients often cannot move themselves, and it is up to us as nurses to move them every few hours in order to prevent skin breakdown. Sometimes called decubitus ulcers, these lesions are notoriously difficult to heal. Initially persistent erythema can develop into necrotic ulceration involving muscle, tendon and bone. Pressure ulcers can be caused by the following:

- simple pressure exceeding that of the blood pressure at the venous or arterial end of capillaries;[48]
- shearing when the patient is dragged up the bed, destroying the micro-circulation in the underlying tissue. In serious cases, lymphatic vessels and muscle fibres can also become torn;[49]

- friction, causing stripping of the stratum corneum, which leads to superficial damage.[50]

Specific areas of the body are at risk for the development of pressure sores. These include the following:

- sacral area – when lying supine;
- coccygeal area – when lying supine;
- ischial tuberosities – when lying laterally;
- greater trochanters – when lying laterally.

Inactivity, immobility and advanced age can contribute to the incidence of pressure sores, but they are also more common among patients with decreased levels of consciousness. Norton and Waterlow produced 'at-risk' scales to show that the type of patient found in a critical-care unit is more likely to be at risk from pressure area sores than other types of patient.[51]

Pressure area sores can be graded according to their severity, and need different treatments for each stage.[52] The degrees of severity range from unbroken skin with simple redness to destruction of skin and the underlying tissue. Once the skin has broken down, careful treatment of the ensuing wound is paramount to prevent infection. Wounds may be categorized as follows:

- dry and clean;
- wet, oozing but clean;
- open and contaminated.[53]

Turner describes an appropriate material for wound dressing as: 'a material which, when applied to the surface of a wound, provides and maintains an environment in which healing can take place at the maximum rate'.[54] I would think that the antimicrobial properties of essential oils diluted in a soothing carrier oil would fit this description.

When the skin is red and sore but still intact, floral waters can be used to soothe the skin and to reduce surface heat. Chamomile and lavender can be useful at this stage. When the skin is broken, a compress using floral waters can be used. However, when the wound has deepened, it is kinder to use a mixture of carrier oil (or gel) and essential oil to prevent the compress sticking to the sides of the wound and increasing the trauma. *Calophyllum inophyllum* (palm kernel) carrier oil is particularly beneficial because of its anti-inflammatory action and gentle analgesic effects. Rosehip (*Rosa rubignosa*) carrier oil is also useful in the treatment of pressure area sores. Aloe vera gel would be an another excellent choice, particularly as it is so effective in the treatment of burns, which show a similar healing pattern to pressure area sores.[55]

Below are some suggestions for suitable essential oils, phytols and hydrolats. Only 1–5 drops of essential oil should be used in a carrier oil or phytol. For specialized carrier oils, please see the section on carrier oils.

Suitable essential oils would include the following:

- *Lavandula angustifolia* (lavender);
- *Chamaemelum nobile* (Roman chamomile);
- *Boswellia carterii* (frankincense);
- *Pelargonium graveolens* (geranium).

Suitable phytols (infused herbal oils) would include the following:

- *Echinacea purpurea* (echinacea);
- *Hypericum perforatum* (St John's wort);
- *Calendula officinalis* (calendula).

Suitable floral waters (hydrolats) to use would be:

- *Rosmarinus officinalis* CT borneol (rosemary);
- *Myrtus communis* (myrtle);
- *Sambucus nigra* (elderflower);
- *Rosa damascena* (rose).

Suitable essential oils for the treatment of infected pressure sores would include the following:

- clary sage (*Salvia sclarea*) against *Klebsiella*;[25]
- German chamomile (*Matricaria recutitia*) against *Staphylococcus aureus* and *Proteus vulgaris*;[56]
- lemongrass (*Cymbopogon citratus*) against *Shigella, E. coli, Staphylococcus aureus* and *Bacillus subtilis*;[57]
- juniper (*Juniperus communis* var. *erecta*) against *Pseudomonas* and *Staphylococcus aureus*;[58]
- marjoram (*Origanum majorana*)[59-61] against *Clostridium, Streptococcus, Proteus, E. coli* and *Salmonella*.

DERMATOLOGY

The skin is the largest organ of the body. It is also a stress barometer which provides the outside world with an indication of the serenity or confusion within.

Much of dermatology is concerned with putting topical drugs on to the skin. However, it has recently been accepted that skin problems may be linked to stress and diet. Possibly two of the most difficult conditions that nurses will encounter are eczema and herpes.

Eczema

Eczema is a 'common itching skin disease characterized by reddening (erythema) and vesicle formation which may lead to weeping and crusting.'[45] Atopic eczema is associated with hay fever and asthma, and affects up to 20 per cent of the population. Orthodox medicine does not consider that outside agents are the primary contributing factors. However, the word 'dermatitis' is frequently used interchangeably with the word 'eczema'. Some dermatitis is definitely due to outside influences producing contact dermatitis (one of the commonest skin problems among doctors is contact dermatitis in response to latex). Substances which can exacerbate eczema include wool, lanolin, some metals found in jewellery, biological washing powders, rubber and cleaning agents which remove grease from the skin.[62]

Seborrhoeic dermatitis involves the nose, lips eyes and scalp and is associated with a yeast infection of *Pityrosporum*.

The traditional treatment for eczema involves the use of corticosteroid creams. More holistic orthodox approaches also encompass dietary exclusions of foods such as dairy products, yeast and food additives, and topical irritants such as those listed above.

Whilst aromatherapy may aid the treatment of eczema, either by reducing stress or by acting at a topical, anti-inflammatory level, if the underlying problems contributing to the condition (which could be dietary sensitivity or contact sensitivity) are not removed, the condition will not improve greatly. *Eczema could be made worse if an essential oil is chosen to which the patient is sensitive. For this reason, patch testing should be mandatory for all eczema patients who wish to try aromatherapy. In addition, a careful case-study, including details of potential antagonists (especially herbal teas, flowers, pollens and cosmetics) should be tabulated.*

Listed below are some essential oils which are considered to be beneficial, followed by a discussion of the reasons why they might aid the treatment of eczema:

- *Lavandula angustifolia* (true lavender);
- *Matricaria recutitia* (German chamomile);
- *Cyperus scariosus* (nagar matha);
- *Boswellia carterii* (frankincense);
- *Foeniculum vulgare* (fennel);
- *Juniperus communis* (juniper);
- *Symphytum officinale* (comfrey) (phytol – an infused oil).

Lavandula angustifolia (true lavender) is very useful because of its recognized cicatrisant and cytophyllactic actions. It was, after all, this essential oil which caused the renaissance of aromatherapy and proved itself in so many ways to Gattefosse.[63]

The almost antihistamine-like action of *Matricaria recutita* (German chamomile) essential oil, coupled with the strong anti-inflammatory effect of its three sesquiterpenes, azulene, bisabolol and farnasene,[64] make this essential oil very useful in the treatment of eczema. Its anti-inflammatory effects have been well researched, and it is used in some pharmaceutical preparations. The chemotype which contains alpha-bisabolol is thought to be the most effective.[65]

German chamomile was tested together with a steroid and a non-steroid (hydrocortisone and benzydamine, respectively) preparation on mice. Although it was not as effective as hydrocortisone, it was as effective as benzydamine.[66] However, in another study on humans, Kamillosan cream, which contains German chamomile, was found to be as effective as hydrocortisone in 161 patients.[67] German chamomile was also found to be effective in wound healing of patients following dermabrasion of tattoos.[68]

Although, classically, German chamomile has been used to treat inflammatory conditions and Roman chamomile has been used to treat antispasmodic conditions, Roman chamomile does also have a role as an anti-inflammatory.[15] Roman chamomile might appear to be more acceptable than German chamomile because it is not dark blue and it smells less pungent, but the two chamomiles have very different constituents.

A little known essential oil, *Cyperus scariosus* (nagar matha in Sanskrit) which is a grass-like herb, showed anti-inflammatory activity in rats within 3 hours of its application. The inhibition of granulation tissue formation was thought to be comparable to that achieved with hydrocortisone.[69] This essential oil is not yet available in the UK.

Resins such as *Boswellia carterii* (frankincense) have traditionally been used in India and Africa to treat inflammatory conditions.[70] In a study of the anti-inflammatory effects of 75 species of plants on artificially induced inflammation in rats, *Foeniculum vulgare* (fennel), *Symphytum officinale* (comfrey) and *Juniperus communis* (juniper) decreased inflammation by up to 50 per cent. As comfrey (an infused oil) also has anti-ulcer properties,[71] it would appear that it could form a useful base for the essential oil mix. Balsam and skin problems were the subject of a doctoral thesis by Descouleurs, written as long ago as 1896.[63]

Gattefosse reported that *Cedrus atlantica* (cedar) was used to treat skin disorders in an Algerian hospital in 1899, with great success.[72]

Herpes

By 'herpes' I mean herpes simplex 1 and 2, which include the sexually transmitted disease that appeared to reach epidemic proportions in the 1980s. Once the disease has been contracted, the patient is infected for life.

The painful clusters of blisters reappear, usually in the same area, with agonizing regularity – often weekly. The outbreaks can be triggered by stress, heat, hormonal changes and occasionally by diet. Although the blisters often occur in the genital area (either internal or external), they may also be found on the thighs.

Extremely contagious at the blister stage, herpes can remain dormant for months or years in the spinal cord, ready to migrate down the sensory nerves to the skin. Current orthodox treatment is with Acyclovir, which often leaves a metal-like taste in the patient's mouth.

There has been a certain amount of anecdotal evidence that essential oils, applied to the area when the initial tingling begins, can prevent the blisters from forming. There is also some evidence that, when such oils are applied to the blisters, the pain and itching are relieved.

Research conducted in 1978 showed the following essential oils to be efficacious in tissue cultures:[73]

- *Juniperus communis* (juniper);
- *Melissa officinalis* (melissa);
- *Laurus nobilis* (bay laurel);
- *Eucalyptus globulus* (eucalyptus);
- *Piper cubaba* (cubebs);
- *Rosmarinus officinalis* (rosemary).

Melissa was the subject of a study at the Mayo Clinic in 1964, and was found to be efficacious against fertilized embryonic chicken eggs impregnated with herpes simplex.[74] This research was investigated further in 1967, when it was found that the tannin in melissa could have been the active component.[75] This research has recently been extended to the human system, when a multicentre clinical trial in Germany found melissa to be effective. A total of 115 patients took part in the study, which involved the use of dried extracts of melissa made up into a cream which was applied 2 to 4 times daily for 5 to 10 days. A significant improvement was observed on day 2, and on day 5 over 50 per cent of the patients were symptom-free.[76]

In another study, anti-herpetic activity was investigated in the tannins found in essential oils. This paper alludes to the anti-herpetic activity of buds of *Syzygium aromatica* (clove).[77]

For those patients suffering from herpes who wish to try an alternative to orthodox drugs, topically applied diluted essential oils may bring great relief. Ask your patient to apply a dilution of 5 to 10 per cent essential oil in carrier oil to the external blisters. For vaginal blisters use a 1 to 5 per cent. The mixture is best applied using a Q-tip or cotton bud. My students have reported that one drop each of undiluted tea tree and true lavender applied to unbroken blisters on external mucosa have reduced both the pain and the itchiness of herpes, and produced a faster healing time in 100 per cent of the cases in which this treatment was tried.

ENDOCRINOLOGY

The endocrine system is the regulator of homeostasis.[78] This balance is maintained through hormones. The word 'hormone' comes from the Greek *'hormaein'*, meaning 'to excite'. In certain instances the nervous and endocrine systems can regulate each other's activities, as well as acting together to bring about changes in physiology. Endocrine cells in the body occur in clusters in the endocrine glands. These glands secrete hormones directly into the bloodstream. As hormones regulate our metabolism, growth, development and reproduction, it is clear that they are a fundamental necessity to life. However, hormones also govern our stress response. It is at this level that aromatherapy is most likely to affect the endocrine system.

However, as all areas governed are so closely interlinked, it could be postulated that there might be a 'knock-on' effect on other glandular activities, including the following:

- the pineal gland which regulates production of melatonin (a dark/light mechanism which affects how we sleep);
- the pituitary gland, which is the master endocrine gland and is divided into two lobes – the anterior lobe which governs our growth hormones, thyroid hormones, adrenocorticotrophic hormone (ACTH) and reproductive hormones, namely luteinizing hormone (LH) and follicle-stimulating hormone (FSH), and the posterior lobe which secretes vasopressin (antidiuretic hormone) and oxytocin (which stimulates contraction of the uterus during labour);
- the thyroid gland, which secretes thyroxine and governs our metabolic rate;
- the parathyroid which controls calcium and phosphate levels;
- the adrenal cortex, which produces corticosteroids;
- the adrenal medulla, which produces adrenaline and noradrenaline;
- the pancreas, which secretes insulin and glucagon;
- the female gonads, which produce oestrogen and progesterone, and the male gonads, which produce testosterone.

Whilst there is no suggestion that aromatherapy could have the same impact as orthodox drugs on the endocrine system, there *is* a possibility that they could still have some therapeutic effects.

Hormones play an important role in the mechanisms involving prosta-glandins. Three classes of prostaglandins – prostaglandin A (PGA), prostaglandin E (PGE) and prostaglandin F (PGF) – have been isolated and identified from a wide range of tissues (it is thought that aspirin exerts its anti-inflammatory action by inhibiting PGE synthesis). Eugenol, carvacrol, thymol and gingeol have also been shown to influence PGE.[79, 80]

All prostaglandins are intimately involved in endocrine regulation by influencing adenyl cyclase and adenosine 3,5-phosphate (cyclic AMP) activity within the cell.[78] Anything that interferes with that cellular activity could be said to affect the hormonal system and thus the endocrine system. PGAs cause an immediate fall in blood pressure and an increased venous supply to the coronary and renal systems.[78] It is known that some essential oils can interfere with the release of calcium at the cellular level. This blocking mechanism has been demonstrated for essential oils which contain menthol, anethole, eugenol and thymol.[81] These essential oil components are found in peppermint, fennel, aniseed, star aniseed, bay, clove, Spanish marjoram, rose, winter and summer savory, sweet marjoram, thyme and oregano.[82, 83]

Premenstrual syndrome and menopausal problems are related to the endocrine system. They affect many millions of women every day.

Premenstrual syndrome (PMS)

PMS became a household name in 1987 when Anna Reynolds was charged with the murder of her mother and jailed for life. Four months later, a petition signed by 6000 people launched an appeal for her release. On 23 June 1988, the appeal court reduced the murder charge to one of manslaughter on the grounds of PMS, and Reynolds was released. This was the first time that a woman had been allowed to plead diminished responsibility due to 'the time of the month'.

Women have known for many years that they can become irrational, irritable, weepy and occasionally violent a few days before their menstrual period. No one quite knows why this is so, or why some women are more affected than others. There is no orthodox treatment apart from antidepressants. However, one wonders whether a woman's menstrual cycle is taken into account when planning surgery or admission to hospital – probably not. What are the allowances made for women in hospital who suffer from PMS?

If we, as nurses (many of us being women), are caring for our patients in a holistic way, we should be looking at the possibility of reducing PMS whenever it occurs. This would mean improving the comfort level of our patient, and reducing her sense of powerlessness. These are both acceptable nursing diagnoses.

Aromatherapy can, in some instances, produce very reasonable results in PMS if regular treatments are given over a period of several months. The essential oils chosen are usually a combination of those thought to have oestrogen-like properties, such as fennel (*Foeniculum vulgare*) and clary sage (*Salvia sclarea*),[84] and those thought to have hormone-like properties, such as Scots pine (*Pinus sylvestris*)[25], and myrrh (*Commiphora myrrha*).[25] Belaiche, who devoted a whole volume to female problems, also suggests the use of sage, hyssop, thyme or geranium.[85] Essential oils rich in citral (an aldehyde found in lemongrass, melissa and verbena) can also sometimes prove to be beneficial due to their potential androgenic action.[86]

Depending on the patient's needs, an essential oil can be added to the 'balancing' essential oil which will help to alleviate the symptoms of the imbalance. For example, if a woman is showing symptoms of depression and is weepy, an essential oil with an antidepressant action such as bergamot[82] or rose[27] could be added. If she is violent and irrational, a sedative such as angelica[25] or ylang ylang could be used.[87] Geranium is an excellent balancer, and has the added bonus of inhibiting platelet aggregation,[88] thereby possibly preventing the extensive clotting during menstruation which so often accompanies premenstrual syndrome.

Personally, I have had some success using tarragon in conjunction with oestrogen-like essential oils on women who have displayed aggressive PMS – one patient actually admitted 'going for my husband with a knife'. Although tarragon (*Artemisia dracunculus*) has fallen out of favour recently due to its estragole fraction, the research that gave rise to this view involved administering fairly large doses of estragole orally to rats over a period of 12 months.[6]

Menopausal problems

The menopause is the natural cessation of a woman's fertility. Once looked upon with secret delight as the end of menstruation and its accompanying messy problems, the menopause now seems to be viewed by many women with dismay and despair. Osteoporosis may be the reason that many women give for taking hormone replacement therapy (HRT), but one wonders if this is always the case. Many very young-looking older women are quick to admit that HRT also makes them feel as well as look younger.

However, cessation of oestrogen production does not happen overnight, and it is the interim imbalance which appears to be so difficult to live with and to regulate. Patients in hospital are more likely to have this delicate balancing act upset, as they are removed from their normal environment and routine. Menopause is part of being a woman, and therefore caring for our patients should include providing support during this difficult time. The main symptoms of the menopause are hot flushes, night sweats, insomnia and palpitations. Essential oils that could be used in a hydrosol spray applied directly to the face during a hot flush include rose,[85] cypress[56] or clary sage. Essential oils that could be used for oestrogen support include fennel,[89] sage,[25] aniseed,[90] geranium[91] and the ubiquitous rose.

For night sweats cypress – with its recognized deodorant effect and hormonal properties – might also be comforting.[56] For insomnia, any of the gently relaxing and sedative oils could be added, but try also root of *Angelica angelica*.[92]

In striving to alleviate PMS and menopausal problems we are caring for our patients in a truly holistic manner, using Koldjeski's caring theory as a framework for our nursing.[93] Whilst both of the above conditions occur exclusively in women and, one could argue, border on gynaecology rather than endocrinology, perhaps a mention of diabetes and the use of essential oils might be in order.

Diabetes

Rosmarinus officinalis (rosemary) was shown to suppress the insulin response in a glucose tolerance test in rabbits when plasma glucose levels remained at 55 per cent for 2 hours. Rosemary also caused hyperglycaemia in rabbits with artificially induced diabetes.[94] Although these studies were conducted on animals and involved intramuscular injections, perhaps it might be wise to avoid the use of rosemary in diabetic patients.

Another study showed that *Eucalyptus citriodora* (lemon-scented gum) had a hypoglycaemic effect on rabbits.[95] Valnet states that geranium has anti-diabetic properties.[56] Ylang ylang is another essential oil thought to be useful in diabetes,[25,82,96] although I personally have found no evidence to substantiate this view.

GYNAECOLOGY

Women have periods whether they are in hospital or not, and if they suffer from dysmenorrhoea, it is often much worse when they are away from home. Similarly, thrush or other vaginal infections are embarrassing to deal with when away from home.

Thrush, anaerobic vaginitis and trichomonas

Vaginal thrush, caused by *Candida albicans,* is a common nuisance factor in many women's lives. Sometimes a side-effect of antibiotics, often occurring during pregnancy or after an illness, thrush is messy, uncomfortable and embarrassing. It can reappear with depressing regularity. Over-the-counter preparations can be purchased, although some forms of thrush have become resistant to many of the orthodox preparations that are on the market.[97] However, there is an essential oil which may eradicate this fungal infection permanently, and within only a few days.[98] It is called tea tree.

Anaerobic vaginitis is extremely difficult to treat conventionally, and is caused by a microbe which can only survive in the absence of oxygen. Often the presence of this microbe can produce symptoms of profound itching capable of reducing a woman to tears. Trichomonas is caused by a parasitic flagellate protozoan, *Trichomonas vaginalis*, which produces inflammation and a pungent discharge. Tea tree is also effective against anaerobic vaginitis and trichomonas.[99]

However, the correct chemotype of the correct species *must* be used. Tea tree is the name of all species of *Melaleuca, Leptospermum, Kunzea* and *Baeckea* plants.[100] In other words, specifying tea tree is not enough, as it covers several hundred different plants. In New Zealand, *Leptospermum flavescens* is also known as tea tree – this is a completely different genus, although it belongs to the same family (Myrtaceae). The tea tree that is used to treat vaginal infections is *Melaleuca alternifolia* CT terpineol (there is another chemotype of the same species which contains cineol, an oxide, which can produce discomfort when applied to the mucous membrane). *Melaleuca alternifolia* CT terpineol contains a high level of the alcohol terpineol. (Chemotypes are covered more fully in the section on chemistry.)

A mixture of this 'tea tree' can be diluted in a carrier oil (2 to 3 drops of essential oil only) and applied to the vagina on a tampon. The simplest method is to mix the essential oil and carrier oil on a saucer and then roll the tampon in the mixture until it is saturated. The tampon should be changed three times a day for a new tampon in a fresh dilution of carrier oil with 2 to 3 drops of tea tree. The tampon needs to kept *in situ* overnight. Systemic absorption from the vagina can be very rapid and effective, so large doses should not be given vaginally. This is a very safe and effective method of eradicating thrush, and I have never known it to have adverse side-effects if the vaginal lining is not raw.

Having audited the effect of this treatment on many patients and colleagues over the last 10 years, I feel confident that the correct tea tree will (nine times out of ten) completely remove the thrush within 3 days, regardless of how long the patient has had the infection. This method of treatment can also be very effective against anaerobic vaginitis and trichomonas.[99] Incidentally, recent research both in Australia and in the UK has shown this particular *Melaleuca* to be effective against 66 isolates of methicillin-resistant *Staphylococcus aureus* (MRSA); 64 isolates were methicillin-resistant and 33 isolates were mupirocin-resistant.[101] However, a word of caution should be given here. Tea tree is very painful if applied to an abrasion (feeling somewhat like lemon on a cut), so if the candida infection has exposed raw areas in the vaginal wall, then *Lavandula angustifolia* diluted in carrier oil should be used instead, and applied in exactly the same way on a tampon for 1 or 2 days until the excoriated area has healed. The tea tree mix can then be used.

There are those who may consider that even discussion of the antibacterial properties of essential oils exceeds our nursing mandate. However, if as nurses we feel that we could improve the comfort level of a patient and reduce their powerlessness (because we have specific knowledge which can help to remove the problem causing the discomfort and powerlessness), is it ethical, as nurses, to withhold that information? This is not to say that we are 'treating' the patients, but merely giving them the information so that *they* may make an informed choice for themselves and treat themselves.

Thrush is uncomfortable, and often makes the sufferer feel powerless to cope with it. Trichomonas smells unpleasant, and the sufferer is embarrassed and frequently complains of 'feeling dirty'. Anaerobic vaginitis is accompanied by unbearable itching. Tea tree does not smell particularly pleasant, and it does not remove stress, but it has proven antibacterial and antifungal properties, and it is very effective against thrush, trichomonas and anaerobic infections.[99] It can also be purchased very easily because it is not a prescription drug. As a nurse, I feel that this kind of advice *is* part of nursing, but, of course, we remain accountable for our advice.

Tea tree has grown from a cottage industry in Australia to a multi-million business with a turnover of $40 million (Australian dollars).[102] New Zealand's tea trees, manuka and kanuka, are being investigated by the New Zealand government with a view to assessing whether they can reach the world potential of Australia's tea tree, *Melaleuca alternifolia* CT terpineol. However, at this point, no clinical trials have been carried out, and therefore the best choice for vaginal infections is considered to be Australia's *Melaleuca alternifolia* CT terpineol.[98]

Dysmenorrhoea

The menstrual cycle is delicately balanced, and can easily be thrown out of equilibrium by stress, illness or a poor diet. Using aromatherapy, there are three ways to approach dysmenorrhoea – with essential oils known for their antispasmodic properties, those with oestrogen-like properties, and those with analgesic properties.

Topical application will focus attention on the affected area of the body (unlike taking a tablet), and brings great comfort. Compresses allow essential oils to be absorbed slowly through the skin, rather like a slow-release time-capsule. A hot-water bottle has been an effective remedy for period pains for decades. Placed on top of the compress, it will allow more rapid absorption of the essential oil, as well as giving the added comfort of heat. Of course, some of the essential oil will also be inhaled, producing a more instant effect. However, the whole process of tending a painful area topically brings with it strong placebo and mind–body links which can only enhance the efficacy of the therapy. By using aromatherapy in this way, nurses are trying to help the body's own self-healing mechanisms.

As well as compresses, the effect of gentle massage can really help those painful cramps. Try 1 to 5 drops of geranium (*Pelargonium graveolens*) diluted in a carrier oil, and gently rub it into the lower abdomen and lumbar area. The best geranium oil comes from Reunion Island, and is usually called Bourbon – it is also the most expensive. For optimum results, it should be applied morning and evening. For severe dysmenorrhoea, add 1 to 2 drops of high-altitude *Lavandula angustifolia* (true lavender) to enhance the anti-spasmodic effect. Other antispasmodic oils that can be tried (traditionally those which contain large numbers of esters) include the following:

- *Chamaemelum nobile* (Roman chamomile);[25]
- *Citrus aurantium* var. *amara* (petitgrain);[103]
- *Eucalyptus citriodora* (lemon-scented eucalyptus);
- *Rosmarinus officinalis* (rosemary)[104] (avoid a ketone chemotype);
- *Salvia officinalis* (sage).[104]

Roman chamomile contains more esters than any other essential oil (up to 310 esters, including those from angelic and tiglic acid), and it is thought to be one of the most antispasmodic essential oils available.[105] It is also a recognized analgesic.[106] Geranium is thought to encourage regular ovulation,[85] and has been used for generations to balance oestrogen levels through its action on the adrenal cortex.[91]

Analgesic essential oils include the following:

- *Lavandula angustifolia* (true lavender) – possibly the most famous of all essential oils. Ensure that you use the real thing, not a lavendin (*Lavandula hybrida*);
- *Cymbopogon citratus* (West Indian lemongrass) – the analgesic effect is thought to be due to myrcene (a terpene).[42] East Indian Lemongrass (*Cymbopogon flexuosus*) does not contain myrcene;[107]
- *Mentha piperita* (peppermint) – the analgesic effect is well described in Gobel's study.[108]

Nursing is about nurturing, and there can be nothing more nurturing than tending someone in pain. Severe dysmenorrhoea can bring with it nausea.

Inhaling a little essential oil of peppermint may help to alleviate this. Aromatherapy seeks to work alongside conventional medicine wherever nursing feels that it might be of benefit to patients.

IMMUNOLOGY

Immunology is a rapidly growing field, this growth possibly having been precipitated by the AIDS epidemic and nurtured by mind–body medicine. Now we *know* that how we feel affects how we are, and of particular importance to the use of aromatherapy in nursing (or medicine) is the knowledge that stress has a negative effect on our health, which includes our immune system. However, it was only 10 years ago that an editorial in an American journal ridiculed such an idea, stating 'that it is time to acknowledge that our belief in disease as a direct reflection of mental state is largely folklore'.[109]

The immune system is highly complicated – a sensitive balancing act linked by nerve cells which receive directions from and send directions to the brain. The organs of the immune system produce lymphocytes. These white blood cells include T-cells (so called because they mature in the thymus) and B-cells, which circulate antibodies. Antibodies are tiny proteins belonging to a family of immunoglobulins. Antibodies will 'key' on to the surface of an antigen (a foreign invader), each antibody recognizing and 'keying' on to a specific antigen.

T-cells do not produce antibodies. There are four different types of T-cell, and they attack foreign invaders in different ways.

- *Killer cells (KC)* are constantly on the alert in the bloodstream, looking for foreign invaders. When they find them, the killer cells attach themselves and release toxic chemicals to destroy the invaders. Just as in the case of antibodies, killer cells are programmed only to kill one thing, whether it is an infective agent, a cell that has been infected, or transplanted tissue.
- *Non-killer cells (NKC)* are also constantly on the alert. These cells can attack a broad range of targets – both tumour and infection.
- Helper cells stimulate B-lymphocytes to produce antibodies.
- Suppressor cells shut off the helper cells when enough antibodies have been produced.

For optimum health, helper and suppressor cells should be in balance. AIDS patients have a deficiency of helper cells, whereas people with autoimmune disease have too many helper cells.

The basic role of the immune system is to defend the body. To do that, it needs to know what is body and what is not. B-lymphocytes tell the body if it has been invaded, but there is another arm to our defence system, namely our cellular response, which involves the T-lymphocytes.

People who have an underactive immune system will constantly succumb to infection. People with an overactive immune system will be prone to allergies and autoimmune diseases as the body begins to attack itself.

Psychoneuroimmunology is the study of the reaction between the nervous system and the immune system. In an article published in the *Lancet*, stress was linked to a depressed immune system.[110] Research has shown that changes in hormone and neurotransmitter levels alter human immune responses.[109] Research also indicates that stress can affect the immune response;[111] increase susceptibility to the common cold;[112] adversely affect conception;[113] increase the incidence of skin disease[114] and affect a patient's perception of pain.[115]

It is accepted that aromatherapy elicits the 'feel-good' factor. Therefore there is reason to suggest that aromatherapy may enhance our immune system by utilizing the positive effects of smell and touch.

Peneol suggests that the effects of phenols could be compared to those of human immunoglobulin M (IgM). IgM is secreted for a short period when the immune system encounters a pathogenic organism. Immunoglobulin G (IgG) is secreted for long-term defence. Peneol believes that the action of IgG is mirrored by the behaviour of monoterpenic alcohols.[116]

Berkarda has reported on the ability of coumarins to increase lymphocyte transformation values in cancer patients.[117] This suggests that coumarins found in other essential oils might also have an effect on the immune system. Coumarin is found (although only in small quantities) in lavender. Perhaps this is why Rovesti stated that lavender stimulated lymphocytosis, although Lapraz is quoted as saying that the presence 'of essential oils in the bloodstream produces leucocytosis'.[118] Price cites Roulier, who suggests that the following essential oils could help to balance the immune system:[119]

- *Syzygium aromaticum* (clove);
- *Lippia citriodora* (true verbena);
- *Melaleuca viridiflora* (niaouli);
- *Pogostemon patchouli* (patchouli).

Other essential oils that are thought to elevate levels of lymphocytes include *Matricaria recutitia* (German chamomile), which increases the number of B-lymphocytes,[120] and *Citrus bergamia* (bergamot), which is thought to be an immune stimulant.[119] Philippe Mailhebiau writes that *Thymus vulgaris* CT thymol has strong immunostimulant properties and is less hepatotoxic than *Satureja montana* CT thymol.[121]

Of the immune dysfunctions most commonly encountered by nurses, perhaps the most difficult to treat are rheumatoid arthritis and HIV/AIDS.

Although there is no suggestion that aromatherapy can 'cure' rheumatoid arthritis or AIDS (and this would be well beyond a nurse's brief anyway), it is possible that aromatherapy might enhance the effects of orthodox treatment. A nurse can improve the comfort of her patient and alleviate feelings of hopelessness by utilizing the anti-inflammatory and analgesic properties of certain essential oils for rheumatoid arthritis, and by using the antibacterial, antiviral and antifungal properties to support HIV and AIDS treatment. In this way a complementary package could be created to support the patient and provide true holistic nursing cover.

Rheumatoid arthritis

A combination of application methods is usually beneficial, e.g. a morning compress and evening bath (which can be a hand or foot bath). It is important to choose the application method which suits your patient. As rheumatoid arthritis affects specific joints, these areas of the body lend themselves to the use of compresses – a method of application which is gaining in popularity again.

As well as being of great topical comfort and focusing attention on the affected area of the body (rather than taking a pill), compresses allow essential oils to be absorbed gradually through the skin, rather like a slow-release time-capsule. Of course, some of the essential oil will also be inhaled, producing a more instant effect. However, the whole process of preparing and treating an injured or painful area of the body carries with it strong placebo and mind–body links, which can only enhance the efficacy of the treatment.

By using aromatherapy in this way we are trying to assist the body's own self-healing mechanisms, drawing on the anti-inflammatory and analgesic properties of essential oils as well as their ability to reduce stress.

Inflammation is caused by an increased flow of blood to the affected area, bringing with it heat, swelling and pain.[64] It can therefore be useful to create a mixture of essential oils that could address each of these symptoms.

Essential oils with some anti-inflammatory properties include the following:

- *Matricaria recutitia* (German chamomile) (bisabol and chamazulene being responsible for the anti-inflammatory actions);[66]
- *Helichrysum italicum* subsp. *serotinum* (helichrysum) – double-bonded ketones give this essential oil a remarkable ability to reduce contusions;[25]
- *Rosmarinus officinalis* CT borneol (rosemary) – rosmarinic acid, ursolic acid and apigenin are thought to produce the anti-inflammatory effect.[71] Franchomme and Peneol suggest avoiding CT verbenone (a ketone) as it

may be neurotoxic.[25] Arguably CT borneol (an alcohol) is safer. Perhaps CT cineole (an oxide) is best kept for patients with infections rather than inflammation. *Do not use rosemary on clients with hypertension, as it is thought to increase blood pressure;*

- *Eucalyptus globulus* (eucalyptus) – recognized for its anti-inflammatory action.[71]

Essential oils that can help to reduce pain include the following:

- *Lavandula angustifolia* (true lavender) – possibly the most well known of all essential oils. Ensure that you use *L. angustifolia* and not *L. latifolia* (often the hospital pharmacy will provide both, each labelled lavender!);
- *Cymbopogon citratus* (West Indian lemongrass) – the analgesic effect is thought to be due to myrcene (a terpene).[42] East Indian lemongrass (*Cymbopogon flexuosus*) does not contain myrcene;[122]
- *Mentha piperita* (peppermint) – the analgesic effect is well described in Gobel's study.[108]

Rheumatoid arthritis is usually eased by cooling, unlike osteoarthritis, which is eased with heat. Your patient will know which he or she finds most comforting. I have found that using a cold (or hot) compress can augment the effect of essential oils. If your patient says that heat helps to relieve the pain, it can be useful to add a drop of an essential oil which has a rubefacient effect and brings heat into the affected area.

Rubefacient essential oils include the following:

- *Piper nigrum* (black pepper);
- *Zingiber officinale* (ginger).

In all cases, it is important to allow your patients to help with the selection. Let them smell the mixture before you apply it – after all, they will have to live with it! Be gentle if you choose to use a massage technique.

HIV and AIDS

There has been a temendous increase in research into plants which could be of value in the treatment of patients with AIDS and HIV. Some of the research has involved specific plants which could inhibit reverse transcriptase production of specific tumours.[123] Other research has concentrated on other antitumour and anti-HIV agents.[124] Many of these studies have shown encouraging results, although the research is still in its preliminary stages.[125–128]

Opportunistic infections remain the most common cause of morbidity and death in people with HIV.[129] There is some evidence that the following opportunistic infections indicative of AIDS[130] may respond favourably to essential oils (the specific essential oils, with research references are listed subsequently):

- candidiasis;
- cryptococcosis;
- herpes simplex;
- tuberculosis;
- mycobacteriosis;
- (Kaposi's sarcoma).

The studies were mainly conducted *in vitro*, so caution is needed before a nurse could recommend using an essential oil for its potential role in treating opportunistic infections. However, many of the essential oils are ones that nurses using aromatherapy would already be considering either for their aesthetic appeal or for their use in stress management. They include the following:

- *Lavandula intermedia* CT grosso (lavandin) – effective in the treatment of non-tubercular opportunistic mycobacteria (NTM);[131]
- *Melaleuca alternifolia* CT terpineol (tea tree) – effective against methicillin-resistant *Staphylococcus aureus*[101] and *Candida albicans*;[98, 132]
- *Lippia alba* – effective against *Trichophyton mentagrophytes*;[133]
- *Rosmarinus officinalis* (rosemary) – effective against cryptococcal meningitis, cryptococcal pneumonia and systemic infections of mycobacterium;[134]
- *Cymbopogon martini* (palma rosa), *Thymus vulgaris* (thyme), *Santalum album* (sandalwood), *Vetiveria zizanioides* (vetivert) and *Origanum majorana* (marjoram) – all effective (to varying degrees) against cryptococcal infections;[135]
- *Origanum majorana* (marjoram) – effective against the TB bacillus at 0.4 per cent;[56]
- *Ravansara aromatic* (ravansara) – effective against parasitic infections;[136]
- *Eucalyptus globulus* (eucalyptus) – effective against herpes[77] and *Cryptococcus nerformans*,[135] this eucalyptus enhances the activity of streptomycin, isoniazid and sulfetrone in Mycobacterium TB;[137]
- *Melissa officinalis* (melissa) – thought to be effective against *Candida albicans*.[138]

The following have been found to be effective against herpes in tissue cultures:[73]

- *Juniperus communis* (juniper);
- *Melissa officinalis* (melissa);
- *Laurus nobilis* (bay laurel);

- *Eucalyptus globulus* (eucalyptus);
- *Piper cubaba* (cubeb);
- *Rosmarinus officinalis* (rosemary);
- *Melissa officinalis* (melissa);[75, 139]
- *Syzygium aromatica* (clove).[77]

A multicentred clinical trial has substantiated the findings that *Melissa* is helpful to herpes sufferers.[76]

There is increasing evidence that plants contain a wide variety of substances that may inhibit cancer formation.[140] Some studies on animal tissue have suggested that certain essential oils have anticarcinogenic properties.[141-143] Although it should be emphasized that there is no evidence in humans yet, the following essential oils are all regularly used for their other therapeutic properties (there is no suggestion that these essential oils – or indeed any – will make a tumour disappear; the objective is only to present some evidence that certain essential oils *might* have some use in preventing cancer formation in humans, and therefore Kaposi's sarcoma, but that we do not really know the answer yet):

- *Anthemis nobilis* (Roman chamomile);
- *Eucalyptus citriodora* (eucalyptus);[144]
- *Cymbopogon citratus* (lemongrass).[145]

Patients with AIDS and HIV are especially appreciative of touch and smell. I have found that *Boswellia carterii* (frankincense) is particularly useful, and call it my 'key-opener', as it frequently appears to help even the most defensive patient to open up – often with tears of release. *Citrus aurantium* (petitgrain) has a wonderful smell which most patients like. It is also antibacterial, especially against *Staphylococcus aureus*.[146] If your patient dislikes a flowery smell, perhaps *Origanum marjorana* (sweet marjoram) might be more acceptable. This essential oil has a lovely 'green' smell, is excellent for muscle pain and is effective against several bacterial infections, including *Clostridium*, *E. coli*, *Proteus*, *Salmonella* and *Streptococcus*.[59]

In-vitro studies mean that the essential oils have been tested in a non-living system. *In-vitro* systems are the first line of research, followed by animal tissue, then live animals, and finally humans. Many question the relevance of testing in animals, because the only 'animal model in which everything works just the same as a human being is the same human being'.[147]

However, there is no reason to suppose that essential oils might not have similar actions in a human. In a life-threatening scenario, it could be argued that it would be unethical not to suggest trying aromatherapy to alleviate any and all symptoms. Of course this would have to be with the patient's consent and their consultant's consent. It would also be important to ensure that there were no contraindications to using that particular essential oil in that particular way. If you are already relaxing your patient by using aromatherapy, why not choose an essential oil which might help their immune system as well as their anxiety level?

ONCOLOGY

Cancer is the general term applied to a series of malignant diseases which may affect different parts of the body.[148] Cancer has been around for a million years – traces were found in mummies from the Great Pyramid of Gizeh.[149] Humans do not have a monopoly on the disease, as higher animals also suffer from cancer.

The main orthodox treatments for cancer are surgery, radiation and chemotherapeutic agents. These treatments have saved lives, but sometimes the treatments have been hard to endure. However, plant materials have been used to treat malignant diseases for centuries. It would be impossible to list them all, and most of them have involved whole plants. It is fascinating how the same plants kept being cited all over the world. For example, having discovered that *Sanguinaria canadensis* (bloodwort) had been used by the Native Americans, Dr Fell completed a study of 25 cases of breast cancer at the Middlesex Hospital in 1857. He states that all of his cases went into remission.[150] However, it is difficult to establish if this really happened, although *Sanguinaria* has a long history of use in Russia for the treatment of cancer.[149]

It is well known that the Madagscan periwinkle (*Catharanthus roseus*) contains several alkaloids which have been useful in treating cancer, including vinblastine and vincristine.[148] However, more recently, an infused oil (*Centella asiatica*) called Gotu Kola or South African Pennywort, has featured in an *in-vitro* study of cultured cancer cells. *Centella* appeared to destroy 100 per cent of the cultured cancer cells. When the study was conducted on mice, *Centella* appeared to double the lifespan of mice with tumours. In both instances *Centella* had virtually no toxic effect on normal human lymphocytes.[151] *Centella asiatica* is an infused oil (phytol). Phytols are often used in aromatherapy, and are supplied by many essenial oils distributors.

Cancer affects approximately one person in three.[152] The side-effects of some conventional treatments for cancer can be very hard to endure. Until recently I had a small aromatherapy private practice in England. My patients came by doctor's referral or word of mouth. Some of them had cancer, and my role was one of support. The cancer patients were mainly undergoing

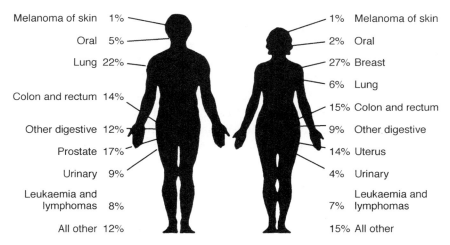

FIGURE 8.1 Incidence of cancer by site and sex. Reproduced from Silverberg, E. and Holleb, A. (1975) *Cancer Incidence by Site and Sex*, with the kind permission of the American Cancer Society, Inc.

chemotherapy and radiotherapy following surgery and, without exception, they found the going very tough. Many expressed their despair about the fact that conventional medicine did not seem to be concerned with the side-effects, only with the efficacy of the treatment.

A pilot survey conducted in 1995 showed that a wide variety of cancer patients sought complementary care therapy.[153] In a study involving two London hospitals, 16 per cent of the patients who had received complementary therapies said that they had wanted them in order to gain emotional support and hope.[154] Well, if there is only time to save a life, so be it, but perhaps aromatherapy can help during the 'dark times', and enhance not only the quality of life of these patients but also the quality of their care. This should be the bedrock of nursing – enhancing quality of care – and it goes right back to the beginning, with Florence Nightingale annointing the foreheads of her patients with lavender as she did her rounds.

There has been some controversy about the use of aromatherapy on cancer patients, with some suggestion that massage could actually spread the disease.[155] However, a study and rigorous review of the published literature indicates that massage would not be contraindicated.[156] I was also glad to read a letter from Bernie Siegal, MD, stating that massage therapy was not contraindicated in a cancer patient.[157] However, deep massage is not what aromatherapy massage is all about. In fact, I have a problem with aromatherapy being called 'massage' at all, as it should basically be more akin to stroking. I feel that if there was another name for it, the confusion that arises between the two therapies would be reduced. However, massage over the actual tumour site should be avoided.

Nausea, constipation, depression, exhaustion, shooting pains, 'feeling my bones might break', lymphoedema, post-radiation burns and insomnia are possibly the most common side-effects of radiotherapy and chemotherapy. Of these symptoms, I have selected nausea, post-radiation burns and lymphoedema, my purpose being to suggest that aromatherapy represents an acceptable enhancement to nursing and, in the words of Dobbs, 'may enrich our interventions and bring comfort and better health to patients with cancer'.[158]

Nausea

One-third of patients with cancer experience nausea and vomiting.[159] Nausea is common during radiation or chemotherapy treatment, and 24 to 75 per cent of patients develop anticipatory nausea and vomiting during the course of repeated chemotherapy.[160] Patients frequently report that everything tastes different. They also say that they are very sensitive to smells, often smelling something which they had not noticed before, or feeling great distaste for a smell which had not bothered them previously. Whilst conventional medicine can be used in the form of anti-emetics, there are also essential oils which could help to reduce nausea. These include the following:

- *Mentha piperita* (peppermint);[161, 162]
- *Zingiber officinale* (ginger);[163]
- *Elettoria cardamomum* (cardamom).[164, 165]

Just a few drops of one of these oils on a tissue can bring relief. Sipping hot water with a sliver of root of ginger can also frequently bring relief from nausea, and is a well-known remedy for morning sickness during pregnancy.

Post-radiation burns

Although certain essential oils are thought to give radiation protection, it is best not to put anything on the skin during the actual radiotherapy. However, when therapy has finished, gentle application to the site can bring rapid relief and help to promote healing.

Carrier oils to choose could include the following:

- *Calophyllum inophyllum* (tamanu) – this is a black sticky carrier oil with skin-healing properties (see section on carrier oils);
- *Rosa rubiginosa* (rosehip) – useful for dehydrated skin;
- *Aloe barbadenisi* (aloe vera gel) – this has been the subject of detailed

research.[166] It has been reported to change a deep thermal burn to a second-degree burn within 48 hours: the wound also healed without gross scarring.[167, 168] Use with a carrier oil, as it is too drying on its own.

Essential oils could include the following:

- *Lavandula angustifolia* (lavender) the classic treatment for burns;[63]
- *Matricaria recutitia* (German chamomile) – good for burns;[162]
- *Chamaemelum nobile* (Roman chamomile).[169]

Infused oils could include the following:

- *Centella asiatica* (gotu kola) – useful in the treatment of ulceration/wounds;[170]
- *Symphytum officinale* (comfrey) – classic treatment to promote skin healing.[169]

A mixture of one drop of each essential oil in 50 per cent tamanu and 50 per cent rosehip (or aloe vera gel) can be very helpful in reducing erythema and tenderness following radiotherapy. *Rosa damascena* was also used in an ointment to treat radiodermatitis and radionecrosis, with apparently good results.[171] However, I personally would not use rose in oncology, except in the terminal stages. Rose is accepted as being the most 'female' essential oil, used throughout the centuries for 'women's problems'.[171] This indicates that it might have oestrogen-like properties, although I have found no evidence for this, and my grounds for avoiding rose in oncology are at best founded on superstition.

Lymphoedema

Lymphoedema occurs frequently following mastectomy, but is also fairly common following lumpectomy if there has been removal of lymph glands. It stands to reason that the lymph will have more difficulty in returning excess interstitial fluid to the blood circulation if there has been a reduction in the number of lymph pathways. Although the large lymphatic vessel walls are contractile (so progress is in one direction only), when one or more of the lymph glands have been removed through surgery or damage, lymph accumulates in the subcutaneous tissue, causing the affected limb to become swollen and tender.[172]

Lymph contains large protein molecules, and build-up of protein in the tissue leads to chronic inflammation and, over a period of time, to thickened, leathery-looking skin. After the initial phase of soft skin and pitting, chronic lymphoedema is characteristically non-pitting. Because of chronic inflammation, local immunity is compromised, with subsequent bouts of cellulitis and poor resistance to insect bites or minor cuts.

Lymphatic drainage must be carried out regularly, as there is no pumping action by the lymphatic system itself. Normal lymphatic drainage relies on the muscular activity that occurs during exercise to move the lymph in the right direction. When this no longer happens, the lymph needs a little extra help. However, because the problem occurs at a subcutaneous level, the pressure needed is extremely light. This is one instance where aromatherapy massage or straight massage are contraindicated. The pressure of an ordinary massage can cause spasm in the lymph vessels, temporarily suspending the lymphatic flow.[173]

Lymphatic drainage is a completely different technique, which needs to be learned. Perhaps the most well-known and accepted method is the Vodder method, which was developed in Austria 50 years ago. However, essential oils and phytols can still play an important ancillary role.

Rather than a massage stroke, which tends to be a two-way directional movement, with both hands working in opposite directions, lymphatic drainage works in one direction only – the direction of flow of the lymph – towards the main lymph ducts, away from the peripheries and towards the thoracic duct. Regular sessions, daily if possible, can reduce the size of a lymph-enlarged limb quite dramatically. The arm will feel lighter and more supple, the elbow will become more clearly defined, and there will be more tactile sensation.

However, as the skin loses its elasticity and infections become more frequent, aromatherapy could provide some support in manual lymphatic drainage therapy, although in general this kind of therapy does not use essential oils.

Base oils to choose would include the following:

- *Centella asiatica* (gotu kola) – useful in the treatment of ulceration and wounds;[170]
- *Oenothera biennis* (oil of evening primrose) – enhances skin care;[174]
- *Passiflora incarnata* (passionflower) – improves skin elasticity.[174]

In this particular instance, essential oils could be used to help to protect the engorged limb from bacterial or fungal infection. Choose an essential oil that the patient likes, and preferably one which does not have an astringent action like *Cupressus sempervirens* (cypress). Essential oils which are kind to the skin and which have antibacterial or antifungal actions actions include the following:

- *Lavandula angustifolia* (lavender);
- *Boswellia carterii* (frankincense);[175]
- *Origanum majorana* (sweet marjoram).[59]

Essential oils to avoid in oncology

I accept that I am possibly being over-cautious, but I would avoid essential oils with oestrogen-like properties, as many tumours (particularly breast tumours) are oestrogen dependent. This would rule out essential oils such as fennel and aniseed, which contain anethole,[176] clary sage, which contains scareol, sage, which contains viridifloral,[25] and geranium, which is thought to balance oestrogen.[91] I have serious doubts about rose, which is a classic 'woman's' essential oil and much used during the menopause by women who feel that it has an advantageous effect. I admit that my doubts are not grounded on any scientific data.

Benefits of aromatherapy for cancer patients

Aromatherapy is used to enhance the quality of life of cancer patients. In a study at the Marie Curie Centre in Liverpool, patients received a massage with or without Roman chamomile. The group that received the aroma-therapy massage was found to have statistically significantly improved quality of life and reduced anxiety.[46] In a study conducted in order to assess the acceptability of using aromatherapy in palliative care, doctors, nurses, paramedics and volunteers were reported to be extremely enthusiastic about the concept.[177]

Finally, the following essential oils are thought to have anti-carcinogenic properties:

- *Cymbopogon citratus* (lemongrass);[145]
- *Anethum graveolens* (dill);[178]
- *Carum carvi* (caraway).[178]

In summary, aromatherapy should not be thought of as a cure for cancer, but as a way to 'enrich interventions and bring comfort and better health to patients with cancer'.[179] Such actions demonstrate caring. Perhaps this is the caring referred to by Orem as 'a moral idea of nursing'.[93]

PAEDIATRICS

There is a Chinese saying that 'Children get illness easily, illness quickly becomes serious', and another saying that 'Children easily ill, easily cured'. There is no doubt that, Chinese or not, children in hospital are very vulnerable. They do indeed deteriorate and improve rapidly, and they need a tremendous amount of nursing love and support, particularly if their family cannot visit. Although children are more adaptable than adults, and often face very intimidating procedures with wide-eyed interest and no apparent fear, many do display behavioural problems just because they have become institutionalized.

Aromatherapy is a natural thing to a child, whose early life revolves around smell and touch. It is known that babies identify their mothers through the mother's smell.[180] This is easy to understand when one realizes that babies are born with structurally mature olfactory systems.[181] Young children up to the age of 5 years are not repelled by smells which most adults would dislike, e.g. faeces. However, by the age of 7 years many children are beginning to establish similar tastes in smells to adults.[182] Children also display the facility of 'learned memory' early on, gravitating towards the smell of a perfume worn by a mother, rather than another unknown perfume.[183] So familiar smells will be more acceptable to children than other smells. This is particularly important in the case of children from other cultures, who may respond to smells which Western children might not identify with, e.g. spices.

Most of us find it an instinctive action to cuddle and stroke a child. Aromatherapy takes that instinct a little further and adds some extra therapeutic value. Parents and relatives can be taught very easily how to massage a sick child gently, and relish the feeling of being empowered to do something in a situation which most parents fear. This experience of empowerment can be made more potent by the addition of an aroma with which both mother and child are familiar, and which they both like. Gentle aromas can soothe a child, but the emphasis is on gentleness – it is necessary to use only half the normal number of drops required for an adult. Children are extremely aware of smell, and are often far more sensitive to it than adults.

It is important to bear in mind that some children may have been subjected to abuse and will not be receptive to touch, finding it more threatening than comforting. If this is the case, then merely using the appropriate aroma can still be beneficial. Children quite like to be involved in choosing a smell that they like, especially if the choice is small – more than four essential oils will demand too much effort from a sick child. Sometimes a choice of just two will make aromatherapy acceptable, whereas if only one smell is offered it might be refused. However, it is important never to insist – children are patients with patients' rights, no matter how old they are. Remember also the Children Act which was introduced in 1991, and states that 'the child's welfare is paramount'.

Of the possible problems which might be helped by aromatherapy, I have chosen hyperactivity and pyrexia of unknown origin (PUO). There is no suggestion that aromatherapy could replace orthodox medicine, but merely that aromatherapy might enhance nursing care within orthodox medicine. It might also bring comfort to both child and parent (if the parents are present), and give a sense of empowerment to staff. Caring for sick children is an emotionally draining experience for many nurses, and caring for a dying child is one of the most daunting tasks faced by any health professional.[184]

Hyperactivity

Hyperactivity in children who have become hospitalized is common. This form of excitable behaviour is different to attention deficit disorder (ADD), which is a recognized mental disorder.[45] Whilst there has been some research on ADD which suggests that many different contributing factors are involved, including sensitivity to the yellow dye tartrazine, no definite cause has been found.

Every child will make his or her own unique response to being hospitalized. Some become withdrawn, some become placatory and others become hyperactive. It is the hyperactive individuals who can become a source of irritation to staff and other children. It is this form of hyperactivity which aromatherapy can sometimes help. The cause underlying the behaviour is often the strange environment (and smells), which makes a child feel threatened. Hyperactivity is a means of asking for more attention. Slow rhythmic touch with a familiar smell may soothe a child and reduce his or her need to be hyperactive.

Essential oils to consider could include the following:

- *Chamaemelum nobile* (Roman chamomile);
- *Citrus reticulata* (mandarin);
- *Lavandula angustifolia* (lavender);
- *Citrus aurantium* subsp. *amara flos* (neroli);
- *Origanum majorana* (sweet marjoram).

A foot massage is usually acceptable to a sick child. If he or she is ticklish, applying a little more pressure should help. Teaching parents to massage their sick child is one of the most rewarding things I have ever done. A mother's touch, no matter how unfamiliar she is with any technique or stroke, is what a child will usually recognize and respond to. Gentleness and slow strokes are what matters. This is particularly important to remember if the child is unconscious. If the mother wears a lot of bangles, do not ask her to remove them, as her child will remember how they sound and how they feel. This is a case where familiarity really does bring content.

Sometimes the smallest amount of a compound in an essential oil can have a profound effect. One example is the smell of rose caused by an oxide which is present at a concentration of only 0.1 parts per million. There is a compound which is present at trace levels in citrus oils, honeysuckle and jasmine, called indole.[185] In large amounts, indole would make us gag. For example, it contributes to the smell of rotting meat. However, indole has a remarkable relationship with tryptophan, and appears to aid its synthesis.[186] Tryptophan is found in various foodstuffs, e.g. chicken, milk, bananas and rice, and is the chemical precursor of serotonin, the 'feel-good' neuro-chemical.[187] Using an essential oil containing a trace of indole and encouraging a child to drink a glass of milk might produce a reduction in hyperactivity.

Pyrexia

When children have high temperatures, the main danger is one of febrile convulsions, and I am sure that we have all tepid-sponged patients in our time, carefully bringing down the temperature 0.5 degrees at a time in order to prevent shock. Tepid-sponging a child brings with it additional problems, as the child is unlikely to be co-operative, and may well demand blankets and covers for what he or she feels is profound cold, not profound heat. Tepid-sponging requires skill and perseverance. There are three essential oils that might enhance tepid-sponging, namely chamomile, lavender and peppermint. However, instead of using essential oils, it is best to choose a floral water or a hydrosol. These are far weaker, much safer and, because they are already water-based, can easily be added to the tepid water ready for sponging.

Chamomile has been used for hundreds of years to treat fevers[169] and for soothing children.[106] Trevalyan and Booth reported it to be a febrifuge.[188] The aroma is very gentle and, because the amount of essential oil in a floral water is very low, it is safe for young children. It is important to use a true floral water produced by distillation, and not a water to which a synthetic chemical has been added.

Lavender can help to take the heat out of a burn, effectively cooling the skin. Peppermint contains menthol which, when applied to an infant's nostrils, can cause apnoea and collapse.[6] However, peppermint is an extremely common flavouring, and is regarded as completely safe at the correct therapeutic dosage.[189] When applied to the skin, peppermint causes local blood vessels to dilate, producing a cooling effect. Perhaps this is why it is an ingredient of so many anti-sunburn preparations.

Rankin-Box writes that 'the use of aromatherapy in nursing has great potential'.[190] I believe she is right. One of those potential uses could be the addition of floral waters to tepid-sponging of children as a safe and useful enhancement of nursing care.

PALLIATIVE AND TERMINAL CARE

Palliative care may involve care of the terminally ill – the dying – but it is not the same as terminal care. Terminal care is just that – care of a person who is in the immediate process of dying. Palliative care means caring for someone who may not get better, but who is nevertheless not at death's door, and may live for many years.[191] Palliative care involves alleviating the effects of disease without curing.[192]

Palliative care also involves reducing the suffering of those whom orthodox medicine cannot cure, and is a great challenge to nursing. One could argue that this is nursing's finest hour, when the whole foundation to nursing, namely *caring*, is allowed to be the rationale behind what we do for our patients. The philosophy of caring is non-reductionistic.[193] One could argue that it is noticeably holistic and therefore it is hardly surprising that aromatherapy is used and accepted so readily in palliative care. In total 90 per cent of cancer patients spend their last year of life in their own home,[194] although, during that last year many of them will be admitted to a hospital for a short time.

Whilst terminal care involves basic nursing skills such as eye and mouth care, attention to pressure areas and prevention of dehydration, palliative care is more involved with the process of helping patients to live fully for as long as possible. Living fully means experiencing joy, and nursing care should be concerned with this as well as with alleviating suffering. It is recognized that suffering can be emotional as well as physical. One of the greatest emotional shocks a person can receive is the knowledge that he or she has a terminal illness. This sets off an internal process of mourning, with the associated feelings of numbness, anger, depression and finally acceptance.[195] Many remain stuck in the second stage with the question 'why me?' Perhaps the answer to this could be found in the following quotation:

The Pathless Path

There is no answer,
There never has been an answer.
There never will be an answer.
That's the answer.   Gertrude Stein[196]

Our society does little to honour the process of mourning – there is no rite of passage. The idea of mourning something other than death itself is given little support, but patients in palliative care are mourning the death of their future. They know that there will be no happy ending, and although we all have to die sometime, realization of the proximity of death comes as a bitter blow to most patients. There is no way of knowing (outside a hospital) if a person has a limited time to live, unless they choose to tell you. Many do not, because they feel they cannot. Some find it difficult to put into words, some are fearful of an uncertain response (pity and forced jollity being equally unacceptable), so fear can keep patients locked into a world of their own, unable or unwilling to communicate.

Gentle touch and beautiful smells can cross these barriers. Touch communicates a sense of acceptance to such patients, many of whom may have feelings of self-disapproval.[197] Touch and smell often penetrate the despondency of a patient who is struggling to accept that life is no longer going to be as he or she had hoped. Touch is an important commodity during palliative care, when patients can often feel more 'skin hunger'.[198] It opens up dialogue, whilst smells nudge memories. Together they can help patients who may struggle with feelings of anger, denial, guilt and frustration by allowing them to verbalize those feelings and communicate at a deep level.

Attractive smells give pleasure and can relax a patient sufficiently to allow him or her to open up. Aromatherapy using touch allows a patient to experience pleasure, relaxation and acceptance simultaneously. Trust can be built up at a deep level between nurse and patient. This level of intimacy allows nurses to show their profound love of humanity in a deeply moving way and provide 'comfort care' to their patients – a recognized criterion of nursing art.[199] Many nurses seek to give this level of care, stating that they feel it is 'the greatest thing in nursing'.[200]

Palliative care should embrace the whole family, who may be trying to 'remain brave'. Smells are not easily hidden, and beautiful smells are an easy way to begin dialogue with family members. It is not unusual for aromatherapy to act as the catalyst, allowing patient and relative to begin talking to one another at a useful level. This period before a patient enters the terminal stage is important for a peaceful death. It is a time to clear old scores and resolve past disagreements. It is a time of completion, so that the process of dying, when it finally occurs, can be as peaceful and dignified as possible.

Aromatherapy can aid the management of pain and nausea in a complementary way, but perhaps its greatest strength lies in its ability to facilitate communication at an emotional and spiritual level, giving feelings of comfort and pleasure. For this reason, the choice of essential oils should rest with the patient. Concentrate on offering a selection to choose from which could give the patient pleasure. If he or she is particularly withdrawn or depressed, an uplifting essential oil known for its gentle antidepressant properties, such as bergamot (*Citrus bergamia*), would be appropriate. However, at this particular stage of illness we are offering aesthetic aromatherapy, rather than targeting specific problem areas.

Terminal care

The process of dying is recognizable.[201] Bodily functions cease and the peripheral temperature drops as the circulation fails, leaving the skin mottled and discoloured. Thirst is often the last craving, with food refused. Many dying patients breathe through their mouths, which can become dry and cracked. Often their eyes are open, even though they may be asleep or unconscious. Rattling in the throat occurs when secretions collect in the throat and the patient is too weak to cough. Although the patient may be unaware of the sound, it is frequently distressing for relatives in the same room. A change in position may help, but some nurses use aromatherapy to alleviate this problem, gently massaging the feet of dying patients with essential oils.[202] Cheyne-Stoke breathing also often occurs prior to death. The patient may be aware that someone is with them, even though they appear to be deeply unconscious. It is recognized that hearing is the last sense to go, so what is said in front of a dying patient is important.

Many people have a fear of dying alone. Although when patients are at the point of death they may well have been unconscious for some time, it is important to really 'be' there for them. Gently talk to them, tell them you are present for them, but give them permission to go. Touch and smell remain important, and aromatherapy using touch is a wonderful way to say goodbye.

Pleasant smells are of particular importance in terminal nursing. The smell of death is something most nurses can recognize. Certainly if there are any fungating lesions, the smell in a patient's room can be quite unpleasant, and patients remain aware of both smell and touch almost until the end.

Other small but highly effective ways to use aromatherapy in terminal nursing include incorporating floral waters in mouth and eye care. Currently, nursing uses antiseptic lotions which can be uncomfortable or burn mouths that are fragile and sensitive (P. Gravett, transcript from *Medicine Now* broadcast on BBC Radio 4 on 23 July 1995). Floral waters, or hydrolats, are ideal to use, as they are water based, dilute and very gentle.[203] Chamomile and cornflower floral waters are useful and gentle for eye care, and linden flowers, myrtle and orange blossom for mouth care. The floral water should be diluted in warm water. Floral waters provide a gentle way of using extremely diluted essential oils. Wounds can be cleansed with floral waters, as they are antiseptic, and floral waters can be added to compresses or dressings, and are a soothing way to wipe a dying face. Floral waters will leave the delicate scent of an essential oil behind. It is important to use true floral waters, and not synthetic blends added to water.

Relatives learn more from what nurses do than from what they say.[204] There is a need to involve relatives and some can be encouraged to massage their loved one's hands or feet gently. Help them to choose a particular blend of aromas that has meaning for their loved one. Perhaps the patient was particularly fond of their rose garden, or maybe they always potted geraniums. Perhaps they travelled extensively and enjoyed the scent of orange blossom and ylang ylang. Maybe they lived in foreign countries and walked through forests of eucalyptus or sandalwood. Perhaps they had a special herb garden. Their favourite smells can be mixed together in a 'farewell blend'. This highly personal blend can be used constantly during the dying process, and will become identified with the person. Following death, this personalized 'farewell blend' can give tremendous comfort to relatives.

I believe that a soul does not die, but rather it moves on, and just as we welcome a newborn child into this world, we should welcome a soul into their death. Whatever your beliefs, by caring for your dying patient in this way, using their favourite floral or herbal smells, you are celebrating this transition in the most holistic way possible. This is nursing at its finest.

Thank you, my friend
For sharing your dying.
I can be with you
To catch a glimpse of the life you are leaving
And the life to which you return.
In the process, I can accompany your tumult,
Your fear, resistance,
And hope.
Thank you my friend
For sharing your soul.

Dorothea Hover-Kramer.[205]
(reproduced with kind permission of the author)

RESPIRATORY CARE

Of all the departments in a hospital, perhaps the one dealing with respiratory problems is the most obvious candidate for aromatherapy, for when we inhale to smell, we inhale to breathe as well. The high solubility of monoterpenes (which occur in most essential oils) in the blood suggests a high respiratory uptake.[206]

Living in a city I have become very aware of air pollution, especially in the long hot summer of 1995, when the very air seemed to retain a used smell that felt heavy. In fact, for over 30 years, environmental influences have been thought to be linked to arterial blood pressure as well as to chest problems.[207]

Asthma and chronic bronchitis have increased by 30 per cent. Asthma in particular has increased significantly during the last 15 years.[208] Respiratory conditions are the single largest cause of spells of certified sickness absence in the UK. Three in ten people consult their doctor at least once a year about a respiratory disease, the most common complaints being upper respiratory tract infections. Diseases of the respiratory tract are thought to be a cause of some long standing illnesses. Ten per cent of all prescriptions are for drugs to treat a respiratory problem.[209]

Nurses have been using *Eucalyptus radiata* subsp. *radiata* and *Styrax benzoin* (benzoin) for many years to treat respiratory infections.[210]

There are two chronic respiratory problems which are becoming endemic in England, namely recurrent bronchitis and tuberculosis.

Chronic bronchitis

Recurrent chest infections, or chronic bronchitis, are on the increase. Each outbreak of the disease begins with an initial dry cough followed by a mucolytic stage, with copious amounts of phlegm being coughed up. The underlying problem is one of infection, and this can be viral or bacterial.

Essential oils have been used in cough medicines for many years.[211] However, it is thought that the expectorant action of a cough medicine is due to the local action of essential oils on the lining of the respiratory tract during exhalation, after the medicine has been swallowed.[212] Research suggests that inhaled expectorants can have an effect even at a subliminal level.[213] In this particular instance, it was cedar leaf. In one study, the expectorant effect of inhaled nutmeg oil was thought to be due to its camphene content.[212]

Camphene is also found in the following:

- *Cedrus atlantica* (atlas cederwood);
- *Cymbopogon nardus* (citronella);
- *Cymbopogon citratus* (lemongrass);
- *Foeniculum vulgare* (fennel);
- *Cupressus sempervirens* (cypress);
- *Eucalyptus dives, E. globulus* and *E. radiata* (eucalyptus);
- *Lavandula latifolia* (spike lavender);
- *Boswellia carterii* (frankincense);
- *Zingiber officinale* (ginger);
- *Citrus aurantium* var. *amara* (petitgrain);
- *Piper nigrum* (black pepper);
- *Rosmarinus officinalis* (rosemary);
- *Pinus sylvestris* (Scots pine).[214]

Boswellia carterii (frankincense) and *Pinus sylvestris* (Scots pine) are frequently used to treat chest infections.[214,215] An ointment containing menthol and camphene was found to be effective in reducing bronchospasms by 50 per cent when it was insufflated through the respiratory system of animals, but was only slightly effective when applied cutaneously.[216] Applying essential oils to an airway via nasal ointment has also been shown to be effective in stimulating airway secretory glands and reducing mucus. However, caution is needed, as in another trial involving children who had been inadvertently given nose-drops containing menthol or eucalyptol (constituents of essential oils) instead of saline drops, adverse effects ranging from irritated mucous membrane to tachycardia developed.[217] This study does illustrate how using a component of an essential oil instead of the whole oil can often have a detrimental effect.

In a randomized trial involving 182 institutionalized patients, 'essence' drops containing mint, clove, thyme, cinnamon and lavender appeared to reduce the frequency of bouts of chronic bronchitis.[218] This could be because some essential oils are known to purify the air by destroying *Staphylococcus aureus* and *Streptococcus pyogenes* within hours. These essential oils are also thought to be an effective way of preventing ailments such as bronchitis.[219] The essential oils in this study which were most effective were clove, lavender, lemon, marjoram, mint, niaouli, pine, rosemary and thyme.

The advantage of breathing in vaporized essential oils is the avoidance of the *'first pass'* effect. However, pulmonary excretion of cineol, menthol and thymol was demonstrated following rectal application in rats, although the percentage exhaled was extremely small.[220]

An essential oil with expectorant properties may be unable to help fight the infection, in which case the cause of the symptom is not being addressed. An aromatogram would be needed to culture the bacteria and find which essential oil was sensitive. There are specialist pathologists who can do this and supply the relevant essential oil (see Appendix 3 and Chapter 7 on infections). In many instances the sinuses are the site where the infection lingers between bouts.[221] Many infections that are resistant to antibiotics can be alleviated with the use of the correct essential oils.[101]

General respiratory essential oils include the following:

- *Origanum majorana* (sweet marjoram);[222]
- *Lavandula angustifolia* (lavender);
- *Melaleuca viridiflora* (niaouli);[96]
- *Pinus sylvestris* (Scots pine);
- *Rosmarinus officinalis* (rosemary);
- *Thymus vulgaris* (thyme);

- *Cedrus atlantica* (cedarwood);
- *Eucalyptus globulus/radiata* (eucalyptus);
- *Cupressus sempervirens* (cypress).[223]

Essential oils thought to be effective against *Streptococcus aureus* infection[224] (common in coughs and colds) include the following:

- *Thymus vulgaris* (thyme);
- *Cinnamomum zeylanicum* (cinnamon);
- *Lavandula angustifolia* (lavender);
- *Origanum majorana* (marjoram);
- *Satureja montana* (winter savory).

Eucalyptus globulus (at 2 per cent dilution) will kill 70 per cent of ambient *Staphylococcus aureus*. Duke writes that, in Cuba, essential oil of *Eucalyptus globulus* is used to treat all lung ailments.[92]

'A nurse's responsibility associated with problems of respiratory function includes preventing problems, reducing or eliminating contributing factors to respiratory problems, monitoring respiratory status and managing acute respiratory dysfunction'.[225]

Tuberculosis

Tuberculosis (TB) is a mycobacterial disease. The most common form is pulmonary TB, which is spread by droplet infection with Koch's bacillus. Sometimes the bacilli can spread to other parts of the body, setting up nodular lesions called tubercules.[45] TB was relatively well controlled in the UK by bacille Calmette-Guerin (BCG) vaccine, and numbers fell to 10 in 100 000 people.[226] However, the incidence of the disease has increased over the last 10 years, and this trend is thought to be directly related to the growing immigrant community who are not vaccinated in their country of origin, and also to the spread of AIDS. Recently, multiple-resistant TB has reared its ugly head. Although there still are antibiotics to treat this form of TB, those antibiotics are expensive, have side-effects and are slowly becoming ineffective.

Before the advent of *para*-aminosalicylic acid (PAS) and isoniazid, patients with TB were sent to sanitoriums, often high in the mountains and frequently close to forests, because it was thought that breathing fresh mountain air and walking beneath pine trees would aid recuperation.

There is no suggestion that aromatherapy could replace conventional treatment for TB. However, if we can enhance a patient's quality of life with essential oils, perhaps we should use those which might also have some effect on the infection as well.

Valnet was one of the first doctors to document the use of aromatherapy in the treatment of TB. He found that hyssop neutralized the TB bacillus at a concentration of 0.2 parts per 1000.[56] This finding was borne out by an Egyptian study by Hilal.[227] Hyssop is eliminated through the lungs (it is contraindicated in epilepsy and has a pronounced hypertensive action).[56]

There are a number of papers which suggest that essential oils might be effective against TB in humans. Most of the research has been conducted on animals.

Some essential oils that could be used to prevent cross-infection or to complement orthodox treatment include the following:

- *Eucalyptus globulus* (blue gum);[137]
- *Melaleuca viridiflora* (niaouli);[137]
- *Origanum majorana* (marjoram);[56]
- *Centella asiatica* (centella)[92] (centella is an infused oil);
- *Juniperus communis* (juniper).[92]

Cupressus sempervirens (cypress) and *Pinus sylvestris* (Scots pine) are also thought to be effective against TB.[228]

Eucalyptus globulus enhances the activity of streptomycin, isoniazid and sulfetrone in the treatment of Mycobacterium TB,[137] and therefore might provide a useful enhancement to nursing care.

Finally, *Lavandula* × *intermedia* CT gross has been found to be effective against non-tubercular opportunistic mycobacterum (NTM), which is common in AIDS.[131]

REFERENCES

1. **Cousins, N.** 1993: cited in *Healing Words* by Larry Dossey. Harper Collins.

2. **McCormick, E.** 1993 *Healing the heart*. London: Optima.

3. **Summers Dunnington, C., Johnson N.J.** *et al.* 1988: Patients with heart rhythm disturbances: variables associated with increased psychologic distress. *Heart and Lung* **17**, 381–9.

4. **Rowe, L.** 1989: Anxiety in a coronary care unit. *Nursing Times* **45**, 61–3.

5. **Vlay, S.C. and Fricchione, G.L.** 1985: Psychological aspects of surviving sudden cardiac death. *Clinical Cardiology* **8**, 237–42.

6. **Tisserand, R. and Balacs, T.** 1995: *Essential oil safety*. London: Churchill Livingstone.

7. **Morris, N., Birtwistle, S. and Toms, M.** 1995: Anxiety reduction. *International Journal of Aromatherapy* **7**, 33–9.

8. **Perez Raya, M.D., Utrilla, M.P. and Navarro, M.C.** 1990: CNS activity of *Mentha rotundifolia* and *Mentha longifolia* essential oils in mice and rats. *Phytotherapy Research* **4**, 232–5.

9. **Agshikar, N.V. and Abraham, G.J.** 1957: The effect of *l*-menthol on the systemic blood pressure. *Journal of the American Pharmaceutical Association* **46**, 82–4.

10. **Thomas, J.G.** 1962: Peppermint fibrillation. *Lancet* **Jan 27**, 222–3.

11. **Wagner, H. and Sprinkmeyer, L.** 1973: Pharmacological effect of balm spirit. *Deutsche Apotheker-Zeitung* **113**, 1156–66.

12. **Buchbauer, G., Jirovetz, L. and Jager, W.** 1993: Fragrance compounds and essential oils with sedative effects upon inhalation. *Journal of Pharmaceutical Sciences* **82**, 660–64.

13. **Buchbauer, G., Jirovetz, L. and Jager, W.** 1991: Aromatherapy: evidence for sedative effects of the essential oil of lavender after inhalation. *Zeitschrift fur Naturforschung* **46**, 1067–72.

14. **Woolfson, A. and Hewitt, D.** 1992: Intensive aromacare. *International Journal of Aromatherapy* **4**, 12–13.

15. **Rossi, T., Melegari, M. and Blanchi, A.** 1988: Sedative, anti-inflammatory and anti-diuretic effects induced in rats by essential oils of varieties of *Anthemis nobilis*: a comparative study. *Pharmacological Research Communications* **20 (Suppl. V)**, 71–4.

16. **Jager, W., Buchbauer, G. and Jirovetz, L.** 1992: Evidence of the sedative effect of neroli oil, citronella and phenylethyl acetate on mice. *Journal of Essential Oil Research* **4**, 387–94.

17. **Hardy, M., Kirk-Smith, M.D. and Stretch, D.D.** 1995: Replacement of drug treatment for insomnia by ambient odour (letter). *Lancet* **346**, 701.

18. **Nacht, D.I.** *et al.* 1921: Sedative properties of some aromatic drugs and fumes. *Journal of Pharmacology and Experimental Therapeutics* **18**, 361–72.

19. **Buchbauer, G., Jager, W., Nasel, B.** *et al.* 1994: The biology of essential oils and fragrance compounds. *Proceedings of the 1994 Aromatherapy Symposium*. Windsor: Empress.

20. **Roberts, R.** 1991: Preventing PPD after surgery. *Nursing* **4**, 28.

21. **Wilson-Barnett, J. and Carrigy, A.** 1978: Factors influencing patients' emotional reactions to hospitalization. *Journal of Advanced Nursing* **3**, 221–9.

22. **Layne, O.L. and Yudofsky, S.C.** 1971: Postoperative psychosis in cardiotomy patients. *New England Journal of Medicine* **284**, 518–20.

23. **Egerton, N. and Kay, J.H.** 1964: PPD and relationship problems. *British Journal of Psychiatry* **110**, 433–9.

24. **Stevenson, C.** 1994: The psychophysiological effects of aromatherapy massage following cardiac surgery. *Complementary Therapies in Medicine* **2**, 27–35.

25. **Franchomme, P. and Peneol, D.** 1991: *Aromatherapie exactement*. Limoges: Jollois.

26. **Dunn, C., Sleep, J. and Collett, D.** 1995: Sensing an improvement: an experimental study to evaluate the use of aromatherapy, massage and period of rest in an intensive care unit. *Journal of Advanced Nursing* **21**, 34–41.

27. **Rovesti, P. and Columbo, E.** 1973: Aromatherapy and aerosols. *Soap, Perfumery and Cosmetics* **46**, 475–7.

28. **Passant, H.** 1990: A holistic approach in the ward. *Nursing Times* **86**, 26–8.

29. **Hardy, M.** 1991: Sweet scented dreams. *International Journal of Aromatherapy* **3**, 12–13.

30. **Buckle, J.** 1992: Which lavender oil? *Nursing Times* **5**, 54–5.

31. **Ehrlichman, H. and Halpern, J.N.** 1988: Affect and memory: effects of pleasant and unpleasant odor on retrieval of happy and unhappy memories. *Journal of Personality and Social Psychology* **55**, 769–79.

32. **Seth, G., Kolate, C.K. and Varma, K.C.** 1976: Effect of essential oils of *Cymbopogon citratus* on central nervous system. *Indian Journal of Experimental Biology* **14**, 370–73.

33. **Jobst, K.A., Hindley, N.J. and Pearce, M.J.** 1994: Clinical investigation and therapeutic aspects of Alzheimer's disease. *Continuing Medical Education* **12**, 401–12.

34. **Jobst, K.A., Smith, A.D. and Szatmari, M.** 1994: Rapidly progressing atrophy of medial temporal lobe in Alzheimer's disease. *Lancet* **343**, 829–30.

35. **Henry, J.** 1993: Dementia. *International Journal of Aromatherapy* **5**, 27–9.

36. **Klauser, A.G., Flaschentrager, J.** *et al.* 1992: Abdominal wall massage: effect of colonic function in healthy volunteers and in patients with chronic constipation. *Zeitschrift fur Gastroenterologie* **30**, 247–51.

37. **Barker, A.** 1995: Bowel care. *Aromatherapy Quarterly* **No. 44**, 7–10.

38. **Barker, A.** 1994: Pressure sores. *Aromatherapy Quarterly* **No. 41**, 5–7.

39. **Hitchin, D.** 1993: Wound care and the aromatherapist. *Journal of Tissue Viability* **3**, 56–7.

40. **Macdonald, E.M.L.** 1995: Aromatherapy for the enhancement of the nursing care of elderly people suffering from arthritis. *Aromatherapist* **2**, 26–31.

41. Sheppard-Hanger, S. 1995: Phytochemical index. In *The aromatherapy practitioner reference manual. Volume 11.* Tampa, FL: Atlantic Institute of Aromatherapy, 486–531.

42. **Lorenzetti, B., Souza, G.E., Sarti, S.J.** *et al.* 1991: Myrcene mimics the peripheral analgesic activity of lemongrass tea. *Ethnopharmacology* **34**, 43–8.

43. **Bohlin, L.** 1995: Structure-activity studies of natural products with anti-inflammatory and immunomodulatory effects. In *Phytochemistry of plants used in traditional medicine.* Oxford: Oxford Science Publications, 137–63.

44. **Deans, S.** 1991: More life in your years. *International Journal of Aromatherapy* **3**, 20–22.

45. **McFerran, T.** 1996: *A dictionary of nursing,* 2nd edn. Oxford: Oxford University Press.

46. **Wilkinson, S.** 1995: Aromatherapy and massage in palliative care. *International Journal of Palliative Nursing* **1**, 21–30.

47. **Shipotchliev, T.** 1969: Pharmacological research into a group of essential oils and their effect on the motor activity and general state of white mice in separate applications. *Chemical Abstracts* **70**, 180.

48. **Pritchard, A.P. and Mallett, J. (eds).** 1992: *The Royal Marsden Hospital manual of clinical nursing procedures*, 3rd edn. Oxford: Blackwell Scientific Publications.

49. **Waterlow, J.** 1988: Prevention is cheaper than cure. *Nursing Times* **84**, 69–71.

50. **Johnson, A.** 1989: Granuflex wafers as a prophylactic pressure sore dressing. *Care – Science and Practice* **7**, 55–6.

51. **Waterlow, J.** 1987: Calculating the risk. *Nursing Times* **83**, 58–60.

52. **David, J.A.** *et al.* 1983: Normal physiology from injury to repair. *Nursing* **2**, 296–7.

53. **Gustafsson, G.** 1988: Guidelines for the application of disinfectant in wound care. *Nursing RSA Verpleging* **3**, 8–9.

54. **Turner, T.D.** *et al.* 1985: Semi-occlusive and occlusive dressing. *Royal Society of Medicine International Congress and Symposium Proceedings.* London: Royal Society of Medicine.

55. **Zawahry, E.E.** 1973: Leg ulcers, acne vulgaris, seborrhea and alopecea. *International Journal of Dermatology* **Jan/Feb**, 68–73.

56. **Valnet, J.** 1993: *The practice of aromatherapy.* Saffron Walden: C.W. Daniel.

57. **Onawunmi, G. and Ogunina, E.** 1986: A study of the antibacterial activity of the EO of lemongrass. *International Journal of Crude Drug Research* **24**, 64–8.

58. **Janssen, A.M. and Chin, N.L.J.** 1986: Screening for antimicrobial activity of some essential oils. *Pharmaceutisch Weekblad Scientific Edition (Utrecht)* **8**, 289–92.

59. **Ross, S.A., El-Keltaw, N.E. and Megella, S.E.** 1980: Antimicrobial activity of some Egyptian aromatic plants. *Fitoterapia* **51**, 201–5.

60. **Deans, S. and Svoboda, K.P.** 1990: The antimicrobial properties of marjoram (*Origanum majorana*) volatile oil. *Flavour and Fragrance Journal* **5**, 187–90.

61. **Deans, S., Svoboda, K., Gundidza, M. and Brechany, E.** 1992: Essential oil profiles of several temperate and tropical aromatic plants: their antimicrobial and antioxidant activities. *Acta Horticulturae* **306**, 229–33.

62. **Gascoigne, S.** 1993: *Manual of conventional medicine for alternative practitioners. Volume 1.* Richmond: Jigme Press.

63. **Gattefosse, M.** 1992. *Gattefosse's aromatherapy* (translated by Tisserand, R.). Saffron Walden: C.W. Daniel.

64. **Mills, S.** 1991: *Out of the earth*. London: Viking Arkana.

65. **Carle, R. and Gomaa, K.** 1992: The medicinal use of *Matricaria flos*. *British Journal of Phytotherapy* **2**, 147–53.

66. **Tubaro, A., Zilli, C. and Redaeli, C.** 1984: Evaluation of anti-inflammatory activity of a chamomile extract topical application. *Planta Medica* **50**, 147–53.

67. **Aertgeerts, P., Albring, M., Klaaschka, F.** *et al.* 1985: Comparative testing of Kamillosan cream and steroidal (0.25% hydrocortisone, 0.75% fluocortin butyl ester) and non-steroidal (5% bufexamac) dermatologic agents maintenance therapy for eczematous diseases. *Zeitschrift fur Hautkrankheiten (Berlin)* **60**, 270–7.

68. **Glowania, H.J., Raulin, C. and Swoboda, M.** 1987: Effect of chamomile on wound healing – a clinical double-blind study. *Zeitschrift fur Hautkrankheiten (Berlin)* **62**, 1267–71.

69. **Gupta, S.K., Sharma, R.C.** *et al.* 1972: Anti-inflammatory activity of the oils isolated from *Cyperus scariosus*. *Indian Journal of Experimental Biology* **10**, 41.

70. **Duwiejua, M., Zeitlin, I.J.** *et al.* 1992: Anti-inflammatory activity of resins from some species of the plant family Burseraceae. *Planta Medica* **59**, 12–16.

71. **Mascolo, N., Autore, G.** *et al.* 1987: Biological screening of Italian medicinal plants for anti-inflammatory activity. *Phytotherapy Research* **1**, 28–31.

72. **Tisserand, R.** 1992: The book that launched aromatherapy. *International Journal of Aromatherapy* **4**, 20–22.

73. **May, V.G. and Willuhn, G.** 1978: Antivirale Wirkung waBriger Pflanzenextrakte in Gewebekulturen. *Arzneimittel-Forschung (Aulendorf)* **28**, 1–7.

74. **Cohen, R.A., Kucera, L.S.** *et al.* 1964: Antiviral activity of *Melissa officinalis* (lemon balm) extract. *Proceedings of the Society for Experimental Biology and Medicine* **117**, 431–4.

75. **Kucera, L.S. and Herrmann, E.C.** 1967: Antiviral substances in plants of the mint family: tannin of *Melissa officinalis*. *Proceedings of the Society for Experimental Biology and Medicine* **124**, 865–9.

76. **Wobling, R.H. and Leonhardt, K.** 1994: Local therapy of herpes simplex with dried extract from *Melissa officinalis*. *Phytomedicine* **1**, 25–31.

77. **Takechi, M., Tanaka, Y.** *et al.* 1985: Structure and anti-herpetic activity among the tannins. *Phytochemistry* **24**, 2245–50.

78. **Anthony, C.P. and Thibodeau, G.A.** 1983: *Textbook of anatomy and physiology*. St Louis, MO: Mosby.

79. **Bennett, A. and Stamford, F.** 1988: The biological activity of eugenol, a major consituent of nutmeg, on prostaglandins, the intestine and other tissues. *Phytotherapy Research* **2**, 124–9.

80. **Wagner, H., Wierer, M.** *et al.* 1986: *In vitro*-Hemmung der Prostaglandin-Biosynthese durch etherische Ole und phenolische Verbindungen. *Planta Medica*, 184–7.

81. **Melzig, M. and Teuscher, E.** 1991: Investigations of the influence of essential oils and their main components on the adenosine uptake by cultivated epithelial cells. *Planta Medica* **57**, 41.

82. **Sheppard-Hangar, S.** 1995: *The Aromatherapy practitioner's reference manual. Volume 1.* Tampa, FL: Atlantic Institute of Aromatherapy, 469–531.

83. **Budavari, S. (ed.)** 1996: *The Merck Index*, 12th edn. Whitehouse Station, NJ: Merck & Co. Ltd.

84. **Zondeck B. and Bergmann, E.** 1938: Phenol methyl esters as estrogenic agents. *Biochemical Journal* **32**, 641–5.

85. **Belaiche, P.** 1979: Syndrome premenstruel. In *Traite de phytotherapie et d'aromatherapie. Volume 3.* Paris: SA Maloine, 60–64.

86. **Balacs, T. and Tisserand, R.** 1995: *Essential oil safety.* London: Churchill Livingstone.

87. **Buccellato, F.** 1982: Ylang survey. *The Perfumer and Flavorist* **7**, 9–10.

88. **Tzeng, S.H., Ko, W.C.** *et al.* 1991: Inhibition of platelet aggregation by some flavonoids. *Thrombosis Research* **64**, 91–100.

89. **Marini-Bettolo, G.B.** 1979: Plants in traditional medicine. *Journal of Ethnopharmacology* **1**, 303–6.

90. **Albert-Puleo, M.** 1980: Fennel and anise as estrogenic agents. *Journal of Ethnopharmacology* **2**, 337–44.

91. **Holmes, P.** 1993: *The energetics of Western herbs.* Berkeley, CA: NatTrop.

92. **Duke, J.** 1985: *Handbook of medicinal herbs.* Boca Raton, FL: CRC Press.

93. **Leddy, S. and Pepper, J.M.** 1993: *Conceptual bases of professional nursing.* Philadelphia: Lippincott.

94. **Al-Hader, A.A. and Hasan, Z.A.** 1994: Hyperglycemic and insulin release inhibitory effects of *Rosmarinus officinalis. Journal of Ethnopharmacology* **1**, 112–17.

95. **Revoredo, N.L.** 1958: Hypoglycemic action of *Eucalyptus citriodora. Monitor de la Farmacia y de la Terapeutica* **64**, 37–8.

96. **Price, S.** 1995: *Aromatherapy for the health professional.* London: Churchill Livingstone.

97. **Goldway, M., Teff, D., Schmidt, R.** *et al.* 1995: Multidrug resistance in *Candida albicans. Antimicrobial Agents and Chemotherapy*, 422–6.

98. **Belaiche, P.** 1985: Treatment of vaginal infections of *Candida albicans* with essential oil of *Melaleuca alternifolia. Phytotherapie* **15**, 13–15.

99. **Pena, E.F.** 1962: *Melaleuca alternifolia.* Its use for trichomonal vaginitis and other vaginal infection. *Obstetrics and Gynecology* **19**, 793–5.

100. **Guenther, E.** 1972: *The essential oils.* Malabar, FL: Krieger.

101. **Carson, C.F., Cookson, B.D., Farrelly, H.D. and Riley, T.V.** 1995: Susceptibility of MRSA to the essential oil of *Melaleuca alternifolia*. *Journal of Antimicrobial Chemotherapy* **35**, 421–4.

102. **Cooke, A. and Cooke, M.D.** 1994: *The Cawthron Report: an investigation into the antimicrobial properties of manuka and kanuka oils. Report Number 263*. Nelson, New Zealand: Cawthron Company.

103. **Reiter, M. and Brandt, W.** 1985: Relaxant effect on the trachea and ilea of smooth muscle of the guinea pig. *Arzneimittel-Forschung (Aulendorf)* **35**, 408–14.

104. **Taddei, I., Gachetti, E. and Taddel, P.** 1988: Spasmolytic activity of peppermint, sage and rosemary essences and their major constituents. *Fitoterapia* **LIX**, 463–8.

105. **Evans, W.C.** 1994: *Trease and Evans' pharmacognoscy*, 13th edn. London: Baillière Tindall.

106. **Wren, R.C.** 1988: *Potter's new cyclopaedia of botanical drugs and preparations*. London: Churchill Livingstone.

107. **Boelens, M.** 1994: Sensory and chemical evaluation of tropical grass oils. *Perfumer and Flavorist* **19**, 24–45.

108. **Gobel, H., Schmidt, G. and Soyka, D.** 1994: Effect of peppermint and eucalyptus oil preparations on neurophysiological and experimental algesimetric headache parameters. *Cephalagia* **14**, 228–34.

109. **Glaser, J.K. and Glaser, R.** 1993: Mind and immunity. In *Mind–body medicine*. New York: Consumer Books.

110. **Cohen, N. and Felten, D.** 1995: Psychoneuroimmunology: interactions between the nervous system and the immune system. *Lancet* **345**, 99–103.

111. **Kiecolt-Glaser, J.K. and Glaser, R.** 1991: Stress and the immune system: human studies. In Tasman, A. and Riba, M.B. (eds), *Annual Review of Psychiatry, Volume 11*. Washington, DC: American Psychiatric Press, 169–80.

112. **Cohen, S., Tyrrel, D.A.J. and Smith, A.P.** 1991: Psychological stress and susceptibility to the common cold. *New England Journal of Medicine* **325**, 606–12.

113. **Domar, A.D., Seibel, M.M. and Benson, H.** 1990: The mind/body program for infertility. A new behavioural treatment approach for women with infertility. *Fertility and Sterility* **53**, 246–9.

114. **Panconesi E. (ed.)** 1984: *Clinics in Dermatology, Volume 2. Stress and skin diseases: psychosomatic dermatology*. Philadelphia: JB Lippincott.

115. **Turk, D.C.T. and Nash, J.M.** 1993: Chronic pain. New ways to cope. In *Mind–body medicine*. New York: Consumer Reports Books, 11–31.

116. **Peneol, D.** 1993: The immune system of mankind. *Aroma 1993 Conference Proceedings*. Hove: Aromatherapy Proceedings.

117. **Berkarda, B.** *et al.* 1983: The effect of coumarin derivatives on the immunological system of man. *Agents and Actions* **13**, 50–52.

118. **Mitchell, S.** 1993: Dementia. *International Journal of Aromatherapy* **5**, 20–23.

119. **Roulier, G.** 1990: *Les huiles essentielles pour votre sante.* St Jean-de-Braye: Dangles.

120. **Wagner, H.** 1985: *Economic and medicinal plant research. Volume 1.* London: Academic Press.

121. **Mailhebiau, P.** 1995: The thymus folder. *Les Cahiers de l'Aromatherapie* **1**, 38–60.

122. **Boelens, M.** 1994: Sensory and chemical evaluation of tropical grass oils. *Perfumer and Flavorist* **19**, 24–45.

123. **Kusumoto, I.T., Shimada, E.** *et al.* 1992: Inhibitory effects of Indonesian plant extracts on reverse transcriptase of an RNA tumour virus. *Phytotherapy Research* **6**, 241–4.

124. **Cardellina, J.H. and Boyd, M.R.** 1995: Pursuits of new leads to antitumour and anti-HIV agents from plants. *Proceedings of the Phytochemical Society of Europe.* Oxford: Oxford Science Press, 81–93.

125. **Nakashima, H., Murakami, T. and Yamamoto, N.** 1992: Inhibition of human immunodeficiency viral replications by tannins and related compounds. *Antiviral Research* **18**, 91–103.

126. **Mahmood, N., Moore, P.S. and De Tommasi, N.** 1993: Inhibition of HIV infection by flavonoids. *Antiviral Research* **22**, 189–99.

127. **De Tommasi, N., De Simone, F. and De Feo, V.** 1991: Phenylpropanoid glycosides and rosmarinic acid from *Momardica balsamina.* *Planta Medica* **57**, 201.

128. **Schols, D., Wutzler, P. and Klocking, R.** 1991: Selective inhibitory activity of polyhydroxycarboxylates derived from phenolic compounds against human immunodeficiency virus replication. *Journal of Acquired Immune Deficiency Syndrome* **4**, 677–84.

129. **Torres, G.** 1993: Treatment issues. *Gay Men's Health Crisis Newsletter of Experimental Aids Therapies* **7**, 1–2.

130. **Pratt, R.** 1995: *HIV and AIDS: a strategy for nursing care.* London: Edward Arnold.

131. **Gabrielli, G., Loggini, F., Cioni, P.L.** *et al.* 1988: Activity of lavandino essential oil. *Pharmacological Research Communications* **20 (Suppl. V)**, 37–41.

132. **Belaiche, P.** 1985: Treatment of skin infections with the essential oils of *Melaleuca alternifolia. Phytotherapy* **15**, 15–17.

133. **Fun, C.E. and Svendsen, A.B.** 1990: The essential oils of *Lippia alba.* *Journal of Essential Oil Research* **2**, 265–7.

134. **Soliman, F.M., El Kashoury, E.A. and Fathy, M.M.** 1994: Analysis

and biological activity of the essential oil of *Rosmarinus officinalis* L. from Egypt. *Flavor and Fragrance Journal* **9**, 29–33.

135. **Viollon, C. and Chaumont, J.P.** 1994: Antifungal properties of essential oils and their main components upon *Cryptococcus neoformans*. *Mycopathologia* **128**, 151–3.

136. **De Blasi, V.** *et al.* 1990: Amoebicidal effects of essential oils *in vitro*. *Journal de Toxicologie Clinique et Experimentale (Paris)* **10**, 361–73.

137. **Kufferath, F. and Mundualgo, G.M.** 1954: The activity of some preparations containing essential oils in TB. *Fitoterapia* **25**, 483–5.

138. **Larrondo, J.V. and Calvo, M.A.** 1991: Effect of essential oils on *Candida albicans*: a scanning electron microscope study. *Biomedical Letters* **46**, 269–72.

139. **Cohen, R.A., Kucera, L.S.** *et al.* 1964: Antiviral activity of *Melissa officinalis* (lemon balm) extract. *Proceedings of the Society for Experimental Biology and Medicine* **117**, 431–4.

140. **Xheng, G., Kenney, P. and Lam, L.** 1992: Anethofuran, carvone and limonene: potential cancer chemopreventative agents from dill weed oil and caraway oil. *Planta Medica* **58**, 338–41.

141. **Wattenberg, L.W.** *et al.* 1989: cited in Xheng, G., Kenney, P. and Lam, L. 1992: Anethofuran, carvone and limonene: potential cancer chemopreventative agents from dill weed oil and caraway oil. *Planta Medica* **58**, 338–41.

142. **de la Puerta, S. and Garcia, M.D.** 1993: Cystostatic activity against HEp-2 cells and antibacterial activity of essential oil from *Helichrysum picardii*. *Phytotherapy Research* **7**, 378–80.

143. **Zheng, G., Kenney, P.M. and Lam, L.K.T.** 1992: Myristicin: a potential cancer chemopreventive agent from parsley leaf oil. *Journal of Agricultural and Food Chemistry* **40**, 107–10.

144. **Muanza, D.N., Eduler, K.L., Williams, L. and Newman, D.J.** 1995: Screening for antitumor and anti-HIV activities of nine medicinal plants from Zaire. *International Journal of Pharmacology* **33**, 98–106.

145. **Zheng, G.Q., Kenney, P.M.** *et al.* 1993: Potential anticarcinogenic natural products isolated from lemongrass oils and galanga root oil. *Journal of Agricultural and Food Chemistry* **41**, 153–7.

146. **Jansses, A.M., Chin, N.L.J.** *et al.* 1986: Screening for antimicrobial activity of some essential oils. *Pharmaceutisch Weekblad Scientific Edition (Utrecht)* **8**, 289–92.

147. **Mansfield, P.** 1996: Animal experiments are an obstacle to health. *Holistic Health* **8**, 4–7.

148. **Dewick, P.M.** 1989: Tumour inhibitors from plants. In Evans, W.C. (ed.), *Trease and Evan's pharmacognosy*, 13th edn. London: Baillière Tindall, 634–56.

149. **Lewis, W.H. and Elvin-Lewis, M.P.F.** 1977: *Medical botany.* New York: Wiley-Interscience.

150. **Fell, J.W.** 1857: *A treatise on cancer and its treatment.* London: J. Churchill.

151. **Foster, S.** 1995: Anti-cancer effects of Gotu Kola (*Centella asiatica*). *HerbalGram* **36,** 17–18.

152. **Stevenson, C.** 1996: Disease. In Vickers, A. (ed.) *Massage and aromatherapy.* London: Chapman & Hall, 193–202.

153. **Clover, A., Last, P. and Fisher, P.** 1995: Complementary cancer therapy: a pilot study of patients, therapies and quality of life. *Complementary Therapies in Medicine* **3,** 129–33.

154. **Downer, S.M., Cody, M.M. and McCluskey, P.** 1994: Pursuit and practice of complementary therapies by cancer patients receiving conventional treatment. *British Medical Journal* **309,** 86–9.

155. **Goodman, S. (ed.)** 1995: Book review: massage for people with cancer. *Positive Health* **Aug/Sept,** 26.

156. **McNamara, P.** 1994: *Massage for people with cancer.* London: Wandsworth Cancer Support Centre.

157. **Seigal, B.** 1996: Letter to the editor. *Massage Therapy Journal* **35,** 12–13.

158. **Dobbs, B.Z.** 1985: Alternative health approaches. *Nursing Mirror* **160,** 41–2.

159. **Finlay, I.** 1995: The management of other frequently encountered symptoms. In Penson, J. and Fisher, R. (eds), *Palliative care for people with cancer.* London: Edward Arnold, 57–80.

160. **Bovbjerg, D.H., Redd, W.H. *et al.*** 1990: Anticipatory immune suppression and nausea in women receiving cyclic chemotherapy for ovarian cancer. *Journal of Consulting and Clinical Pathology* **58,** 153–7.

161. **Briggs, C.** 1993: Peppermint: medicinal herb and flavouring agent. *Canadian Pharmacology Journal* **126,** 89–92.

162. **Williamson, E.M. and Evans, F.J. (eds)** 1988: *Potter's new cyclopedia of botanical drugs and preparations.* Saffron Walden: C.W. Daniel.

163. **Mowrey, D.M.** 1982: Motion sickness and psychophysics. *Lancet* **March 20,** 655–7.

164. **Nadkarni, K.M.** 1992: *Indian Material Medica, Volume 1.* Prakashan: Bombay Popular.

165. **Cabo, J., Crespo, M.E.** 1986: The spasmolytic activity of various aromatic plants from Granada: the activity of the major components of their essential oils. *Plantes Medicinales et Phytotherapie* **20,** 213–18.

166. **Aloe Vera Research Institute** 1993: *Medical Research in Aloe vera.* West Valley City: Aloe Vera Research Institute.

167. **Rovath, B.** 1959: Burns and aloe vera. *Industrial Medicine and Surgery* **28,** 364–8.

168. **Crew, J.E.** 1959: Aloe vera. *Minnesota Medicine* **20,** 670–73.

169. **Grieve, M.** 1931: *A modern herbal.* Harmondsworth: Penguin.

170. **Foster, S.** 1995: Anti-cancer effects of Gotu Kola (*Centella asiatica*). *HerbalGram* **36,** 17–18.

171. **Brud, W.S. and Szydlowska, I.** 1991: Bulgarian rose otto. *International Journal of Aromatherapy* **3,** 17–19.

172. Badger, C. 1995: Lymphoedema. In Penson, J. and Fisher, R. (eds), *Palliative care for people with cancer.* London: Edward Arnold, 81–90.

173. **Idoux, M.** 1996: Treatment for lymphoedema following mastectomy or lumpectomy. *Holistic Nurses' Association Newsletter* **3,** 4–5.

174. **Earle, L.** 1991: *Vital oils.* London: Vermilion.

175. **Duwiejua, M., Zeitlin, I.J., Waterman, P.G.** *et al.* 1993: Anti-inflammatory activity of resins from some species of the plant family, Burseraceae. *Planta Medica* **50,** 12–16.

176. **Albert-Puleo, M.** 1980: Fennel and anise as estrogenic agents. *Journal of Ethnopharmacology* **2,** 337–44.

177. **Arnold, L.** 1995: The use of aromatherapy and essential oils in palliative care: risk versus research. *Positive Health* **Aug/Sept,** 32–4.

178. **Zheng, G., Kenney, P. and Lam, K.T.** 1991: Anethofurna, carvone and limonene. Potential cancer chemopreventive agents from dill weed oil and caraway oil. *Planta Medica* **58,** 338–41.

179. **Penson, J. and Fisher, R.** 1995: *Palliative care for people with cancer.* London: Edward Arnold.

180. **Russell, M.J.** 1976: Human olfactory communication. *Nature* **260,** 520–22.

181. **Humphrey, T.** 1940: The development of the olfactory and the accessory olfactory formations in human embryos and fetuses. *Journal of Comparative Neurology* **73,** 431–68.

182. **Engen, T.** 1974: Method and theory in the study of odor preferences. In Johnston, J. (ed.), *Human response to environmental odors.* New York: Academic Press, 121–41.

183. **Schleidt, M. and Genzel, C.** 1990: The significance of mother's perfume for infants in the first weeks of their life. *Ethology and Sociobiology* **11,** 145–50.

184. **Hodson, D.** 1995: The special needs of children and adolescents. In Penson, J. and Fisher, R. (eds), *Palliative care for people with cancer,* 2nd edn. London: Edward Arnold, 198–229.

185. **Collin, G. and Hoeke, H.** 1993: *Ullman's encyclopedia of industrial chemistry. Volume 14,* 5th edn. Weinheim: VCH.

186. **Clark, G.S.** 1995: An aroma chemical profile: indole. *Perfumer and Flavorist* **20,** 21–31.

187. **Parish, P.** 1991: *Medical treatments: the benefits and risks.* Harmondsworth: Penguin Books.

188. **Trevalyan, J. and Booth, B.** 1994: *Complementary medicine for nurses, midwives and health visitors.* London: Macmillan.

189. **Briggs, C.** 1993: Peppermint: medicinal herb and flavouring agent. *Canadian Pharmacology Journal* **126,** 89–92.

190. **Rankin-Box, D.** 1995: *Nurses' handbook of complementary therapies.* London: Churchill Livingstone.

191. **McCusker, J.** 1983: Where cancer patients die: an epidemiological study. *Public Health Reports* **98,** 170–6.

192. **Fowler, H.W. and Fowler, F.G.** 1964: *The Concise Oxford Dictionary of Current English,* 5th edn. Oxford: Oxford University Press.

193. **Drew, N. and Dahlerg, K.** 1995: Challenging a reductionistic paradigm as a foundation for nursing. *Journal of Holistic Nursing* **13,** 334–7.

194. **Doyle, D.** 1986: Domiciliary care – a doctor's view. In *International Symposium on Pain Control.* London: Royal Society of Medicine, 61–7.

195. **Childs-Gowell, E.** 1992: *Good grief rituals.* Raleigh, NC: Station Hill Press.

196. **Stein, G.** 1995: The pathless path. In Dossey, L. (ed.), *Healing words.* HarperSanFrancisco.

197. **Pratt, J. and Mason, A.** 1981: *The caring touch.* London: Heyden, 80.

198. **Simon, S.B.** 1976: *Caring, feeling, touching.* London: Argus Communications.

199. **Kolcaba, K.Y.** 1995: Comfort as process and product, merged in holistic nursing art. *Journal of Holistic Nursing* **13,** 117–31.

200. **Montgomery, C.L.** 1996: The care-giving relationship: paradoxical and transcendent aspects. *Alternative Therapies* **2,** 52–7.

201. **Newbury, A.** 1995: The care of the patient near the end of life. In Penson, J. and Fisher, R. (eds), *Palliative care for people with cancer.* London: Edward Arnold, 178–98.

202. **Tattam, A.** 1992: The gentle touch. *Nursing Times* **88,** 16–17.

203. **Kusmerik, J.** 1996: Floral waters. *Aromatherapy Quarterly* **No. 49,** 5–7.

204. **Dossey, B.** 1994: Dynamics of consciousness and healing. *Journal of Holistic Nursing* **12,** 4–10.

205. **Hover-Kramer, D.** 1993: Thank you my friend. *Journal of Holistic Nursing* **11,** 115–16.

206. **Falk, A., Gullstrand, E.** *et al.* 1990: Liquid/air partition coefficients of four terpenes. *British Journal of Industrial Medicine* **47,** 62–64.

207. **Cruz-Coke, R.** 1960: Environmental influences and arterial blood pressure. *Lancet* **Oct 22,** 885–6.

208. **Newman-Taylor, A.** 1995: Environmental determinants of asthma. *Lancet* **345,** 296–9.

209. **Lung and Asthma Information Agency,** 1995: *Factsheet.* London: Department of Public Health Sciences, St George's Hospital Medical School.

210. **Stevenson, C.** 1995: Aromatherapy. In Rankin-Box, D. (ed.), *The nurses' handbook of complementary therapies*. London: Churchill Livingstone, 52–8.

211. **Boyd, E.M.** 1954: Expectorants and respiratory tract fluid. *Pharmacological Review* **6**, 521–42.

212. **Boyd, E.M. and Sheppard, P.** 1970: Nutmeg and camphene as inhaled expectorants. *Archives of Otolaryngology (Chicago)* **92**, 372–8.

213. **Boyd, E.M. and Sheppard, E.P.** 1968: The effect of steam inhalation of volatile oils on the output and composition of respiratory tract fluid. *Journal of Pharmacology and Experimental Therapeutics* **163**, 250–56.

214. **Sheppard-Hanger, S.** 1995: *The aromatherapy practitioner reference manual. Volume 11*. Tampa, FL: Atlantic Institute of Aromatherapy.

215. **Abdel Wahab, S.M., Adoutabl, E.A., El-Zalabani, S.M.** *et al.* 1987: The essential oil of *Olibanum*. *Planta Medica* 382–4.

216. **Schafer, D. and Schafer, W.** 1981: Pharmacological studies with an ointment containing menthol, camphene and essential oils for broncholytic and secretolytic effects. *Arzneimittelforschung* **31**, 82–6.

217. **Melis, K., Bochner, A. and Hanssens, G.** 1989: Accidental nasal eucalyptol and menthol instillation. *European Journal of Paediatrics* **148**, 786–8.

218. **Ferley, J.P., Poutignat, N.** *et al.* 1989: Prophylactic aromatherapy for supervening infections in patients with chronic bronchitis. Statistical evaluation conducted in clinics against a placebo. *Phytotherapy Research* **3**, 97–100.

219. **Bardeau, F.** 1976: Use of essential aromatic oils to purify and deodorise the air. *Chir Dent Fr* **46**, 53.

220. **Grisk A. and Fischer, W.** 1969: Zur pulmonalen Ausscheidung von cineol, menthol und thymol bei ratten nach rektaler applikation. *Zeitschrift fur Arztliche Fortbildung (Jenä)* **63**, 233–6.

221. **Belaiche, P.** 1979: *Traite de phytotherapie et d'aromatherapie. Volume 2*. Paris: Maloine SA Editeur.

222. **Culpepper, N.** 1826: *The complete herbal*. Deansgate, Gleave & Son.

223. **Lawless, J.** 1992: *The encyclopedia of essential oils*. Shaftesbury: Element.

224. **Belaiche, P.** 1979: *Traite de phytotherapie et d'aromatherapie. Volume 1*. Paris: Maloine Editeur.

225. **Carpenito, L.J.** 1993: *Nursing diagnosis: applications to clinical practice*, 5th edn. Philadelphia: Lippincott.

226. **MacSween, R.N.M. and Whaley, K. (ed.)** 1992: *Muir's textbook of pathology*. London: Edward Arnold.

227. **Hilal, S.H.** *et al.* 1978: Investigation of the volatile oil of *Hyssopus officinalis*. *Pharmaceutisch Weekblad Scientific Edition (Utrecht)* **19**, 177–84.

228. **Schnaubelt, K.** *Aromatherapy Course. Part 3*. San Rafael, CA: Pacific Institute of Aromatherapy.

Part 3

The future

9

TRAINING

ACCREDITATION, VALIDATION AND CERTIFICATION

There are several misunderstandings about training courses in aromatherapy and what those trainings mean.

Accreditation

An accredited course means that an external board has approved the content of the course. Accreditation is a word commonly used with prior learning. For example, a nurse wishing to apply to register for a higher degree may be asked what other courses she has completed so that she can be 'accredited' with this prior learning, thereby reducing the number of credits she still has to complete. Academic credit is recognition of learning expressed in terms of a number of credit points (4 credit points are equivalent to 1 week of full-time study at a particular level). Accreditation also takes into account the level at which the learning occurred. For example: level 0 = foundation level; level 1 = certificate level; level 2 = diploma level; level 3 = degree level; level 4 = postgraduate level.

Validation

Validation means that what has been claimed by the course to be included (methodology, course outline, learning outcomes, levels, etc.) has been agreed upon by an external board, usually of academic status. This external board validates the course, thereby verifying its content. Universities can validate new courses which are outside their areas of expertise by setting up validation committees to study the documentation and approve (or fail to approve) a new course. In other words, an academic external body has given the course a stamp of approval.

Certification

A certification can mean one of two things:

- that a student has attended a course (although he or she may not have learned anything);
- that a student has attended a course and passed the required examinations.

The term 'certified' usually implies that a student has passed the required examinations and therefore, in the mind of the certifying board (which may or may not be the school that set the examination) is competent in that subject. In America, a certified person is often described as *licensed* to use that training, e.g. a certified lawyer or accountant. However, in the field of aromatherapy there is no body either in the UK or in the USA that can *license* an aromatherapist. The closest thing in the UK is a self-regulating body called the Aromatherapy Organization Council (AOC), who set a core curriculum for aromatherapy training.

TRAINING FOR NURSES

The Royal College of Nursing (RCN) has issued guidelines for nurses who wish to use aromatherapy. These state that a nurse 'should know her subject and have received training'. There is no suggestion that the course should be nursing based. However, if aromatherapy is to be used to enhance nursing (which is what happens at the moment), perhaps it should be nursing based.

The guidelines issued by the RCN include the following:

- supervised practice;
- anatomy, physiology, pathology and pharmacology;
- a practical and theoretical examination;
- a holistic approach;
- supervised clinical practice;
- counselling/communication and self-development skills training;
- appropriately qualified teachers;
- support for the trainee therapist;
- a sensible tutor/pupil ratio;
- basic management and business skills included.

The above list is taken from the RCN document, *Choosing a complementary therapy*.[1]

Choices of training

Aromatherapy training can be divided into three types as follows:

- professional;
- academic;
- nursing.

Professional: AOC recognized

AOC-regulated schools require a minimum of 60 hours of massage, 40 hours of anatomy and physiology and 80 hours of aromatherapy. This training, which takes 1 to 2 years, part-time, contains required core subjects such as client care and modesty, hygiene and sterilization and managing a business, which may not be required by a nurse.

Many of the techniques taught in the massage section will not be used in nursing care, e.g. tapotement, hacking, cupping and mechanical massage. In fact, many nurses will not use massage at all, pointing out that they do not have the time. An AOC course may provide very little information about the use of *clinical* aromatherapy, which is what is required for a nurse to be competent and able to use aromatherapy safely in a hospital setting. So there is one main point at issue – what do nurses need to know, and at what level?

Academic: university validated

An academic training (which has been validated through a university) may only provide theoretical knowledge. The hours do not have to conform with AOC rules. However, insurance from an AOC-regulated organization or the RCN may not be possible after this training.

One interesting academic option that is currently available is a university-validated hospital-based course. The theory and practice of essential oils course at the Royal London Homeopathic Hospital, London is validated through South Bank University. This modular course is accredited with 30 credits at level 2, and is made up of nine individual days each of 5 hours, producing 45 hours in total. Entry requirements are evidence of a massage course of at least 50 classroom hours in duration. By holding the course in a hospital the implicit suggestion is made that some *clinical* experience will be involved.

The University of Greenwich has another type of course leading to a Diploma in Higher Education in Complementary Therapy: Aromatherapy. This course is held part-time over a period of 1 year. The compulsory components of the course are complementary therapies in health care, aromatherapy, and therapeutics of aromatherapy oils. The brochure states that the course will not certify the nurse to work independently, i.e. there is no professional certification.

Nursing: ENB awards

The English Board of Nursing and Midwifery currently has a course outline (A49) which is a course in complementary therapies in nursing, midwifery and health visiting. The course includes two modules of aromatherapy at level 3. The course is modular, with two pathways lasting a minimum of 30 weeks. This means that anyone holding an ENB A49 will have received that training.

Diploma in Higher Education (complementary therapies)

Three courses advertised in the Royal College of Nursing Education Prospectus 1995/1996 list aromatherapy as an elective module. The module (level 3) can be taken as part of the BSc(Hons) in Health Studies which comes under the Education and Health Studies Programme. It is also an elective module in the BSc in Nursing Studies and the BSc in Midwifery Studies. This is interesting in view of the fact that the use of essential oils in pregnancy is a controversial subject. The elective is entitled 'Aromatherapy Applied to Practice'.

The information states that 'At Level 3, this module aims to help you enhance your caring role with the use of essential oils, application of massage techniques and the development of a professional relationship'. The entrance requirements are that students have completed the course on Introduction to Complementary Therapies (level 2), or Massage Applied to Practice (level 3). The brochure points out that most 30- or 40-point modules involve about 50 hours of time-tabled teaching over 33 weeks and an estimated 5 hours of study per week.

Several of these types of training course are run in the UK. They are open to health care professionals with a nationally recognized qualification and current registration. The resulting qualification will allow that health professional to use complementary therapies (including aromatherapy) within their health care practice, but will not give that individual licence to practise independently. This training may be accepted by the RCN but not by the AOC, in other words, there is no 'professional' qualification.

Middlesex University is in the process of setting up a joint programme, at certificate or diploma level, based on the accreditation of prior learning. The proposal will be facilitated by the National Centre for Work-Based Learning at Middlesex University. This centre will work with the AOC's guidelines and Competence Framework for Holistic Clinical Aromatherapy which has been developed from the AOC's core curriculum and training standards, so this course may produce both an academic and a professional qualification.

Finally, a course in *clinical* aromatherapy for nurses and other health professionals is currently being developed by the School of Health Care

Studies at Oxford Brookes University. This modular Diploma Course in Higher Education/Advanced Studies/BA/Clinical Aromatherapy, which is planned for 1998, seeks to fulfil university validation (academic qualification), AOC requirements (professional qualification) and ENB 49 (nursing qualification). In other words, students could end up with all three qualifications for the one course.

The Diploma in Higher Education will consist of nine advanced modules at levels 2 or 3, of which five are compulsory. The BA course will consist of nine modules at degree level built on to an accredited diploma of nine modules. One of the many unusual and exciting features of this course, apart from its focus on *clinical* aromatherapy, is the opportunity to undertake comparative studies in other international centres.

How to use Aromatherapy in Nursing

Whilst it is pleasing that many courses now appear to be opening up for nurses, perhaps we should remain mindful of something R.H. Lange wrote in the *New York State Medical Journal* in 1993: 'If it sounds too good to be true – it probably is'. We still have to obtain permission to use the information learned on these courses. Much education of hospital managers and doctors needs to take place before clinical aromatherapy can be seen to be an accepted extension of nursing. At the end of the day, aromatherapy has to be perceived to be of real benefit in financial terms as well as in quality-of-life terms, and this means demonstrating both efficacy and safety.

For nurses to be able to use aromatherapy in nursing, *they first need to have a recognized training in aromatherapy*. This means that they will probably have trained with a school recognized by the Aromatherapy Organization Council or the RCN. They will need to approach their employer, usually a hospital trust, with their credentials and renegotiate their contract to include the use of specific 'enhancement' skills. Once this has been agreed, and is written into their contract, they are within their right, as nurses, to use these skills. They can also receive insurance cover from the RCN of up to £3 million (see the RCN and UKCC statements in Appendix 1). However, many Trusts are becoming wary of using essential oils without a set protocol, and nurses should be prepared to create and follow protocols and safety policies for aromatherapy in nursing (see Chapter 6 on COSHH and CHIP).

It is suggested by the RCN that all patients' rights should be addressed – not everyone wants to be touched or massaged, or to smell aromas. Verbal permission must be obtained (written permission is not deemed necessary) and 'as a matter of courtesy' the consultant and nursing colleagues should also be informed (verbal communication with the RCN spokesman).

In a personal verbal communication with an RCN spokesman, the terms used are 'informing', not 'asking permission' as 'nurses have responsibility for their nursing role'. In other words, blanket baths are not prescribed, so if aromatherapy is deemed to be part of a nurse's remit, it does not need to be prescribed either. However, it should be remembered, as is stated in the UKCC document, that nurses will still have accountability for their patients.

The Patient's Charter gave patients the promise of a designated nurse who would be responsible for the planning and implementation of their care. This bill of law gives patients a choice in their nursing care plan, and could prove to be the difference between being washed twice a day or having one aromatherapy treatment and one wash.

In 1994, The Royal College of Nursing produced a continuing education video on aromatherapy for nurses. The video was broadcast by the BBC and showed ways to use aromatherapy within nursing. The video ends with the following sentence: 'A nurse who is well qualified in the understanding of aromatherapy can play a leading part in therapeutic prevention and cure and perhaps give to medicine a little more of the art.'

A nurse, if she uses aromatherapy within her nursing remit, and is a member of the Royal College of Nursing, can be insured to use those aromatherapy skills if she can prove that she has received adequate training. If a nurse uses aromatherapy outside her nursing remit, she will need to have a professionally recognized training which will permit insurance from one of the professional organizations regulated by the AOC.

STRUCTURE OF AROMATHERAPY ORGANIZATIONS IN THE UK

In England there is a structured learning system for aromatherapy which is growing in maturity. Until universities decided to validate courses in aromatherapy, there were only two different methods of training available in aromatherapy:

1. through independent aromatherapy schools;
2. through National Vocation Qualifications (NVQs) – there are two levels of NVQs for aromatherapy:
   (a) through the Health and Beauty Therapy Training Board, which comes under the aegis of the Social Care Forum;
   (b) through the Complementary and Alternative Steering Group (CAST), which comes under the aegis of the Health Care Forum.

Both the Social Care Forum and the Health Care Forum are under the aegis of the Care Sector Forum, which is responsible to the Department of Employment. The Health and Beauty Therapy Training Board (HBTTB) has made it clear that it is *not* concerned with complementary medicine. It was the first to be funded by government to standardize training in aromatherapy, and currently has three levels of training, none of which is acceptable to the AOC (the main body for professional aromatherapy). Many HBTTB training courses in aromatherapy (NVQs) can be found in local colleges such as adult training centres.

However, NVQs in aromatherapy for the Health Forum, which are being written under the eagle eye of the Complementary and Alternative Steering Group (CAST), *will* be concerned with complementary medicine and will involve aromatherapy which is concerned with complementary medicine. At the moment this process is in its elementary stages.

Under the Complementary and Alternative Steering Group (CAST) there are three groups:

- the Council of Complementary and Alternative Medicine (CCAM);
- the Institute of Complementary Medicine (ICM);
- the British Complementary Medicine Association (BCMA).

Council of Complementary and Alternative Medicine (CCAM)

Founded in 1985, the CCAM provides a 'forum for communication and co-operation between professional bodies representing acupuncture, herbal medicine, homeopathy and osteopathy'. The vast majority of CCAM members are non-medically qualified practitioners (NMQPs), and their chairman is Stephen Gordon. Member organizations include the National Institute of Herbal Medicine. This is interesting because many professionals consider that aromatherapy should be part of herbal medicine, although it is not currently part of the curriculum as set by the Institute of Medical Herbalists.

Essential oils frequently have different therapeutic effects to herbal remedies, although many would describe aromatherapy as botanical. In 1994, at a conference hosted by the Office of Alternative Medicine in Washington and entitled *Botanical Medicine – a Place in US Health Care*, the 'expert panel' took some time to reply to the question 'is aromatherapy part of botanical medicine?' The eventual answer was 'yes', although there was some obvious confusion about exactly what aromatherapy was!

Institute of Complementary Medicine (ICM)

Founded in 1981, this organization has a high media profile, led by Michael Endicott. The ICM has done a great deal to raise the public's awareness of the field of complementary medicine. During the early years, the ICM had prestigious offices next to the Royal College of Nursing in Cavendish Square. The organization moved to docklands several years ago, and sadly the information line is now only manned for 2 hours a day. The ICM does not appear to have the support of all of the principal organizations involved in complementary medicine.

British Complementary Medicine Association (BCMA)

This is the new name of the National Consultative Council (NCC) which was launched in 1990, as a result of the work of the British Congress of Complementary and Alternative Practitioners Working Party (BRICCAP).

The BCMA represents 78 organizations within complementary medicine, which include schools, clinics, training establishments and research foundations. In total, 30 different therapies and over 22 000 practitioners are represented. It is the only organization that has a code of conduct common to all of its member organizations. This code takes into account both civil and criminal law, and is supported by disciplinary procedures. It is the first time in the history of complementary medicine that such a code has been agreed upon by so many therapists. The primary aim of the BCMA is to integrate complementary medicine into the nation's health care system.

The Aromatherapy Organizations Council (AOC)

This organization is answerable to the BCMA. Founded in 1991, the AOC is the self-governing body for the aromatherapy profession in the UK. It is also an organization composed of organizations. At the present time, there are 13 associations, 24 training organizations and a further 67 affiliated training organizations in total. The AOC has its own constitution, is democratically governed and represents approximately 5000 aromatherapists in the UK. It is currently seeking charity status.

The most important roles of the AOC are maintaining standards of training and establishing and monitoring dialogue between the aroma-therapy profession and the essential oil trade. From its inception to the present time there have been many discussions about the discrepancy between what the profession felt was required by therapists, namely safe oils, and what was needed by the essential oils trade, which was good profits. As a result of what appeared to be opposing factions, the Aromatherapy Trade Council (ATC) was founded. There is a representative of the ATC on the executive committee of the AOC.

The other aims of the AOC are as follows:

- to unify the profession;
- to establish a common standard of training;
- to act as a public watchdog;
- to provide a collective voice to dialogue with government via the BCMA;
- to offer a mediation and arbitration service in disputes;
- to initiate, support and sponsor research.

Some of the main organizations under the AOC

International Federation of Aromatherapists (IFA)
Initially founded by beauty therapists, the IFA is the oldest established aromatherapy organization. It has had some difficulty in deciding whether to remain under the AOC, and it opted out of the research project initiated by the AOC. The IFA used to have the highest number of therapists, and the current membership of practising aromatherapists is around 1000.

Register of Qualified Aromatherapists (RQA)
Originally this was an initiative of the Institute of Traditional Herbal Medicine and Aromatherapy, but now 70 per cent of the 261 members are from outside this school. The RQA has always imposed a minimum of 200 taught hours, even when many schools still only required 120 hours. It holds regular teaching seminars. Its current membership is around 300.

International Society of Professional Aromatherapists (ISPA)
This organization was founded by Dr George Bennet, an orthodox medical practitioner with an interest in aromatherapy. It is the most recent organization, and makes a clear distinction between clinical practitioners and beauty/cosmetology therapists, emphasizing the need to respect and acknowledge their different requirements and interests. The ISPA is extremely well run. Its register of practitioners informs the public of the different types of therapist, to 'avoid embarrassment'. The ISPA was the first organization to ask for proof of ongoing training (CEUs) and to ask all therapists to take a First Aid training course (nurses are not exempt). Its current membership is above 3000.

The Association of Physical and Natural Therapies (APNT)
Formed in 1986, the APNT represents aromatherapy and several other therapies, including reflexology, touch for health and massage. It has several thousand members, but it is unclear how many of these are aromatherapists.

Institute de Sciences Biomedicales, France (IScB)
Membership of the IScB is only open to students who trained with Pierre

Franchomme and Dr Daniel Peneol (for training in aromatic medicine). Membership closed in 1990. The 1-year course was open to students who had trained in medicine, herbal medicine, chemistry or nursing. Membership is less than 100.

The International Therapy Examination Council (ITEC)

This organization is known world-wide. It is an examination council, not an aromatherapy association. It was formed in 1973 in order to set and maintain standards in the practice of beauty therapy by establishing courses. Over 400 educational establishments world-wide are registered for ITEC courses. The most recent of the ITEC courses is the one in aromatherapy. There is no membership, as the organization is an examining board.

Organizations that are not under the AOC

Institute of Aromatic Therapists (IAT)

Started by Shirley Price and Alan Barker in reponse to the needs of aromatherapists who did not want to use a full body massage, the IAT considers that essential oils can be used in many ways, not just for massage. It stipulates that the training should concentrate on essential oils, with attention being given to chemistry. This is a young organization but one to watch with great interest, as outside the UK aromatherapy is *not* synonymous with massage. Many nurses in the UK also feel that the idea of giving a patient a full body massage can be inappropriate. The IAT is not recognized by the AOC as yet, but this situation might change as more and more nurses start to use essential oils clinically.

HERBAL MEDICINE AND UK LAW

On 3 December 1991 a major Government statement was issued which established that any family doctor could employ, within his or her practice, complementary therapists to offer NHS treatments, provided that the GP remained clinically accountable for the patient. Fundamental mechanisms were put in place to authorize NHS funding, as well as to permit doctors to use the services of complementary therapists. This opened the door to integration and, as Leon Chaitow, editor of the *Journal of Complementary and Alternative Medicine*, wrote in an article, 'integration is now growing at such a pace, which, taking with it the staggering degree of interest being displayed by mainstream medicine, means we really need to consider the best way forward'.

This viewpoint was seconded by a book-report on complementary medicine published by the British Medical Association (BMA) in June 1993.[2]

The report concentrated mainly on 'the big five', namely osteopathy, acupuncture, chiropractic, homeopathy and herbalism, although aromatherapy *is* mentioned, and much of what is required of 'the big five', is relevant to aromatherapists. Of the many comments which stand out as being particularly relevant to aromatherapy, perhaps the following paragraph should be quoted:

It is difficult, at present, for individuals to be certain that the therapist whom they are consulting is competent to practise. Similarly, it is not easy for doctors to ensure that the therapist to whom they transfer care of patients is competent. The present situation, in which anybody is free to practise, irrespective of their training or experience, is unacceptable. Where individuals undergo courses of training designed to equip them for the practice of particular therapies, these should conform to minimum standards appropriate to the responsibilities and domains of that therapy.

The BMA also recommends that a single regulating body be established for each therapy. Such organizations should follow a code of best practice in adopting all of the following: registration, professional standards, training, research, regulation, and monitoring and surveillance.

There is still much to be done before aromatherapy really has its house in order. However, considerable progress has been made by the Aromatherapy Organizations Council, and they are to be commended for this. In the 1960s there was only one aromatherapy training school – now there are around 160 such schools.

One of the weaknesses of the current standardization in the UK is that the different types of aromatherapy have never been agreed upon, although most people involved in the profession accept that there are *many* aspects to aromatherapy. It is arguable that nurses need a different kind of training in order to use essential oils in hospitals.

TRAINING IN THE USA

Outside the UK, there are many distance-learning courses. Of course, essential oils *can* be learned through the post, but to understand about an aromatherapy treatment, experience is needed in both the receiving and giving of such treatment. Touch is a wide-ranging subject to absorb. Nurses are not taught to touch except in a procedural sense. A video will not explain how it feels to give or receive aromatherapy, which is why videos (and distance-learning courses) are not accepted by the AOC. Conveying smell through books is not the same as smelling and discussing the aroma in class.

A core of individuals dedicated to unity and professionalism is beginning to emerge in seeking a national curriculum in the USA, where there is no national regulatory body, and many of the courses are distance-learning ones. At the moment each course certifies it own training, but there are tremendous differences in the length and depth of courses – some only last 2 days! As Susan Earle writes in the winter issue of *Scentsitivity*, the magazine of the National Association for Holistic Aromatherapy (NAHA), 'I do not think having masses of people with two, four or six days of aromatherapy workshops, walking around with certificates claiming to be "certified aromatherapists" is going to do much for the reputation or advancement of aromatherapy'.[3]

In a hard-hitting, but much needed, article she continues, 'I think perhaps aromatherapy would do well if a few or all of those now offering certification take a weekend or two off from signing certificates and get together to develop some standards, some guidelines, some specific areas of study and some clear lines of practice.'

CHANGES IN THE NHS TO ALLOW AROMATHERAPY

The National Health Service has changed greatly in the last few years, allowing an expansion of aromatherapy which a few years ago would have been unthinkable. Contracting out – the ability of hospitals to use their own budget however they wish – was a huge step. Thus hospital managers could employ the number of nurses, doctors and occupational therapists that they felt they needed. The changes also allowed them to contract in specialist skills such as aromatherapy, and to allow nurses to train in and use special skills.

By changing health from a service industry to a business industry, hospitals are being forced to compete to obtain funding from health authorities who allocate funds according to how inexpensive or efficient a hospital is. If a hip replacement costs a certain amount at one hospital, another hospital will try to reduce the cost. Some area health authorities, such as Grampian, are open to complementary medicine, while others are not.

In November 1994 the Conservative Government tried to pass a paper which would ostensibly have outlawed herbal medicine and aromatherapy. Integral to this was the removal of an exclusion clause placed there for the very protection of those two professions. The *European regulations and directives* on licensing procedures for medicinal products, collectively referred to as the 'Future Systems' package of legislation, were in a document which was to be implemented through the Medicine for Human Use (Marketing Authorizations, Pharmacovigilance and Related Matters) Regulations 1994. In simple language, by drawing the UK in line with

Europe we would have lost our ability to buy all herbal products, including essential oils, unless those products had a licence.

European law is very clear, stating that 'no medicinal product may be placed on the market of a Member State unless a marketing authorization has been issued by the competent authorities of that Member State in accordance with this Directive' (Article 3 of Chapter 11 of Directive 65/65 EEC, amended by Directive 93/39/EEC).[4]

Herbal remedies are medicinal products as defined in Directive 65/65/EEC ('any substance or combination of substance presented for treating or preventing disease in human beings or animals').

Herbal remedies are thus subject to the full requirements of the marketing authorizations referred to in Articles 4 and 4a of Directive 65/65/EEC, and in the Annex to Directive 75/318/EEC and in article 2 of Directive 75/319/EEC. Therefore, even without the MCA licence fee of £84 000 for a new licence application, the costs of bringing products up to application status would in themselves be crippling.

The British public rebelled in their thousands. What should have been just a rubber stamp removing herbal medicines, many homeopathic remedies and essential oils at a single stroke was thwarted. MPs were deluged with letters from individuals and organizations. This display of public outrage resulted in a very constructive meeting between the Medicine Control Agency and the herbalists, aromatherapy representatives and manufacturers of herbal medicines.

Following this meeting, a letter was sent to the secretary of the AOC, in which it was stated that 'I am pleased to be able to confirm that aromatherapy products sold through retail outlets are not affected by the new Regulations to be laid before Parliament unless they are marketed as medicinal products with claims, e.g. as having some sort of curative, restorative or preventative effects.'

This issue arose during the preparation of Regulations to be laid before Parliament to introduce the new European medicines licensing system. It was suggested that some kinds of herbal medicines, which are exempt under section 12 of the Medicine Act 1968 from the requirement to have a product licence, might not be exempt under Directive 65/65 as amended by a 1989 Directive.

We have looked into the matter and are satisfied that the current exemption from product licensing requirements can continue. The position of herbal medicines is therefore safeguarded. There is also no change to the existing exemptions and public health safeguards under Part 111 of the Medicines Act 1968, including Section 56.

Essential oils used in aromatherapy are similarly unaffected by the new Regulations. If they are used by aromatherapy practitioners for a medicinal purpose, the current exemptions from licensing will continue to apply. So, although aromatherapists cannot claim to treat disease, they *can* use essential oils as medicines!

The débâcle in Parliament only goes to highlight how easy it would be for the existing exemptions to be removed in future debates, and we must all keep an eagle eye upon the situation if herbal medicine and aromatherapy are not to be removed from our hands in years to come.

1. As a rule, we would not normally consider an aromatherapy product to be licensable where it was used for cosmetic purposes and did not have any medical claims associated with it.
2. In situations where aromatherapy practitioners use essential oils for therapeutic purposes on individual patients, such products would be considered to be 'medicinal products'. However, these products are exempt from the requirement to hold a manufacturer's or product licence under Section 12(1) of the Medicines Act 1968, provided that they fulfil the criteria laid down in that section, i.e.:
   (a) that the remedy is manufactured or assembled on premises of which the person carrying on the business is the occupier, and which he or she is able to close so as to exclude the public, and;
   (b) that the person carrying on the business sells or supplies the remedy for administration to a particular person after being requested by or on behalf of that person and in that person's presence to use his own judgement as to the treatment required.
3. Essential oils used by aromatherapy practitioners as in paragraph 2 above would be considered to be 'herbal remedies'.

(Linda A. Anderson, Medicines Control Agency, Department of Health, 1995, personal communication)

It is interesting to note that similar developments are afoot in America. A Food and Drugs Administration briefing paper dated 23 April 1986 contained the following statement:

Aroma Therapy
A new category of aroma products is being introduced with claims or implications that their use will improve personal well-being in a variety of ways, such as 'strengthening the body's self-defense mechanisms'. What are called 'behavioral fragrance' products are beginning to be marketed. The following may be used to answer questions.

Traditionally, perfumes have been considered cosmetics by the FDA. The Food, Drug and Cosmetic Act defines cosmetics as articles to be introduced into or otherwise applied to the body to cleanse, beautify, promote attractiveness or alter appearance.

On the other hand, articles intended for use in the diagnosis, treatment or prevention of disease, and intended to affect the structure or any function of the body, usually are considered to be drugs – with all 'new drugs' requiring the FDA's pre-market approval.

While cosmetics and drugs are both under FDA's jurisdiction, the legal requirements applying to them differ. A claim that a perfume's aroma is good or beneficial, in general, is a cosmetic claim not requiring FDA approval before the product is sold. But if someone tries to market a scent with labeling 'for treatment or prevention of allergies' or some other condition or disease, presumably this could be found after investigation to be a new drug claim, requiring pre-market approval. The agency will make judgments on a case-by-case basis.

Claims made in advertising but not on product labeling are regulated by the Federal Trade Commission. Room fragrance systems (deodorizers, odour control) are the Consumer Product Safety Commissions' responsibility.

A copy of the paper containing this quotation was shown to the author at the White Plains Aromatherapy Symposium in November 1994.

So similar dilemmas face aromatherapists in both countries: they can practise but they cannot make claims for the products that they use. This is really nonsense, as there is enough anecdotal/historical usage to substantiate the claims, but not enough research, or money to warrant a licence. Although there could be a problem in lumping together herbal products and aromatherapy products, there is an advantage in presenting a larger lobbying force.

The AOC hosted the first Seminar on Essentials oils and Public Safety in November 1992, when it brought together Dr Virginia Murray (toxicologist), The Poisons Unit, Guy's Hospital, Victor Perfitt (Chairman of the British Herbal Medicine Association), Charles Wells (Chairman of the Essential Oil Trade Association (EOTA)) and Tony Balacs (Scientific Editor of the *International Journal of Aromatherapy*).

As a result of this important first step, the Aromatherapy Trade and Industry Committee (ATC) came up with the following voluntary code of practice.

1. Droppers – all bottles on sale to the public should have single-drop dispensers integral to the bottle. A bottle of essential oil with an integral dropper has a built-in safety factor which prevents the contents from being swallowed quickly by an unattended child.
2. Labelling – although detailed information on usage and dilutions of oils can be explained fully in leaflets, the warnings and information below *must* be printed on the label.

(a) Instructions – add five drops of essential oil to 10 ml of carrier oil to give an approximate 2 per cent dilution (15–20 drops per ml).
(b) Keep away from children and from the eyes.
(c) Do not take internally or apply undiluted to the skin.
(d) The quantity supplied, e.g. 5 ml.
(e) The company name and address.
3. All promotional literature should give clear guidelines as to how the aromatherapy products are to be used, including recommended dilutions where necessary.
4. No medicinal claims can be made on labels, promotional material or advertisements regarding products which have not been licensed. No aromatherapy product can make remedial claims if it relates to a specific disease or adverse condition.

The Consumer Protection Act (1987) states that it is a criminal offence to supply unsafe consumer goods in the UK: 'a person shall be guilty of an offence if he supplies consumer goods which are not reasonably safe having regard to all the circumstances'. As with safety regulations, an offence may have been committed even when no one has been injured. Contravention of the General Safety Requirement can result in a fine of £2000, up to 6 months in prison, or both.

In the Act 'safe' is defined as 'reducing to a minimum the risk of death or personal injury'. The General Safety Requirement refers to goods being reasonably safe, taking into account all of the circumstances. These circumstances include 'the manner in which the goods are marketed and instruction or warnings given with the goods'.

The Trading Standards officer can issue suspension notices prohibiting suppliers from selling goods which they believe contravene safety legislation. They can also apply to a magistrate's court for an order that such goods be forfeited and destroyed.

Insurance companies used by aromatherapy organizations give cover of up to £1 million and encompass malpractice, public liability and products liability. All aromatherapists belonging to organizations that are under the aegis of the AOC *must be insured to practise*. In addition, many nurses who use aromatherapy are also covered under RCN insurance for up to £3 million. To date, no claims have been made.

REFERENCES

1. **Royal College of Nursing.** 1993: *Choosing a complementary therapy.* London: Complementary Therapies in Nursing Special Interest Group, Royal College of Nursing Department of Nursing Policy and Practice.

2. **Fisher, F. (ed.)** 1993: *Complementary therapies in medicine*. London: British Medical Association.

3. **Earle, S.** 1994/95: Student's view of certification. *Scensitivity* **4,** 12–14.

4. **EEC** 1965: *Council Directive of 26/1/1965. Approximation of provisions laid down by law of regulations of administrative action relating to proprietary medicinal products*. London: HMSO.

SUMMARY

A good book is not written – it is rewritten – and the best books are never finished – they are 'to be continued'.

By the time this book is printed, aromatherapy and nursing will have moved on and more studies will have been published. Some of the ideas presented here will already be out of date. However, the caring in nursing will *never* be out of date. I believe that there is a valid and important role for clinical aromatherapy within nursing, and I feel that this integration could lift nursing to new heights and form a bridge between orthodox and alternative medicine.

There will be those who will accuse me of being before my time, and who will argue that there has not been enough research. There will be those who will say that, as aromatherapy is not taught in nursing schools, it cannot be seen to be part of nursing. To the first, I reply 'You are right.' To the second, I reply 'Nurses are using aromatherapy *right now*. And nursing courses are already being developed.'

However, we need to keep a clinical focus. We need to remember that we are first and foremost nurses. Then we are more likely to ensure safe practice.

APPENDIX 1

RCN STATEMENT OF BELIEF FOR THE PRACTICE OF COMPLEMENTARY THERAPIES

1. We believe that nurses using complementary therapies as part of their care should know and understand their responsibilities to the patient/client and the United Kingdom Central Council for Nursing, Midwifery and Health Visiting. Further, we believe that the UKCC code sets the professional requirement to be met by all registered nurses using complementary therapies.
2. We believe that all patients and clients have the right to be offered and to receive complementary therapies either exclusively or as part of orthodox nursing practice.
3. We believe that all patients have the right to expect that their religious, cultural and spiritual beliefs will be observed by nurses practising complementary therapies.
4. We believe that all complementary therapies available to patients must have the support of the collaborative care team.
5. We believe that a registered nurse who is appropriately qualified to carry out a complementary therapy must agree and work to locally agreed protocols for practice and standards of care.
6. We believe that the patient/clients, in partnership with the nurse complementary therapist, should determine the suitability of any proposed complementary therapy. Informed, documented consent should be obtained and detailed records kept with the patient/client record.
7. We believe that, where possible, research-based complementary therapy practices should be used. Where this is not possible, then nurse complementary therapists, as accountable professionals, must be able to justify their actions.

8. We believe that nurse/complementary therapists should, where appropriate, be prepared to instruct significant individuals in the patient's/client's life (including the patient/client), so that they can learn basic complementary therapy skills for self-care.

9. We believe that nurse complementary therapists should seek to develop their self-awareness and inter-personal skills, and so enhance their role as reflective practitioners.

10. We believe that nurse complementary therapists have a responsibility to collect detailed information on all therapy sessions and to evaluate the outcomes of therapy on the patient/client.

11. We believe that the practice of complementary therapies by nurses should be the subject of at least an annual review by an appropriately constituted multidisciplinary committee. The review should take into account patient measures of satisfaction and benefit.

APPENDIX 2

PROFESSIONAL ISSUES AND CODES OF CONDUCT: UKCC

The United Kingdom Central Council is responsible for the registration of nurses, midwives and health visitors and issues Codes of Professional Conduct by which registered nurses must abide.

The Council recognizes that nursing is practised in a context of continuing change and development. These changes are the result of advances in research, alterations to the provision of health care, and new approaches to professional practice. Nursing must therefore be dynamic and responsive to these changing needs and must adopt modes of adjustment based on education and experience.

The Council does not and will not regulate complementary medicine, most of which has no statutory regulatory bodies. The following points are offered as guidelines which will help to ensure that clinical practice remains safe.

We are individually responsible for judging whether the qualification in a complementary therapy has produced a level of competence sufficient to use that skill in patient care. Self-evaluation of competence and accountability are vital.

We must acknowledge our limits of personal knowledge, and we may not work beyond the level of that skill.

The Council recommends that every nurse using a complementary therapy gets formal consent to practise from all persons and authorities involved in the patient care, and that at all times we are able to justify the intervention as being in the best interest of the patient.

Independent insurance cover should be obtained, and formal consent of the patient is advised.

APPENDIX 3

ORGANIZATIONS

Aromatherapy Organizations Council
3 Latymer Close
Braybrooke
Market Harborough
Leicester LE16 8LN

Aromatherapy organizations belonging to the AOC

English Societé de l'Institut Pierre Franchomme, France
Belmont House
New Port
Essex CB11 3RF

International Federation of Aromatherapists
Stamford House
2–4 Chiswick High Road
London W4 1TH

International Society of Professional Aromatherapists
ISPA House
82 Ashby Road
Hinckley
Leicestershire LE10 1SN

Register of Clinical Aromatherapists
PO Box 6941
London N8 9HF

Other organizations

Institute of Aromatic Therapists
27 Danehill
Ratby
Leicestershire LE67 8WD

Aromatherapy Alliance of Aromatherapy
PO Box 309
Depoe Bay OR 97341 USA

National Association for Holistic Aromatherapy
219 Carl Street
San Francisco CA 94117 USA

ESSENTIAL OIL DISTRIBUTORS USED BY THE AUTHOR

Butterbar & Sage
7 Tessa Road
Reading
Berkshire RG1 8HH

Essentially Oils Ltd
8 Mount Farm
Churchill
Chipping Norton
Oxfordshire OX7 6NP

The Fragrant Earth Co. Ltd
PO Box 182
Taunton
Somerset TA1 1YR

Quintessence Aromatics Inc.
PO Box 536
Marsing. Id 83639

Rosa Medica
The Barn
Crickahm Wemore
Somerset BS28 4JT

Saffron Oils
Belmont House
Newport
Saffron Walden
Essex CB11 3RF

Shirley Price Aromatherapy Ltd
Essentia House
Upper Bond Street
Hinckley
Leicestershire LE10 1RS

RECOMMENDED READING

Rankin-Box, D. (ed.) 1995: *The nurse's handbook of complementary therapies.* London: Churchill Livingstone.

Trevelyan, J. and Booth, B. 1994: *Complementary medicine for nurses, midwives and health visitors.* Basingstoke: Macmillan.

Tisserand, R. and Valnet, J. (eds) 1980: *The practice of aromatherapy.* Saffron Walden: C.W. Daniel.

Tisserand, R. and Balacs, T. 1995: *Essential oil safety.* London: Churchill Livingstone.

Price, S. and Price, L. 1995: *Aromatherapy for health professionals.* London: Churchill Livingstone.

Lawless, J. 1992: *The encyclopedia of essential oils.* Shaftesbury: Element.

Vickers, A. 1996: *Massage and aromatherapy.* London: Chapman & Hall.

Pratt, J.W. and Mason, A. 1981: *The caring touch.* London: Heyden.

Siegal, B. 1986: *Love, medicine and miracles.* New York: Harper and Row.

Bach, R. 1972: *Jonathan Livingstone Seagull.* London: Turnstone Press.

Williams, D.G. 1997: *The chemistry of essential oils.* Weymouth: Michelle Press.

SUBJECT INDEX

Note: unqualified references to 'oils' should be read as essential oils.

AUTHOR INDEX